quantum EATING
the ultimate elixir

TONYA ZAVASTA

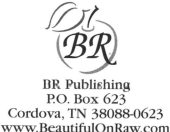

BR Publishing
P.O. Box 623
Cordova, TN 38088-0623
www.BeautifulOnRaw.com

Disclaimer

The information presented herein represents the view of the author as of the date of publication. Every effort has been made to make this book as accurate as possible. It was written with the intention of providing information about the raw food lifestyle and giving the motivation to follow it. If you are not ready to accept full responsibility for your actions, safety, and health, please do not follow these ideas.

The information contained herein is not intended as a diagnosis, cure, or treatment for any disease or ailment. Because changing one's diet for the better often produces initial cleansing reactions, readers are advised to educate themselves adequately and seek advice from a qualified holistic or medical professional when needed. Neither the author nor BR Publishing accepts liability or responsibility for any loss, injury, or damage allegedly arising from any information or suggestion in this book.

Cover design: Gavin Anderson and Dan Denisenko
Layout: Gavin Anderson, Sterling Studios
Editors: Sharron K. Carrell, Bradley Harris, and
         Wendy Griffin Anderson
Photos: Serhiy Balenko, Balenko's Design & Photo

Published by:

BR Publishing
P.O. Box 623
Cordova, TN 38088-0623

Library of Congress Cataloguing-in-Publication Data

Zavasta, Tonya.
    Quantum eating : the ultimate elixir of youth / Tonya Zavasta.
    p. cm.
    Includes bibliographical references and index.
    ISBN-13: 978-0-9742434-5-0
    ISBN-10: 0-9742434-5-0

    1. Aging—Prevention. 2. Nutrition. 3. Beauty,
        Personal.   I. Title.

RA776.75.Z38 2007   612.6'8
                        QBI07-600191

Printed in Canada.

Dedicated to:

Victoria Boutenko, author of Green for Life *and* 12 Steps to Raw Foods, *for seeing the remarkable health potential in my unique raw food experience and encouraging me to share it with the world.*

Acknowledgments

Many people helped me to bring this book to you.

I collected an enormous body of research for this book. I am deeply grateful to **Margaret Aranguren** and **Amy Pendley** for their transcription of this material.

I have been blessed with wonderful editors. They not only edited my work, but taught me a great deal in the process. I am very grateful to **Sharron Carrell.** Without her help, the delivery of this book would have been much more complicated. Sharron often acted as a midwife to help me to give birth to the right words to express my ideas better. Helping me with the first draft, she often said, "I had to translate from Russian." She did an excellent job considering she does not speak any Russian! She used her superb intelligence and editorial brilliance to help me to transform the work on this book into a labor of love.

Bradley Harris's contribution to this book was invaluable. Being my friend for many years, he helped to make the tone of this book more conversational and my presence more tangible. I consider the editorial insights he furnished to be precious gems that made my work sparkle.

I am very fortunate to have had **Wendy Griffin Anderson** proofread the book. A stickler for details, she found glitches that others might have missed. Her final polishing of the text made it shine!

My deepest gratitude goes to **Gavin Anderson,** who did the typesetting and worked on the cover of this book. Gavin exemplified professionalism and infinite patience as he dealt with my never ending requests "to make one more change."

My thanks go to **Branden Canepa** for organizing the recipes chapter and for reading the whole book to flag inconsistencies.

Above all, I am indebted to my **husband** and **son** for their gentle care, generous constructive criticism, and endless good will in helping me to make this book the best it can be.

Finally, I want to thank **all of my readers** and **supporters** over the years, who have inspired me to learn more, teach more, and share more knowledge and wisdom about the raw foods lifestyle.

Contents

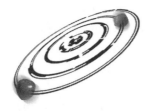

Chapter 1

Introduction:
Tell Me It Can't Be Done,
and Watch Me Do It!

I am a failure, folks. I am a failed mathematician. I am a failed mechanical engineer. And I am a failed high school teacher. I owe these failures, obliquely, along with all the consequences they've brought me, to a strange friend and enemy. Its name? *Food*.

Along came the raw foods revolution and suddenly my failures became surprising virtues and values. Everything I'd done up to this point revealed itself as a precious gift that I would integrate into my new endeavor. From the realm of mathematics came the gifts of logic and deductive reasoning. From engineering, I learned how to research, to dig deep, looking for unorthodox solutions. From teaching ninth graders in an all-boys school, I acquired three vital attributes: perseverance, survival skills, and raw courage.

I'm fortunate to hold advanced degrees in mechanical engineering and theoretical mathematics. But I've spent the last decade devoting every waking moment to researching the benefits and techniques of consuming raw foods. *Why on earth,* I used to wonder, *did I spend so many years studying hard science without using it?* Had I defied my destiny? Wasn't I supposed to be squatting in some underground supercollider facility, holed up with brilliant social misfits, hurling bits of atoms at other bits of atoms, munching on ineptly homemade tuna sandwiches, and playing exotic computer games?

One day I picked up a book on quantum physics. Suddenly, it was *there!* I *knew* it! I had to write a book on Quantum Eating. It all began to make sense — my abundant academic background, the vast experience of my raw food journey, endless research and keen interest in beauty and anti-aging. I've experienced many life changes, including changing countries and careers. But deep down, I somehow *knew* that anti-aging research was central to my life's direction even before I was consciously aware of it.

All my life people told me there were things I just couldn't do. I had to overcome the inevitable prejudice that the world holds against handicapped people. It is as if people feel that a deficiency in your physical appearance makes you deficient in every other way. Some people like to put you down. Especially, it seems, when you're already down. Often, they do so innocently, unintentionally.

When I was a child, because of the bilateral hip problem, my parents were told I would never walk. After years of grueling therapy, I *did* learn to walk without crutches, though I still had a limp. It was then that I experienced, for the first time, the wonderful feeling that comes from accomplishing something that others think *impossible*. As Walter Bagehot put it, "The greatest pleasure in life is doing what people say you cannot do."

When we immigrated to America, I visited orthopedists to find one who would rise to the challenge of my hip disability. It "couldn't be done," they said. So I went to get a second opinion. A third. Ultimately, even a fifth opinion. The sixth doctor was utterly dismissive: "Why are you so hard-headed? You have limped all your life until now. You are going to limp for the rest of it. Just get used to the idea!"

That's all I needed. I stopped pleading with doctors. I began thinking — for myself. I found my own solution. Then I found a doctor with enough courage and vision to go along with my idea. The result: I am an orthopedic miracle!

My high school English teacher told my mother that I would never learn English. She wanted me out of her English class because I was hopeless. I overheard this conversation. From that day I made straight A's. I think my passion for English and the audacity to write books in English sprang from her putdown.

When I was a teenager, my girlfriend told me outright, "If I looked like you, I wouldn't even want to live." My interest in beauty was a direct result of the hurt I experienced that day. It took me many years to find my way to what I now call (to employ one of my trademarks) "Rawsome Beauty." The advantage of Rawsome beauty over in-born beauty is this: In-born beauty fades, but you can be Rawsomely beautiful when you are 40, 50, 60 and beyond. So these days I receive numerous emails from my seminar attendees with generous beauty compliments.

For me, even something as simple as attending a first-time yoga class can become a major obstacle — physically and emotionally. My first encounter with Bikram yoga resulted in a confrontation with the studio's owner. My stringent hip limitations made me unfit for most of the 26 Bikram poses.

Breathing exercises and the shavasana (the "dead body pose") were all I could manage without serious modification. So I came equipped with a strap. Little did I know, bringing a prop and insisting I keep it because of my affliction's severity, was a crime worthy of threats to call the police.

After this encounter I took private yoga classes. Eighteen months later I was back in the same studio. I love it. These days, when I am more flexible, I am able to appreciate the unbendable Bikram rules my instructor imposes. I will soon submit an article about my yoga experience to one of the yoga journals. I am also expected to attach pictures of some of my poses. No matter how hard I have to work to perfect them I promise one day you will see them in print.

Want to make me do something? Just tell me it can't be done. I *like* to solve problems! And I believe every problem has a solution. I believe in doing *whatever* needs to be done to get where you want to be. Exercising stubborn legs for hours a day just to make them do what they're supposed to do, endlessly researching anti-aging practices — either way, I'll take it to the limit. Farmers call it "hoeing to the end of the row." My motto: Whatever it *takes*. You are likely fortunate — your "whatever it takes" may well be much less than mine.

Older people endure the same prejudices as the handicapped. I saw, early in life, a glimpse of what it's like to be old, a glimpse of how older people are treated. I was determined to find a way to avoid decrepitude. And dying young was *not* an option. I thought, *I have to find a way to avoid this fate.* And I did! The result of my research and experience is detailed in my three books. The book you are holding now, *Quantum Eating,* is the last in my trilogy devoted to anti-aging and Rawsome beauty. I strongly advise you to read my first two books before reading this book.

Some ideas you'll read here are different from those in my previous books. I stand by what I said in those books; however, I am developing knowledge and experience and now I am at a different stage of life. New possibilities open, new practices emerge. It's my responsibility — indeed, my joy — to capture them for you in this new book.

There's a wonderfully insightful book by Thomas Kuhn that you should read, if the progress of science excites you. It's entitled *The Structure of Scientific Revolutions*. Kuhn makes a penetrating point: When you're in the middle of a scientific revolution, you normally can't see it — like the calm at the center of the storm. So it is with life. When you're at a crossroads and your life makes a turn, you may not notice it until much later.

In 2005, my husband and I spent Christmas with the famous raw food family of Victoria Boutenko. (For the curious: No, we did not have a raw turkey for Christmas dinner.) Victoria set up a presentation for me in Ashland, Oregon, her hometown. We spent two full days with this radiant family, absorbing fresh raw foods knowledge, sharing green smoothies, and being immersed in their warm, vibrant energy. It was a genuinely life-altering experience. Victoria got interested in my personal regimen of not eating after 2 P.M. She encouraged me to write an article explaining my theory.

I was gripped with the same excitement until I sat down at my keyboard. *Theory?* I wondered. I didn't have a theory. All I knew in that moment was … *my* raw food regimen felt thoroughly *good,* totally *right.* Doing it myself was one thing. But justifying it for others was a different story. Though I'd stumbled upon this life-enhancing practice through my own experience, my analytical mind needed more in order to help me explain it to others. I needed *proof.*

Research in nutrition is contradictory, at times, frustrating. It's like collecting berries (and really, come to think of it, it felt more like collecting a berry here and a berry there, but never a whole quart). Information was scarce. Each book held promise, but each contributed only tiny insights, just snippets of information. Before I knew it, I was getting deeper and deeper into quantum physics. I read more than *three hundred books*. And I gained a deeper understanding of why my own practice with raw foods was so good, not only for me, but for many other people throughout history.

If there is anything that unites all cultures and philosophies, it is the never-ending quest for preserving youth and reversing age. In writing this book, I researched and adapted teachings from Christian, Buddhist, mystic, and animist traditions, as well as findings from eastern and western medicine. Longevity traditions are known in every culture. Collecting pearls of wisdom about long life, I let my studies span centuries, cultures, and endless variations, until I could string them together to create a necklace of knowledge.

Together we will explore all the way from the distant past to the most recent theories in anti-aging research. I have looked into the folk traditions and medical practices of different countries and cultures, devised a strategy to use every one of these different methods that offered real improvements in human well-being. Just like doctors from different specializations — cardiology, endocrinology, neurology, etc. — come together to save a person's life, the wisdom from different parts of the world must be combined to successfully tackle the aging puzzle.

What is Quantum Eating? It is an advanced level in the raw food lifestyle in which you eat 100 percent raw, twice daily and only in the first part of the day. In this book, step by step, I will supply the evidence for why this way of eating provides the utmost in anti-aging benefits. Each chapter discusses a specific topic. But the main point plays out over the course of the whole book, and every chapter adds another piece to the anti-aging puzzle.

Science can be interpreted in different ways. Any research by experiment can never be 100 percent reliable. Nonetheless, I will introduce some research findings that are available. I will attempt to show how some scientific conclusions contradict logic, yet others confirm the wisdom of natural order. These latter findings can be convincing on a macro level, but on a quantum level, I have learned, even logic becomes questionable. So I implore you never to get attached to certain scientific hypotheses or theories — be ready to evaluate them and change entirely as new experiments, especially on your own body, open new secrets to you.

The raw food lifestyle can only be individually experienced — it cannot be authoritatively proven. The best science can achieve is to disprove erroneous concepts. Nevertheless, I researched scientific findings extensively. I quote the available data, and present conclusions I believe scientists' research have arrived at, but never delivered. I have tried to present evidence and disclose flaws in reasoning, so you can judge for yourself whether my interpretations are plausible.

You must gain some degree of raw food maturity to proceed to Quantum Eating.

This book is dedicated to Victoria Boutenko, because without her encouragement I do not think this book would have ever seen the light of day. If you do not know who Victoria Boutenko is, this is a good indication that you may not be quite ready to take this advanced health journey. If your eyes are glazing over, wondering what on earth this woman is talking about, get my first book or other books on the raw food lifestyle and start at the beginning.

Everyone can benefit from not eating at night, but making Quantum Eating your lifestyle and enjoying every minute of it can be accomplished only on the 100 percent raw method. I consider it a great stroke of personal good fortune to have stumbled upon the raw food lifestyle. I advise you to learn and experience it as well.

I'm extremely grateful to Victoria for her persistent nudges. It wasn't until she encouraged me to share the discoveries of my own raw regimen that this new adventure began to unfold. Writing this book has changed my life. My prayer is that it will change yours.

Wearing your favorite old comfortable shoes — that's how it feels to write in your native tongue. Writing this book in English, from the perspective of my mother tongue, Russian, felt like running the Boston Marathon in stiletto heels. My beloved editor Sharron Carrell went to great lengths to fit Cinderella's slipper on this Russian stepsister's foot. My fairy godmother often had to wave her magic wand to find just the right words to express my ideas. If there are still some faults in my English it is because, sometimes, I fought ferociously to keep my authentic footprint, ignoring her better judgment.

I've read that many writers learn to speak perfect English but spend the rest of their lives trying to find something worth saying. Me — I'd rather have something valuable to say even if I say it imperfectly. I write fearlessly. I feel that the information that I have is so powerful that, even if my English stilettos sometimes disrupt my balance, the message itself will get me to the end of the race.

One thing I *do* know about writing ... You must lead people to the truth even if it means baring your heart in the process. It's true that "there is nothing new under the sun." However, it's equally true that each of us is a unique human being with unique life experiences and knowledge. If you filter an idea through your very soul, there is a great chance you'll come up with something original. But this happens only on one condition: You must be completely honest with yourself. You must say what you genuinely feel — even if it contradicts mainstream opinion or you lose some popularity points. I strive to maintain such honesty in this book.

I believe in God. Therefore, I will use the word *God* where I feel it is appropriate. I was reared in the former Soviet Union as an atheist. I earned — and I do mean *earned* — the right to speak the name of God when I came to the U.S. I do so with great pride. If you believe in Mother Nature or the Universe ... fine with me, so long as you allow me to be who I am. You won't find me addressing the Creator as *He/She/It*. Consider: It is not Eenie/Meenie/Miney/Mo who wrote this book, but I, Tonya Zavasta, and you deserve to know where I stand.

I couldn't be "politically correct" if I tried. (And I *have* tried. But politically correct and socially inept proved *not* to be a winning combination.) You will find here no attempt to please everyone. I use *man, men, him,* etc. for persons generally. You'll find both *he* and *she* throughout the book, but never *he/she*. I love English too much already to commit such punctuational atrocities in the name of correctness. If this is socially abhorrent to you, well ... I'm comfortable with your opinion.

We live in a free country. Here I do not even have to hold a license, as I would have had to in the former Soviet Union, to write a book. Write your own book, if you like. Pollute it with meaningless oddities like the Victorians putting ruffles on the legs of their pianos because they thought limbs were obscene. My style is my own; it shouldn't keep you from exploring the validity of my ideas. I am convinced that you can benefit greatly from a good book — even if you do not agree 100 percent with the author.

When I announced at my local raw food group that *Quantum Eating* was about to be released, a lady asked me: Who is going to write the foreword? I was stunned, then speechless (which does not happen to me often). Later I gave it some thought and came to two important revelations.

A foreword is usually written by a compatriot, an expert in the field. I wish there were someone who had gone before me to turn to for advice and clarification. But I am in uncharted waters. What I am presenting here has not been presented by anyone else. My second revelation was that I wished I could have the philosopher-mathematician, Pythagoras, write it. His diet was very similar to the one I advocate in this book. His contemporaries commented on his vitality and especially youthful and beautiful appearance even though sources say he lived to be 100. Since he is currently unavailable, I will struggle on alone. No foreword, but hopefully no backward either.

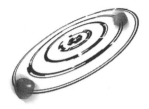

Chapter 2

War Against Aging:
Modern Medicine & Artificial Health

Please understand: It's not that I spend an undue amount of time lounging about at radiator shops. But this one morning, when I'd rather have been peering into the flaxseed bin at our local health food store, I instead found myself at Mel's Radiator Shop, peering into the open hood of my car, at the shop-owner's invitation. "She's gonna be in for some major surgery," Mel said as he spread a quilted pad over the right front fender for me to lean on. The pad wore as much grease as Mel and my car combined, so I stood back a respectful few inches and tried to add a look of interest to my look of dread over the coming bill.

"I just want ya ta know," said Mel, "what yer in for before we start cuttin'. And you know, Miss Tonya, ya got options." I looked closely at Mel. I don't think Mel has ever been any-where near the flaxseed bin, though I suspect he'd spent a great many mornings breakfasting on cold pizza and hot instant coffee laced with real sugar and real partially hydro-genated soybean oil.

"Options?" I said. It was all I could think to say.

Mel wiped some grease on his nose with the back of his hand, which still clutched the radiator's lower drain cap, part number G608A453. He sniffed and looked briefly to the side, in the way movie he-men do when they're about to say something portentous and scene-changing.

"Gunk," he said, nodding sagely.

I do try, when it comes to expanding my English vocabulary. I got through graduate school unscathed. I can pronounce those great, lovely, Latinate polysyllables with a full measure of unassailable articulation, plus a touch of Russian accent that adds a certain zest and, for some, even a little charm. I can define *prestidigitation,* and use it in a sentence. I could natter competently for hours on *disestablishmentarianism,* and never appear *disingenuous.*

But "gunk" — short as it is — was a word beyond the frontier of my own lexicon. Still ... I couldn't let *Mel* know that.

"Gunk," I said.

"Gunk," Mel said. And nodded. And waited.

"What *kind* of gunk?" I ventured. Surely, I thought to myself, even "gunk" must exhibit *some* typology.

Mel bent down on one knee. Not good, I saw from his wince. He leaned, reached, grunted. And, though reaching blind, he found the spot. He'd palmed the radiator's lower drain cap, and this time stuck his index finger under my nose. What hung and dripped there seemed to resemble one of the nastier substances mentioned in the Book of Revelation.

"Gunk," he said, and nodded, waiting for my acknowledgment.

"Gunk," I said. I began nodding, too.

Mel started in. "Yeah, Miz Zee," he said. "You just gotta lotta gunk in there. You know — corrosion and crap and stuff. You get that gunk, it goes all through, winds around inside them coils, around, around she goes, and pretty soon you got yerself ..." His voice trailed off.

"What?" I asked.

"You got yerself one gunked-up radiator, little lady," said Mel. "Probably terminal," he said.

I wanted to sound wise, yet economical with words. I said: "So … ?"

"Two options," Mel said. "First, like I was tellin' ya, the big surgery. The whole enchilada, *with* the refried beans," he said. Mel knows I'm an aficionado of good nutrition. He's tried these food metaphors before. "New radiator," he said. "Rip 'er out, shove a new one in. Slap some hoses and hose-clamps on, fire this sucker up, you're good to go in two, three hours, you never look back."

I thought back to the surgeons who'd so skillfully equipped me several years ago with a pair of artificial hips. I wondered: If my own doctors had employed Mel's vocabulary and syntax, might I have opted for the wheelchair after all?

Mel jerked me into the present again. "OR," he said grandly, twirling his gunk-stained index finger in the air, "there's your non-invasive surgery." He was, as they say, on a roll. A great big kaiser roll, it seemed, as he went on and on. "Yessirreebob, we gonna try a rad flush. But not just *any* rad flush —"

"I should think not," I said.

"No, ma'am." He hoisted a neon-orange plastic gallon jug of … *something*. "Brand new. Works like the devil," he said.

"Oh, *good*," I said.

"Now no guarantees, but I've seen this stuff save a lotta cars, even cars that have been abused, ya know. Just like your Drano at home, you pour down your sink when you get your corn husks stuck in your garbage disposal. You know, them docs," he said, relaxing and lighting a grease-stained cigarette as he leaned against a faded no smoking sign. "Them doctors get a lotta their ideas from us, you know," he said. "Your human body — just like a car: Take care of her, she'll work like the dickens. You don't, you die, simple as that. And the number one thing about your car?" Mel asked.

After quite a long wait, I realized the question wasn't rhetorical. I started to answer, but he filled it in for me.

"Gunk," he said. "Pure gunk. There's nothin' ages a car faster 'n bad juice, neglect, and lettin' that gunk build up. We're in a war," he said. "A war against gunk. Just keep her gunk-free, and you'll be spending a lot less time with me, and a whole lot more time just livin'. Know what I mean?"

I believe, in fact, that I do.

We *are* engaged in a war on aging. For cars and humans. Mel may be greasy, but Mel's right about that.

The effects of the CR (Caloric Restriction) diet — sometimes called the CRON (Caloric Restriction Optimum Nutrition) diet — on animals point to impressive, life-changing results for humans. Of that there can be no doubt. Surely, then, we're winning the war.

But, as in all wars, there are loyal soldiers … and not. Dedicated workers … and not. People *with* the program … and not.

Gerontologists, you see, are not happy with the diet-based program. There's no money in it. Instead of promoting a nutritionally charged, low-calorie lifestyle, gerontologists are looking for two other factors to arrest aging. Drugs are one avenue the gerontologists take. The other is the avenue we shall call "procedures": a drug or procedure to arrest aging.

These two avenues are the major themes in the anti-aging studies outlined in a book some of you may have read: *The Scientific Conquest of Death: Essays on Infinite Lifespans.* The book's list and analysis of proposed solutions to aging left me in a strange and rather mixed state of mind — I might call it "anguished awe."

Drugs, for some gerontologists and some futurists, are "the only answer." Anti-aging medicine worthy of the name does not yet exist. Certainly, it would seem, none such *could* exist for at least fifteen to twenty years. But let us see if what is coming is optimistic enough.

Scientists agree that aging will never be cured in the sense that a bacterial infection is cured. Amoxicillin kills bacteria — disease dead — we're done. But it's different with aging. Aging is, after all, terminal. Therefore, we need not clutch desperately at cures, in the way Juan Ponce de Leon searched for a literal Fountain of Youth. (There *is* a physical Fountain of Youth, you know, the very one Ponce de Leon thought he had found. It's in Florida ... it doesn't work, never has, and is mostly visited by rapidly aging tourists.)

Instead, we must think of aging in the way we think of AIDS, or diabetes, or some kinds of epilepsy. Like these diseases, aging cannot, so far as we know or can rationally predict, be 'cured.' But it *can* be controlled.

One direction in which to seek such control is the development of new drugs. Antibiotics ... pain-killers ... corticosteroids ... anti-depressants ... in fact most pharmaceutical interventions are composed of chemicals that transmit signals to the body. These signals instruct one or another of the body's systems to delay, stop, or reverse symptoms related to a given pathology. These pharmacological instructions are fairly simple: A pain-killer 'tells' neurons to stop transmitting pain signals ... Corticosteroids 'tell' the immune system to diminish its response.

Curing aging is intended to be approached the same way. But the symptoms of aging are many — virtually innumerable. These symptoms are complex. And they occur all over the body. Thus the pharmaceutical approach to aging, having to wage war on so many fronts, will require transmitting much larger amounts of information to many more receptors, for many more specific purposes, than is presently the case. This, in turn, means more medication.

Since a *single* drug or treatment will not be enough to treat all the varied symptoms and systems involved in aging, literally thousands of pharmaceuticals and other medical treatments will be needed to give us our hoped-for 'immortality.' Some life, that — you'll live to be a hundred and eighty-six years old, but you won't be able to venture more than a hundred and eighty-six feet from your local drugstore.

Nanotechnology is another emerging frontier of development. Here the game is different. In nanotechnology, the game isn't 'treating' a disease or symptom. It isn't a game of masking a symptom, or of 'management' or 'coaching.' Nosirreebob, as Mel would say. It's a much stranger game that's afoot in the case of the nanotechnology soon to be revealed to us. Nanotechnological solutions are about no less a feat than this: improving the human body by reshaping its very biological features.

If you're over forty and have ever watched a lick of American television, you've seen the image. I'm talking, of course, about *The Six Million Dollar Man*. Lee Majors starred in this cheesy seventies sci-fi series. You recall the opening scenes … a frightful aircraft crash … the medicos' providential proclamation: "We can rebuild him. We *have* the technology!" To work they go, replacing lungs, heart, limbs, muscles, and more — and doing it more quickly than you can slap a radiator hose in a Dodge. The result: A square-jawed, handsome American movie-man, made to run at fifty miles an hour through the magic of speeded-up film.

The human body consists of about seventy trillion cells. Each cell contains about ten thousand times as many molecules as the Milky Way galaxy contains stars. The process of reducing biological aging entails letting loose a variety of kinds of procedures on each of the cells in your body. It's magnificent, this vision. "We *have* the technology." Well, we have the *idea*. They're working on the technology, and it is, already, beginning to get slightly past the drawing board. First, a tiny spherical device will be sent to enter every tissue, to remove accumulating metabolic toxins. As these toxins continue to re-accumulate (as they have all your life) you'll need a whole-body cleanout to prevent further aging, maybe once a year. As every mechanic knows, your real enemy is good old "gunk."

Second, chromosome replacement therapy will be used to correct accumulated genetic damage and mutations, cell by living cell. This, too, may be repeated every so often, and conceivably could become nearly as routine as a radiator flush.

Third, using cellular repair devices, we will be able to repair structural damage at the cellular level that the cell cannot repair by itself, and we'll do so on a cell-by-cell basis.

Tiny machines. Grand ideas. And all with one carefully calculated price: You will be attached at the hip to your newest doctor — the nanosurgeon.

If this seems futuristic ... just listen further.

They are talking about radically reengineering our bodies. They want to redesign our biological system through engineering on a molecular scale. They are so deeply ambitious as to want to reconstruct — indeed, redesign — our biological heritage.

Who's "They"? you ask. You know ... *They* ... with a capital 'T' ... The omnipotent, omnipresent, always looming in the dark "They." "They" are capable of a great deal. "They" brought you the transatlantic cable and the Forth Rail Bridge. "They" brought you penicillin. "They" brought collagen injections. "They" brought the land mine. And "They" brought Chernobyl.

They claim we will no longer need the present version of our digestive system at all.

They are looking forward to disconnecting the eating of food from the function of delivering nutrients into the bloodstream. We won't need to bother with extracting nutrients from food at all: Nutrients will be delivered to the body by other means. At the same time nutrients will be delivered to the bloodstream, using a completely separate process. The possibility exists that all the food we eat would pass through a digestive tract that has been disconnected from any possible absorption into the bloodstream.

They realize this would place a burden on our colon and on our bowel functions. So they propose to dispense with the function of elimination all together.

At present, you see, a trip to the restroom doesn't cost you anything, beyond soap, towel, toilet paper, and the little lavender toilet paper cover Aunt Nettie knit to hide the unsightly spare roll. There's no way to bill for a restroom trip, you see. In America, pay toilets never did net much more than a dime a time. And "They" require profits more worthy of a medical degree than a janitorial school certificate.

But what a wonder this newly re-engineered waste removal system would be. Now, gentlemen — no more reading your wife's lingerie catalogue as you enjoy a brief respite from the world's noise and haste. Now, you'll have to go to a specialist in filth removal. No crude "rad flush" here, good people. They are planning to accomplish this feat of sanitation using special elimination nanobots, each acting like a tiny garbage compactor. As the nutrient nanobots make their way from the nutrient garment into our bodies, the elimination nanobots will go the other way. Periodically, we would replace the nutrition garment for a fresh one.

In a car, there's nothing it cannot do without. Fuel filter, fuel pump, starter, alternator, spark plugs, distributor, and even your radiator lower drain cap, part number G608A453 — you name the part, it has to be there. There's a certain design economy, you see, in the way GM and Toyota do things.

"They," however, think less well of God's engineering. "They" think the human body contains some redundant organs. *Besides* the appendix. They want to get rid of some other organs. First on the hit list is the heart. Reason: It has a number of severe problems and it represents a fundamental weakness in our potential longevity. Though artificial hearts are increasingly well developed and are beginning to work well now, that's not good enough for the Brave New Wave of scientists. In *their* view, a more effective approach will be to get rid of the heart altogether. They suggest nanorobotic blood cell replacements that provide their own mobility, so the extreme pressures required for centralized pumping can be eliminated by using nanobots, tiny mechanical devices, to provide oxygen and remove carbon dioxide.

What the new breed wants is to get rid of organs that produce chemicals, hormones, and enzymes that flow into the blood and other metabolic pathways. Since part of the goal is eliminating most of our biological organs, many of these substances may no longer be needed, and will be replaced by other resources required by the nanorobotic system.

Hearts, for these scientists, are merely clever pumps. Muscles and bones arc mere motors and beams. Digestive systems are chemical reactors. They see the solution to aging in the transplanting or replacing of any or all of these parts. To combat biological wear and tear, simply replace each organ, when, or even before, it threatens to fail, with a biological or artificial substitute. "Yes, Miz Zee. We'll just rip that radiator right out, stuff a new one in — you'll be good to go by five o'clock."

That seems to be the fashion in which we're proceeding. And, as those of you concerned with fashion know ... "Accessories are *so* important."

No part of our body will be out of bounds for attaching new accessories. They are searching for ways to replace every part of the body and brain, and thus to repair the body's every defect and flaw — whether the result of aging or simply of God's 'sloppy' design. It seems certain that this will develop in purely cosmetic directions as quickly as in medical ones. Why wait for the anguish of your child's getting a tattoo as a drunken teen? Give her one from birth!

They say it is the limitations of our biology that make our lives so brief. Scientists are now looking into strategies to augment our brains as a means of gaining greater wisdom. Eventually, they want to entirely replace our brains — using nanotechnology, of course. They say they want to deliver us from the limitations of biology in order to achieve immortality.

The goal, ultimately, is to make us more *non*biological than biological.

"Too often, scientific 'facts' turn out to be wrong or misleading — we are told that there is 'no risk' of a Frankensteinian disaster, only to see it come true before our own eyes." — Dr. Nick Lane, honorary senior research fellow at University College, London, in *Oxygen: The Molecule that Made the World*.

Mary Shelley's *Frankenstein* didn't go far enough in its prediction. At least Dr. Frankenstein's monster was made largely of parts we'd recognize.

Science, there's no denying, can take justifiable pride in its many discoveries. What is hard to reconcile, however, is the hubris of science — its egocentricity. Medical science seems at times to be too much impressed with what it *creates,* and too little impressed with what has been *created.*

Education — technical education, most especially — offers no substitute for humility and common sense. Science's pride in its accomplishments must be tempered by man's acknowledgment of our own ignorance about how this human body of ours is so fearfully and wonderfully made. What about the billions of cells that are already doing their work marvelously?

The obvious approach is: Take care of this marvelous instrument. They — to be fair, some of "They" — look for ways to outsmart the body. They therefore undertake a monumental task — to achieve, and to improve upon, what a *healthy* body is already doing perfectly well.

While conventional, technologically oriented medicine embarks upon ever grander, ever more frightening schemes, alternative medicine is talking about more respect for the human body. The concept of a doctor being a healer in a sense of assisting the body to heal itself is the hallmark of alternative medicine, increasingly anathema to technologically oriented medicine. Medical science sees the body as a functioning machine, which can be manipulated when it malfunctions. Science does not see its mission as advocating the need to preserve the body and let it run its course. "No," say those on the technological leading edge of medicine, "Let that body fail and fade, let it even be destroyed." *Then* promise that body that you can do better.

That's the model presented in the book I've been describing all along — *The Scientific Conquest of Death: Essays on Infinite Lifespans*. The scientists in this book marvel about the prospect of freeing us from our biology. But they say not a word about not destroying, about understanding, using well, and preserving that which is already perfect. Not a single word does this volume voice about the need to treasure the ingeniously designed creation that is the human body.

What I do not understand is this: Are they trying to oversimplify the aging process, trying to fool the public into believing that they are close to the breakthrough of engineered immortality, forcing public opinion to accept the foreseeability of serious human life extension, all so that they can procure endless additional funding? Or are these arrogant men and women of science merely teens in that "know-it-all" adolescent stage?

You remember that stage ... You wouldn't be told by a mere mom what you could and could not do with your chemistry set. Things happened. And you went to school for two weeks with no eyebrows.

We put a great deal of faith in new technologies, new surgical procedures, and new pharmaceuticals. We expect miracles from medical science and refuse to see the miracles that take place in the human body.

The complexities of the human body have been reduced to CAT scans, colonoscopies, and mammograms. Our right to health has been taken from us and placed in the hands of the medical profession. Listen to me now. Get ahold of this powerful, shocking truth of modern life ... *You can't have health without a doctor*. It's just not allowed. The exuberance of living vitality and mature beauty have been reduced to antidepressants, annual check-ups, and Botox™ injections. Science, ladies and gentlemen, is only partly to blame. Who else is at fault? We are. *We* have relinquished our responsibility for our own health and subjugated ourselves to medical dependability.

We are bombarded with commercials for new drugs, which are proclaimed as panaceas today, disparaged as poison tomorrow, and litigated on massive scales the day after. The technology that promises to sustain our health creates, instead, both fear and dependency. Even the breakthroughs in medical technology that pledge to give us power to conquer serious diseases leave us helpless in the face of the common cold. Each of us has access to at least some medical care with its numerous devices from the latest research; many have the best health insurance, yet we feel utterly unprotected.

Does medical science hold anything *sacred?* It looks into changing the genetic program at a DNA or epigenetic level. It fragments the human body into smaller and smaller pieces in quest of solving the riddles of *How* to conquer aging and death. Yet all it finds is more *Whys.*

Medical science cries out that poor Johnny needs a liver transplant because of a debilitating genetic condition, yet they will use this technology and shamelessly promote it to millions of Tommys who indulge themselves with ham sandwiches and Hostess Twinkies. Yes, Johnny needed this liver transplant this time. But millions of other recipients simply needed to change their lifestyles. Artificial joints, transplanted organs, pacemakers. What should be an emergency need for a person in critical condition is being projected as the norm for aging. Medical science gives an increasingly artificial health, devoid of genuine vitality, and has practically extinguished the example of the person who is healthy by means of choice and discipline.

We will, I fear, succumb to this vision of the medical establishment. It is by laziness, by sloth and gluttony that we will succumb. Our goal will become to eat whatever we want, without limit, without remorse, without discipline or self-awareness, whatever gives us gastronomic pleasure. Only those who never miss a meal could come up with such ideas. *Little* eating gives *enormous* pleasure. They cannot know the meaning of real pleasure if they want to hold on to the pleasure of a gorged body!

In our never-ending quest for instant gratification we are pursuing addictions of all kinds. Instead of lasting satisfaction, we reinforce old patterns of suffering. Instead of seeking the new and the refreshing, we repeat, *ad nauseam,* our deeply dysfunctional paradigms. We are like a mouse being caught in a trap because it can't resist eating the cheese. The best thing we can do for ourselves is to refrain from the short-term pleasure of cheese in order to have the long-term pleasure of living. *But that is not what medical science is telling us.*

Cripples criticize the upright, the sick condemn the healthy. Medical science is, to a considerable and tragic degree, talking about health and spreading sickness.

Discouraged by traditional medicine, we search for health in alternative health care — acupuncture, herbs, aromatherapy if someone will help us. These practices are not without merit. But we need to help ourselves. We need finally to realize that health and longevity are our business. The human race now stands on the brink of a realization: we must move towards personal responsibility for our health and well being. If we do not, we will cause our own extinction.

I do not know about you, but I'm already fifteen percent titanium, and I'm guarding the rest of this body God gave me. Not that it's a perfect body, by any means. I'm not a runway model. I just do the best I can with what I have.

I'm really a lot less about the exotic than I am dedicated to the plain. To plain common sense. To plain truths. And to plain, simple techniques. Techniques you needn't go farther than your kitchen or your bathroom counter to apply. Techniques that don't have to cost much more than the price of a good juicer or blender at your local health food store. On the personal level, I'm about making *this* little body act as well as it can be made to. I do, as I say, the best I can.

Ladies? Do you remember when that was about the unkindest, most patronizing phrase that could be uttered about a girl or woman? That she "does the best with what she has." The ultimate in female-to-female insult by faint praise. But it's faint praise I'll take, thank you very much.

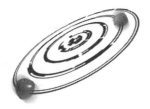

Chapter 3

Ancient Raw Food Roots, or Long-Haired Samian

In my search for anti-aging secrets I looked in the most unusual places. I once read a best-seller by an American psychic. To my surprise, I found the book intelligently written and packed with stimulating ideas. Even without accepting her beliefs, I enjoyed the book. The information was mind expanding and highly educational. But when I came to the section where the author's *Spiritual Guide* told her to eat more protein, waves of disappointment flooded me. I closed the book with a thud. The guide was obviously *misguided*. The author's being mistaken would be understandable — she's only human, I reasoned. But surely one would expect more enlightenment from a spiritual entity. When I hear a *Spiritual Guide* start talking like a poster boy for the Meat and Dairy Council, it certainly shatters my credulity. What's worse, this was a spiritual being muscling in on *my* turf!

I'm a voracious reader. Sometimes I find that special book that changes the paradigm of my thinking. You know the feeling — a method or idea that changes your perspective so profoundly you'll never be the same again. Such was the book *The Miracle of Mindfulness* by Thich Nhat Hanh. Amid this author's genuine jewels of wisdom, I stumbled upon an awkward little pebble. Admittedly, he made the statement only as an analogy in a quite different context. Still, raw food aficionados will cringe with me: "Without enough heat," the author says in his *The Miracle of Mindfulness,* "food will never be cooked. But once cooked … food reveals its true nature and helps lead us to liberation." In an otherwise brilliant text, overflowing with wisdom, I began to wonder, *how could the author have made such a grotesquely false statement?* More often than not, famous thinkers, past and present, see no absurdity in cooking food. No wonder the average person feels a shock upon hearing *No cooking — period!*

History, however, does give us those rare, enlightened individuals to whom we owe our breakthrough in conventional thinking about food. Raw food initiates know key names like Arnold Ehret, Herbert M. Shelton, T. C. Fry, and others from the not-so-distant past. The Bible, in Genesis 1:29, reads: *"God said, Behold, I have given you every herb bearing seed, which is upon the face of all the earth, and every tree, in the which is the fruit of a tree yielding seed; to you it shall be for meat."* Here, for Christians, is clear evidence for raw foods as the Creator's intended diet. Now, this is God talking. What about mortal individuals who promoted raw foods centuries ago? As I searched for the historic roots of the raw foods lifestyle, I developed an intense interest in the life of one particular philosopher — Pythagoras, and not only because he was a mathematician. Another reason, as you might have guessed, is the fact that historical sources point out again and again: he was exceptionally healthy and handsome in his "old" age.

Grade school encounters with geometry introduced Pythagoras to most of us. You may even remember the theorem bearing his name. I am introducing him here for an entirely different reason, however. Books on the history of fasting always acknowledge that Pythagoras made his students fast for forty days to purify their bodies and minds before he would even teach them. This frequent allusion was enough to stir my curiosity. I read every book available about him and was greatly rewarded for my effort. Everything I learned about him left me in awe of this philosophical giant's remarkable personality.

Pythagoras, one of the most prolific but sadly underappreciated geniuses of all time, is the father of Western science, medicine, and philosophy. His is one of the most famous names in the history of philosophy, prior to Socrates and Plato, whose philosophic works were partially derived from his teachings. He is credited with having first used the word *philosophy,* after rejecting the Greek *sophia,* or wisdom, as pretentious. He settled on describing his own pursuit of understanding as *philosophia* — the love of wisdom. It's a subtle distinction, this, but a clue to the man's humility. In contemporary culture, outside of the philosophic world, he is best known as a mathematician. For musicians, he is the father of the Western musical scale.

According to Diogenes Laertius, Pythagoras "was the first person to call the earth round, and to give the name of *kosmos* to the world." Mathematics and the numerical configuration of the universe figured into all Pythagorean thought. All things had a numerical base, something not unlike the molecular theory of today. Despite his impressive contributions to Western civilization, there is another side of Pythagoras which is relevant to contemporary lifestyles but which has been almost completely forgotten.

Pythagoras was one of the very first to advocate vegetarianism and to promote it as a prominent part of his curriculum. According to some sources, he was a raw food eater who convinced many to live on raw vegetables (not including legumes) and water, and to give up eating flesh (including fish). He was ultra-healthy. Evidently *he* never worried about if he getting enough protein. How about fatty acids? He lived for some 90 years, perhaps 100, and would have lived longer had he not, as some suspect, been killed by rivals. He died, in any event, a healthy, mature man.

Pythagoras' influence is much more widely spread than is ordinarily assumed, because many of his teachings have been incorporated into later doctrines. Contemporary vegetarianism depends on a moral and dietary base that would seem to have nothing in common with Pythagoras. But there *is* a connection, though no one has explored it.

As a reformer, the great teacher promoted strong morality. He taught the virtues of friendship, generosity, fidelity, abstinence, and moderation in eating. He opposed the ritual sacrifice of animals, believing that good, simple foods such as unleavened bread, honey and incense would honor the gods as well as would the blood of innocent creatures. Part of this belief came from his parallel belief in the immortality of the soul of both man and beast, and the ultimate reincarnation of both equally. He felt that the slaughter of beasts led to the slaughter of men and that abstaining from flesh was conducive to peaceful existence. Plutarch (A.D. 40–120), in his essay "On Flesh Eating," describes Pythagoras' views on diet as follows:

> "[Y]ou ask me why Pythagoras abstained from eating the flesh of animals, but I ask you, what courage must have been needed by the first man who raised to his lips the flesh of the slain, who broke with his teeth the bones of dying beast, who had dead bodies, corpses, placed before him and swallowed down limbs which a few moment before were bleating, bellowing, walking and seeing? How could his hand plunge the knife into the heart of a sentient creature, how could his eye look on murder, how could he behold a poor helpless

animal bled to death, scorched and dismembered? Does not the very smell of it turn his stomach? Is he not repelled, disgusted, horror-struck, when he has to handle the blood from these wounds, and to cleanse his fingers from the dark and viscous blood stains?"

The mathematician, Euxodus of Cnides (c.390–c.337 B.C.) went so far as to say Pythagoras not only avoided eating meat, but avoided both hunters and cooks whenever possible. (As for me, I avoid only those cooks who are likely to ask me to help them!)

Concerning Pythagoras as vegetarian, John Manas, president of the Pythagorean Society, writes:

"All vegetarians will be interested to know that Pythagoras had established in his philosophical school in Crotone a strict vegetarian system of living. The reason was twofold. No person who applies himself to the study of mathematics, philosophy astronomy, music, healing and other kindred subjects, can afford to fill his system with the impurities, poisons and toxins that the flesh of dead animal bodies carries. Besides this, animal flesh, as is well known to all occultists, is filled with animal magnetism and vibrations of the lowest type. These low vibrations and animal magnetism interfere with the emotional nature of man. The other reason is moral. All life was considered by Pythagoras and the Pythagorean as sacred, and as such no one has the right to take it. Killing in any form, directly or indirectly was considered a crime against the gods — the laws of Nature — and therefore the eating of flesh of a murdered defenseless animal was the same as participating in this murder. For these reasons all their sacrifices to the gods consisted of fruit and flowers. So repulsive to the Pythagoreans was the use of animal flesh as food for the aforesaid reasons, that they used the following characteristic slogan to express their utter disgust of this act:

'The carcass of animals should be avoided as something worse than manure'."

According to Diogenes Laertius, Pythagoras taught:

"No one ought to exceed the proper quantity
of food and drink."

In the ancient Mediterranean cultures, the common diet included bread and honey. But one thing was constant: Very little food was consumed by Pythagoreans. Since the stove had not been invented, bread was unleavened and uncooked. According to history, Pythagoras lived for the most part on bread and honey, with vegetables as dessert. He was also known for fasting. Says one source, "he used to stay in sacred precincts, and was never seen drinking or eating."

Pythagoras traveled widely and reinforced his belief in his chosen lifestyle by adapting traditions from other civilizations. By the time he was 56, he had studied in Babylon, Persia, India and Egypt.

His chronology, as much in dispute as any and all from the ancient world, is roughly:

589 B.C.	Birth
571-567 B.C.	Study and travel
567-545 B.C.	Egypt
545-533 B.C.	Babylon
33-529 B.C.	Samos
529-509 B.C.	Crotone (Crotona)
509-490 B.C.	Metapontum
490 B.C.	Death

In his sixties, Pythagoras settled in Crotone (formerly Crotona), a city in southern Italy, where he founded what today might be called a commune — a combination school and community to promote his lifestyle and teachings. Like all such societies, especially the schools of ancient Greece, the regimen of learning, exercise, and discipline was strictly adhered to. This particular manner of living became known as the Pythagorean Life.

The daily program at Crotone began with the observance of sunrise, a Pythagorean ritual where the white robed Pythagoreans gathered to greet the rising sun, while offering a hymn to the sun god Apollo. After a morning walk, students bathed, engaged in athletics, and then proceeded to the temple, forming groups around the masters of various studies. At noon they gathered for prayers to the heroes, followed by their first noonday meal of bread, honey, and olives. In the afternoon, they performed in the gymnasium, after which they spent some time in meditation on the studies given them in the morning. At sunset, prayers were offered and hymns sung to the gods of the cosmos. The second meal, taken always before sunset, was likewise vegetarian, consisting of maize and raw vegetables. In the evening, younger members read aloud, while the elders critiqued them.

Pythagoras' followers adapted what we would now call a low protein diet, which he believed promoted both physical and moral supremacy. His health regimen was considered responsible for his longevity, vigor, and handsomeness. As a result of his hygienic mode of living, Pythagoras preserved his body at all times in a state of health and vitality. He is said to have been over six feet tall, with a classic, perfectly formed physique, likened to Apollo's. His sheer presence, marked with power and intellect, never waned, but so increased with maturity that even nearing his hundredth year, he appeared to be in his prime. One biographer writes: "He was not sometimes sick and sometimes well, sometimes fit and sometimes lean, but always at the height of physical perfection."

He traveled to India at a time when Gautama Buddha was teaching a similar philosophy. Current accounts have it that Pythagoras appropriated these teachings for his own. But there's no proof to indicate that it happened that way. It may very well be that he exchanged ideas and that a part of the metempsychosis prevalent in Buddhism came from Pythagoras' beliefs. The Hindu prophet's teachings have become the universal source because he was the founder of a great religion. Pythagoras wore the blessing and curse of having been a "Renaissance man" in ancient Greece. DaVinci suffers much the same fate in the perception of the modern world. Both men are compartmentalized by the interests of their biographers.

In *Iamblichus's Life of Pythagoras* by Thomas Taylor, his bibliographer points up the respect Pythagoras enjoyed among his followers: "Such was their reverence for Pythagoras that they considered him as one of the Olympic gods who, in order to correct and improve terrestrial conditions, appeared to his contemporaries in human form, to extend to them the salutary light of philosophy. It was said of him "Never, indeed, came, nor will ever come to mankind greater good than that which was imparted to the Greeks through Pythagoras. Hence, even now, the nickname of 'long-haired Samian' is still applied to this most venerable among men."

Pythagoras' teachings influenced not only the men of his epoch such as Plato and Aristotle, but also Romans like Ovid and Apollonius of Tyana, who lived long, healthy, vital lives by adhering to strict vegetarian diets coupled with abstinence. Apollonius lived exclusively on fruits and herbs. Strictly followed, these essential aspects of the Pythagorean Life contribute to excellent health as gauged by increased vigor of body and brain. Apollonius revived Pythagoras' teachings five centuries later. As a neo-Pythagorean philosopher in the first century, he influenced another generation. These teachings were adopted by the Essenes, a sect of Jews and Greeks. The Essenes, whose communities were based along the shore of the Dead Sea, may well have been influential in the ministry of Jesus.

Shelley and Tolstoy were two of the great figures of the 19th century who studied Pythagoras' teachings. Let me mention also two remarkable 20th century personalities who followed his beliefs — Professors Hilton Hotema and Arnold Ehret. I am particularly interested in their writings about health because they were pillars of health themselves. Though neither acknowledged the contributions of Pythagoras to their lifestyles, they achieved remarkable results in forestalling aging by frugal, mostly raw eating. In so many historically famous cases of superior health and youthful physical appearance in advanced age, eating little seems to be even more important than eating raw.

None of Pythagoras' original writings survive. Much of his philosophical teaching reaches us from Plato through Aristotle. Pythagoras met with unfortunate biographers. It is doubtful whether any of his biographers ever missed a meal intentionally, and, thus, were unable to fully empathize with his teachings. They may have understood certain of his findings that paralleled their own, but they have nothing in common with his basic life premise. One author even refuses to believe that Pythagoras adhered to the rules he advocated for his followers. Obviously, this author never limited his food intake so he thinks anyone who claims to have done so must be lying.

Reading about Pythagoras left me with the feeling that most authors have left out the details about his lifestyle because they did not understand it. Almost every work I consulted touched his eating habits only marginally. I surmise, even, that some authors who sympathize with him have intentionally omitted the details of his peculiar lifestyle as freakish, perhaps worrying that this might detract from his genius. Often, the particularities of his lifestyle are, in written accounts, brushed off as an unfortunate side effect of a great mind.

Another reason Pythagoras is misinterpreted is because he was a polarizing figure, even in his own time. From his own time to ours, some have considered him nothing but a liar and charlatan, while others considered him a great mystic. His contributions to concrete science can't be denied, but his lifestyle has been questioned ever since his own time. The learned men of his time were widely divided about his ideas on diet and living. He was openly ridiculed by many.

Anyone who follows a person's lifestyle knows a great deal more about that person than do those who have no concept of the sensations involved. Though I claim no great level of expertise in the subject of Pythagoras, I do have an advantage over other authors who have written about Pythagoras, precisely because I am closer to his dietary regimen. This aspect alone affords me a deeper insight into his personality.

His dietary practices are considered an exaggeration by many who study him. What is there to exaggerate? Have *you* not been ridiculed and questioned about your personal choices? By following Quantum Eating, we have a connection and camaraderie with one of the most brilliant and innovative men who ever lived!

Some biographers begin with the wrong attitude. They believe that his minimal food consumption had no connection with his brilliance. They picture him as an oddity. Even more, they separate his strict dietary regimen from his extraordinary personality. Actually, *his long-practiced eating habits made him exceptional.* He was able to perform these remarkable deeds partly because of his lifestyle. One follows from another. Eating less and eating simply contributes greatly to developing higher conscience.

The very fact of eating less frees the mind from the unnecessary obsession of deciding what and when to eat next. The average person spends a great deal of time in thinking about, shopping for, preparing and eating food. Worse, they do it three to five times a day! Add working, watching TV, and sleeping, and your life is pretty well shot, without ever having had an idea, let alone an original one.

Pythagoras stands also as the father of modern medicine. He is not generally credited with the ongoing basis of the entire approach to medicine as represented in the Hippocratic oath, but it seems that his teachings were the basis for that famous edict. L. Edelstein references the oath in a brief 1943 publication:

"The oath, then, contains a view which was by no means generally accepted and it is impossible to suppose that all Greek doctors swore it. Yet it was a professional oath, but apparently applicable to a limited group only, which distinguished itself from the majority in its severe view, viz. the Pythagoreans."

The Pythagorean school practiced healing very carefully. They attempted to ascertain the symptoms in relation to the overall problem. They emphasized the preparation of the patient's food. Carefully prepared sustenance was an essential part of their prescription. Clean living and careful eating were the essentials of good health. The use of drugs was limited. Surgery was virtually prohibited — a clear precursor to the Hippocratic directive "First, do no harm."

Pythagoras not only taught his beliefs but performed nutritional experiments on his students. He is known to have written an extensive thesis (which has been lost) on the health and nutritional value of the sea onion. We now know, of course, that sea vegetables are rich in iodine and useful in health treatments. Our knowledge of nutrition has grown to the degree that we now understand that the by-product of foods are molecules referred to as free radicals, which can speed aging and severely damage cellular DNA. All modern anti-aging research can be summarized in one mantra Pythagoras practiced 26 centuries ago: lowering your calories is the surest way to health and longevity.

Many modern scientific breakthroughs were originally promoted by Pythagoras. The history of his life and health shows that, even without modern science, he managed to prove many of these theories simply by "walking the walk." In our time, of course, the looming shadow of capitalism has taken the idea of nutrition-based control of aging and turned it into anti-aging products, including a projected anti-aging beer from a German brewery. Clinics dedicated to the proposition of eternal youth spring up everywhere with vitamin cocktails, hormones and antioxidants. Some such clinics are excellent, but too many are emphasizing every-thing *but* a change of lifestyle. Their attitude is the ultimate promotion of "having your cake and eating it too."

Aristotle says that the Pythagoreans made a distinction between three planes of being: men, gods, and those like Pythagoras, who stand between the two. From my own and others' experience I can say that, even though Quantum Eating, like a Pythagorean diet, will not turn you into "gods," it will make your humanity more intense. It will make your step light and vibrant. It will diminish your interest in the merely material, and instead make you hungry for spiritual growth. The few historical personalities known for con-suming minimal food were all highly spiritual beings.

Minimal, "low protein" eating helps keep your fiber-optic channel to God unobstructed. Should some author's *Spiritual Guide* tell you otherwise, inviting you to boil your broccoli and braise your brisket, be skeptical.

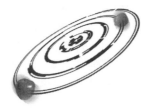

Chapter 4

Follow Me Down the Rabbit Hole Where Things Get "Curiouser and Curiouser"

I can hear you thinking out there ... What does the latest research in physics have to do with the ancient quest for perpetual youth? Answer: Everything! The answer has lain before us for centuries. The concept is simple. Yet *simple* doesn't necessarily mean obvious. In fact, a mind-bending discovery in physics was needed to understand this simple concept.

When you're dealing with big things — macro objects — senses and intuition are good guides. But in the weird wonderland of subatomic particles, your senses don't help. Only advanced mathematics help us make sense of the *micro* universe.

I hear your plea: *I hate math!* But before you throw the book across the room, wait! Get ready to follow me down the rabbit hole. Like Alice, you will find that things get "curiouser and curiouser ..."

"One can't believe impossible things."
"I daresay you haven't had much practice," said the Queen.
"When I was your age, I always did it for half an hour a day.
Why, sometimes I've believed as many as six impossible
things before breakfast!" — Lewis Carroll

Maybe you're thinking this is all way out of your league.
Or maybe you're totally intrigued. Either way — no worries!
I won't leave anyone behind as I explain the exciting new
theories in this book. My aim: to make them easy to grasp,
easy to apply in your daily life.

Remember when personal computers first came out? You
may have resisted learning how to operate one simply
because it was *unknown*. You thought computers were just
for geniuses, wizards. One day your daughter or grandson
mastered the computer, and you began to think — *It can't
be that hard. I made this genius,* you thought. *So I can
learn, too.* Now you're surfing the 'net, collecting baseball
scores, cruising sports and hobby pages, emailing and blog-
ging with the best.

What if I tell you that, if you shy away from quantum
concepts, you're missing on something *much* more profound than just about anything you'll find on the 'net?

Quantum mechanics has hit the mainstream! It's no
longer just for physics professors. Indeed, it's entering our
popular culture. Think of the expression *quantum leap* —
everyone knows it, and even the now-gone TV show of the
same name. Understanding quantum mechanics can improve
your diet, your health, your relationships, your business, your
entire life. The quirky world of quantum physics is a place
we can't — shouldn't, *mustn't* — avoid.

Quantum concepts can be quite abstract, and sometimes
have no analogy in common experience. But we need to
comprehend them, so you might as well learn from me. I've
always been a good teacher, if I do say so myself. (I taught

Algebra to ninth grade boys squirming to get to their next soccer game, and I made it *stick!*) Forget that you're "not mathematically inclined." Don't even *think* about your Attention Deficit Disorder as an excuse. (No matter — if you have it, you'll soon forget mentioning it anyway.) ADD is my specialty. Innumerable parents would tell me that their child had ADD. I'd always begin my lesson by explaining to the student that our educational system is the disorder — not them. Those of my students who understood that — ADD or not — finished with A-grades.

Then, as now, baby steps are the right steps to start. This is going to be simple. I'm going to *make* it simple. Starting with something very comfortable, taking one step at a time, we will safely complete the journey.

I promise I'll make your trip as painless as it can be. But with one condition: You promise to stick with me. As you venture through this book, feel free to re-read a sentence or paragraph as you need to. But never abandon or skip over a passage. Go for the most solid understanding you can reach. I'll do my best to make these concepts comprehensible even to the most science-challenged reader. I have no doubt about the ideas here — after you grasp this material, you'll love it. You'll be looking out toward new horizons. You'll gain access to the magical world of miracles between matter and energy. You'll be rewarded with real insights into the nature of matter and its relation to the human body.

The reader who wields Occam's Razor with both vigor and precision might cringe as I talk about "vibrations" and moving energy. Even though quantum physics says these vibrations are real, feel free to consider them metaphorical or allegorical. However you want to interpret the idea, be sure not to throw the baby out with the bathwater. Trust me — once you get over the twitches and at least consider a new outlook on the world, you will find an epiphany comparable to what the ancients must have felt when they discovered that the Earth is round.

Give me your hand. Let me guide you into the Quantum Age. Your willingness, plus an open mind, will lead you to rebirth, new ideas, new experiences. And a bold new beginning in anti-aging journey.

"Nothing exists but atoms and the void," said Democritus, some 2500 years ago. Materialism was born when this Greek philosopher proposed that all matter is made up of tiny, indestructible units which he called atoms. Newton's laws of motion were once considered the supreme laws of the universe. According to these laws, the physical world was nothing but a gigantic mechanism that worked like a clock. Now you can, of course, disassemble a clock and then put it back together. (Though, come to think of it, I once took apart an alarm clock in attempt to repair it. I still have all the parts. They're in a zip-lock bag in the drawer of my buffet, where they've been since zip-lock bags were invented.) The general opinion, in the world of conventional physics — the kind Democritus and Newton represent — is that an object could in principle be taken apart and put back together, and it would be exactly the same.

The primary feature of the Newtonian worldview is this clockwork universe. This universe is predetermined from the beginning to the end of time. It possesses "objectivity" — the assumption that rocks and planets objectively exist even if we do not directly observe them. Newton's laws give the sense that everything in the material world is predetermined. If you are standing under an apple tree directly beneath a ripe apple, it will hit you on the head sooner or later. Newton's laws reflect order in the visible world of common objects like stones falling, the motion of planets, rockets, cars and bodies.

In the Newtonian world, the assumption is also that not only are things immutable, unchanging, and subject to specific laws but also that the observer (casual or scientific) has no influence on the object of observation. Quantum physicists, however, believe that every act of observation disturbs the particle being observed.

Remember Gulliver among the Lilliputians? Or Alice in Wonderland? Peering into the realm of subatomic particles is just like looking into those literary miniaturized worlds. Opening a bedroom door unexpectedly can create bedlam. (Not to mention emotional cataclysm, dicey reputations, and some pretty nifty topics for neighborhood barbecues. That's "vegetable festivals" in my neighborhood, mind you. But I digress …) It is naïve to think that peering in at these worlds *doesn't* disturb the order of things. It can appear to be a crazy place, this world of the subatomic — but only if those who are looking are big. For subatomic particles, that is how they behave, that is their behavior code.

The weirdness of the quantum world defies common sense. We resist it vigorously. One of the reasons why this view is so difficult to accept is that it has no analogy in our everyday intuition and experience. The macro objects we see every day are not at all visibly disturbed or affected by observation.

When two different researchers observe a cup in a certain position, each researcher's observation affects the object's position so negligibly that it seems they are observing the same cup in the same place, that nothing has been affected by their mere observation. Their agreement on the data lets them conclude that the macro-world of matter is independent of their observation. Laser experiments show that simple solid objects like cups, vases and chairs *do move* by some tiny imperceptible distance between observations. And these infinitesimal amounts can be mathematically calculated. Welcome to the Mad Tea Party — with the teacups taking part!

In the macro, world we take it for granted that when you leave something in the fridge overnight, it will still be there in the morning, in more or less the same form you left the night before. If it does disappear, the only plausible explanation would be that somebody in your family chowed down on it while bingeing at night. Not so in the quantum world. Imagine for a moment that you are very tiny and can directly explore this subatomic world. Now suppose you were to leave something on one shelf — a flaxseed cracker, say — and then later return later to look at what had been left. It would appear that the object had moved to a different shelf or had disappeared entirely — this is the norm, here in subatomic land. An electron behaves by jumping from one orbit to another, without an observer's ever knowing where to look for it in the next instant. Therefore, we can only give an object's probable position, never an exact position.

Quantum physics insists that the human observer is not only necessary in order to observe the characteristics of an object, but that the observer is also necessary to specify the object's characteristics. According to quantum physics, there is no utterly objective world "sitting out there" waiting for us to discover it. We ourselves as observers, through our own individual perception, create and influence what we see as the world.

In the subatomic world you could peer into a refrigerator and see a slice of raw carrot cake, but immediately after that your friend could look into the same refrigerator and see a slice of cheese pizza. You see, reality changes depending on who is looking. If all this sounds like you are creating your own reality, then you've got it!

In the famous illustration of "My Wife and My Mother-in-Law" do you see an old woman or a young woman? Both are present, but you won't be able to see both simultaneously. In the quantum world, it gets even more interesting because there are multiple pictures from which to choose. The *potential* reality is available for our choosing. What we perceive as "reality" depends on the choice we make. Every act we perform is a choice, even if we are unaware that we have made a choice.

Our acts of observation are what we experience in the everyday world. How does an "act of observation" take place? As an observer, you have the choice of how you will view the picture. It is your choice that resolves the paradox. According to quantum physics, all paradoxes dealing with the physical universe are resolved in a similar manner by observation. Quantum physics implies that subatomic processes occur at random and that human intention influences the outcome of experiments.

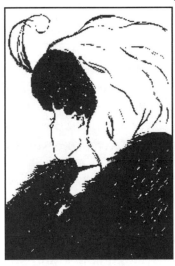

Look at the illustration again. Your act of observation creates the picture in your mind that "it" is a "young woman." Then the image is playing hide and seek with us: one moment it is a young woman, the next an old one. The picture seems to "jump" from one perspective view to another. The alteration is a good analogy of the abstract world of quantum physics. The world, like the phenomenon of the young woman versus the old woman picture, also must be realized in complementary ways. Be aware, too, that the dominant side of your brain or your dominant eye will dictate which picture you see first.

Observation makes it "real." Without observation, no "real" world would be possible.

According to quantum physics, there *is no* reality until that reality is perceived. We create our reality every instant of our conscious lives. We accomplish this construction by choosing among the many alternatives offered to our minds. Thus, at the quantum level of reality, when we choose to "see" what we see, this experience becomes reality.

This notion is called the *Principle of Complementarity*. Complementarity refers to a duality, like the young woman versus the old woman. The complementarity principle reminds us that while we are observing the young woman, the old is not seen but is still there. The same thing happens in quantum reality. When we concentrate on one display of reality, we are not able to see other possibilities. They are there, but invisible. To grasp the reality in it glorious paradoxical nature while observing, we must be able to see its opposite. Most of us can either see the fact or its opposite, but not both at once.

Subatomic particles are not solid little billiard balls, but vibrating swirls of energy that cannot be precisely quantified or understood in their private world. While observing a particle, we can choose to measure the particle's position or its momentum (a quantity defined as the particle's mass times its velocity), *but not both*.

An important law of quantum theory, the *Uncertainty Principle* says that these two quantities can never be precisely measured simultaneously. To gain precise knowledge about the particle's position we must assume it is fixed at least for a split second. To obtain knowledge about the particle's velocity we must assume it is moving. We have to start with one assumption or the other. But never both, because moving and staying still are opposites. We cannot have both — not at the same time. Do you see now that our calculations about the electron or other small particles are based on crude, imprecise knowledge?

To observe an electron, we must reach. We must install the proper measuring equipment. It is up to a researcher to decide whether to measure position or momentum. To install the equipment to measure the one prevents and excludes installing the equipment to measure the other. Moreover, the measurement changes the state of the electron itself.

It's not just a matter of the equipment we have now. Mere invention, mere technical progress, will never let us rise above the *Uncertainty Principle*. This limitation is never going to disappear because it has nothing to do with the imperfection of our measuring methods. This restriction is an integral part of the atomic reality. We cannot measure the particle's position precisely because the particle simply does not have a fixed position that can be measured. If we decide to measure the momentum (velocity multiplied by mass), the particle does not possess an exact velocity to measure.

The very fact of observation changes everything. The universe will never afterwards be the same. To describe what has happened, cross out the old word *observer* and put in its place the new word *participator*. Quantum physics says we are co-creators. Aren't we given a free will to choose? Thus, "reality" is a participatory creation.

The *Principle of Uncertainty* inherent in quantum physics denies us continuity and stability in all things. It goes against our ingrained desire for security. Yes, it takes away continuity. It takes away stability. It takes away predictability. But quantum physics gives a great deal in return. It gives us something more empowering — the ability to create our own reality. Our universe as a whole, and our bodies in particular, follows the laws of quantum physics.

Think of all the possibilities it can give us, if we can only learn to use quantum principles to our advantage.

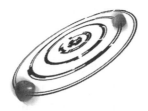

Chapter 5

Quantum Solution
to the Anti-Aging Quest

Many of you have never been to Moscow, but you have a concept of it. Some of you have visited the Russian capital as tourists or with church missions, so you, too, have a different perception. People who live in Moscow have a quite different impression yet of what Moscow is. And I, who am Russian, but never lived in the city, have still another concept. None of our concepts is Moscow. Conceptualized knowledge is infinitely limiting. The universe as a whole, and the human body in particular, is quite different from anyone's concept of it.

Classical Newtonian physics says that the entirety of material creation — largest to smallest, from galaxies to grains of sand to gluons and other exotic subatomic particles — moves in three-dimensional space. Any object's position and trajectory can be described with absolute accuracy under Newton's laws.

Subatomic physics changed everything. The old Newtonian model no longer gives a satisfying account of nature. New models must be found to replace the old. We apply the Newtonian model only to objects comprising huge numbers of atoms, and to speeds far short of the speed of light. The Newtonian model just won't fly when we're talking things as small as the workings within the human body. For us, the Quantum Age is already here!

The medical and nutritional sciences, however, seem to be unaware of the new revolution. Newtonian views of the human body still dominate these disciplines. But nothing in this Newtonian model accurately or fully reflects the real complexity of a human being.

Scientists have traditionally supposed that anything alive still operates according to the laws of Newton. They have assumed that the weird quantum rules apply only in dead, inorganic matter. Modern medicine, biology, chemistry, and even biochemistry depend upon Newtonian mechanics. Because aging is studied through these disciplines, they are looking for a solution where none exists.

The solutions to our problems can no longer be solved by using the machine model of the body. An entirely new pattern of thinking is needed. The mystery of health and longevity lies in quantum physics.

Let's throw no babies out with the bathwater. Quantum mechanics does not show that Newtonian mechanics is wrong. Quantum physics merely shows us that the Newtonian picture is limited. In the same way, this book ventures to show that the medical community's anti-aging aspirations are not wrong — just limited. Nanotechnology, gene therapy, stem-cell research are all three-dimensional solutions for four-dimensional problem. These Newtonian-based techniques, new or old, deal with visible symptoms instead of invisible courses.

Let's walk together now, out through the front door of classical physics, out onto a broad and very green lawn. (No, you won't have to mow it. One of the great benefits of quantum science is that we don't do yard work. We just clean the occasional window, the better to see through.) We'll shift our focus to quantum physics as I apply it to the fields of beauty and aging, showing you the bright possibilities of a radical new perspective on health.

Pretend we are living in Flatland.[1] You are a triangle. You have found yourself in a circular prison that you want to escape. This apparent problem has no real solution in a flat land. But add another dimension to this flat land — height, for example — and your problem is easily solved. With this new dimension of height, you can experience going up and down. Soon you discover you can get over the two-dimensional barrier of the prison wall simply by rising above it. Just go up and over the circle and there you are — outside the circle and *free!*

Adding a new dimension allows for new possibilities. Not just in imaginary worlds, but in the very world we live in. Some problems have no solution in a two-dimensional world. Some problems have no solution even in our three-dimensional world — where *do* those socks that disappear in the dryer go? Aging is that kind of problem. A new dimension offers a new way of solving a problem — a way that seems impossible in our three-dimensional world.

---

1. *The reference here is to a remarkable and delightful work far ahead of its time — Edwin Abbott* Abbott's Flatland: A Romance of Many Dimensions *(1884). Sixth edition. Dover Publications. 1953.*

Our language and mentality knows only three-dimensional 'images' and, therefore, we find it extremely hard to deal with the four-dimensional reality of relativistic physics.

Mathematics describes a world of four or more dimensions, indeed of any number. Most people think of mathematics as dealing with calculating taxes and balancing checks. But that is arithmetic. *Mathematics* deals not only with real numbers, but also with the concepts of multidimensional spaces and infinity, which we have no way of experiencing with our senses.

We tend to define our reality through the five senses — sight, sound, taste, smell, and touch. By doing so, we conclude that the solid, substantial objects in our everyday existence are real. Not so, when you peek into the subatomic world. The fantasy realm of *Alice in Wonderland* is a great nonsense story, similar to our material world, in which the reality "out there" is much stranger than we could ever imagine it to be. Our senses are of no help in dealing with the subatomic world.

Quantum theory transcends sensory experience. As we cut deeper and deeper into nature, we have to abandon more and more of the images and concepts of ordinary language. Our ordinary language pares down word representation with its images from the world of the senses. Senses are no longer helpful when dealing with the micro world. We are at a loss for words to describe observed phenomena. Indeed the very phrase *at a loss for words* implies the words are there — we simply cannot put them together adequately. In this case, the words simply don't exist, because language is based on the world as we know it — and we do not know the micro world.

"The problems of language here are really serious. We wish to speak in some way about the structure of the atoms ... But we

cannot speak about atoms in ordinary language."
— W. Heisenberg

Our senses give us only three-dimensional views of ourselves. Einstein taught us that space and time are not what they seem to the human senses. They should be regarded, he said, as two connected entities within a greater whole called space-time. The four-dimensional space-time world is presented through abstract mathematical formulas, but their visual imagination is limited to the three-dimensional world of the senses.

You are not simply the image you see at one time and one place. In a regular two-dimensional mirror, we see a snapshot of ourselves in one particular time and space. If there were a three-dimensional mirror, we would, perhaps, see a long, accordion image, including a snapshot of every single moment of our lives. Our state, in that instantaneous moment of space-time, is influenced by all the conditions, all the relationships in our prior living and even our future. Remember, when we add another dimension, the future becomes foreseeable. Now we see how unscientific it is, according to the New Physics, to focus on treating just a symptom of a disease, or a sign of aging.

Anti-aging science is on the wrong track! We are four-dimensional. This book confronts the painful limitations of the machine model of the human body. Humans and their organs are still treated, for most purposes, as machinery. Medicine that treats symptoms offers "Flatland" solutions to multidimensional problems. Aging is a four-dimensional problem. It has no solution in three-dimensional space. This book adds another dimension to aging and suggests that aging goes far beyond its mere symptoms or signs.

Just as physicists had to give up their preconceived ideas about the physical world, now it's is your turn to give up yours. Are you ready? Quantum Eating will require a quantum leap in your belief system. When we add time as the fourth dimension, we're forced to look at the constants in our lives — food, water, oxygen, sleep, sunlight, even thought. Quantum Eating will change your perception of everyday activities like eating, breathing, exercising, thinking and living as a whole. At the same time, quantum physics helps us to see that no quick fix found in a doctor's office or a pill bottle can possibly solve the anti-aging problem.

The Second Law of Thermodynamics — the Law of Entropy — states that everything in the universe is running down, or falling into disorder. We now recognize this fundamental law of physics to be just the natural tendency of things to move ever nearer chaos. Take socks, for example. In my house, they seem to begin their cycles of use in the drawer, neatly folded, nicely arranged by color and style. Then, after wearing, they go in the clothes hamper, where they're anything but organized. If I go away for a week and leave my husband, I'll come home to socks on the floor, hanging from the lampshades, etc. I'm thinking of writing a new book called *Entropy and Men*. But I digress ...

When a system that is not alive becomes isolated or is placed in a uniform environment, all motion comes to a rapid standstill as a result of friction. Electric current flows until high and lower potentials become equal. Substances which tend to form a chemical compound do so. Heat gets redistributed and temperature stabilizes. The whole system becomes a dead, inert lump of matter. No observable events occur. The physicist calls this state "thermodynamic equilibrium" or "maximum entropy."

Entropy — the degradation of the matter and energy in the universe to an ultimate state of inert uniformity, a process of degradation or running down or a trend to disorder.

Entropy is bad. Entropy is degeneration. At the same time entropy is a wonderful concept you can use in your daily life. Say you're at your high school or college reunion. You see a rather nasty former classmate. Yes — you know just who I'm talking about! Instead of saying she's showing her age, just sidle up to a friend, point out Ms. Meanie, and say: *Her entropy is showing, don't you think?* Who says science isn't socially useful?

Sickness is positive entropy at work. Dying is reaching your maximum entropy. When someone questions your raw food lifestyle, just say, "I'm reducing my entropy." That will keep them thinking for a while. The good thing is that entropy can be taken away. To signify this situation mathematicians use the minus sign. Entropy, with the negative sign, they call "negative entropy." And now something good and positive is called "negative." Confusing? Mathematicians and physicists seem to enjoy doing that to us! Life, rejuvenation, simply stated, is a form of order or negative entropy. You could tell your next date, "Your negative entropy blinds me." If they understand what you're saying, you may have found a soul mate. If not, well, good riddance.

With aging, a living organism continually increases its entropy — or, you might say, produces positive entropy — and thus tends to approach the dangerous state of maximum entropy — that is, death. The living order somehow manages to escape degeneration at least temporarily. How? The work of Ilya Prigogine, Nobel Prize-winning author of *Order Out of Chaos: Man's New Dialogue with Nature,* shows that this is because living systems are dissipative, open systems. They can release positive entropy, giving up heat, and they can suck in negative entropy from other sources. For plants, the sun is an ultimate source of negative entropy. Plants possess the marvelous ability to harness sunlight, the ultimate source of energy, becoming a condensed sunlight.

Living organisms seem to compensate for the effects of entropy by the very fact of living. Life attracts a stream of negative entropy upon itself. Life retains a high level of orderliness by continually sucking orderliness from its environment. The kind of order humans feed upon is sunlight and plants, harnessed sun energy which serves them as foods. Life is an orderly behavior of matter. As Schrodinger said, life is "order from order." It's like living in a miraculous house that keeps itself clean without a cleaning crew.

Living organisms create "negative entropy" in the opposite sense of the law of degradation. Energy is produced or synthesized within the living organism. The living body postpones aging and decay for a considerable time by metamorphosis. The body absorbs and assimilates the available elements from the environment to sustain itself. The body produces negative entropy through eating, drinking, breathing, and assimilating. The ability to produce this energy declines, causing the breakdown and death of matter. The anti-aging solution lies in this ability to create negative entropy.

Time and reality are closely related. For humans, reality is embedded in the flow of time. You cannot run the body backward to make up for entropy. We cannot replay events in time. Time is a one-way street, like an arrow shot from a bow. The irreversibility of time is itself closely connected to entropy. To make time flow backwards we would have to overcome an infinite entropy barrier. If it were time aging us, there would be no hope. But different people age at different rates. (The most vivid, if not exactly the most scientific, proof of this fact will come to you vividly if you'll perform one simple experiment: Go to your high school reunion.) So it is not time that is aging us — *then what is?*

Aging is the cumulative effect of the abuse your body has taken, both natural and self-inflicted. It did not happen overnight, and it cannot be fixed by a one-time solution. Of course, it took time for you get where you are now, sick and tired, so time will be needed to make you healthy and youthful. But since you will not be re-tracing your steps, the good news is that not as much time will be needed. The cumulative effect of your rejuvenative practices will get you there.

Glaring evidence that this is the correct way is the fact that, during rejuvenating practices such as fasting, you re-live your symptoms briefly, with their duration directly linked to their severity. And a short fast takes off years of abuse.

Quantum physics sees the human body as a dynamic web of interconnected relationships. Your body is a complex controlled feedback system, a self-organizing entity. The information from the smaller units, like cells, travels to the larger units like organs, glands, and tissues, to the circulation and maintenance systems. Different levels of complexity are present in each manifestation. The human body is a complex interlaced with so much "feedback" that study based only on analyses of parts of the body is infinitely limiting.

The human body is infinitely more than reductionistic science can ever envision. Modern physics has confirmed that all concepts we use to describe the human body are limited, that they are not reflections of reality, as we tend to believe. In fact, a profound change of approach, from the intent to dominate and force the body organs and systems into submission to an attitude of cooperation and non-invasiveness, is needed.

The non-linear properties of the human body must be taken into account when searching for a solution to aging. There is no one-time, one-place solution. For example, a surgery or a supplement is not a solution because it is a three-dimensional approach to a four-dimensional problem. When you remove the dimension of time, the promised elixir of youth becomes a fairy tale. So anti-aging possibilities must be lived and experienced every moment of your physical existence.

When it comes to the human body, conceptualized knowledge becomes a huge obstacle in your learning to benefit from the body's extraordinary abilities. Trying to outsmart the human system is futile and foolish. We must simply let the human system *be,* let it do what it is so well designed to do. Do not interfere. It eats, so be sure it has the best food available. It breathes, so be sure it has the cleanest air to breathe. It moves, so be sure it has the opportunity to do it on a daily basis. It thinks, so be sure you have positive thoughts to occupy your brain.

The fact that you are the one who dwells in your body is essential. No visiting doctors or healing specialists can help you here. Practices like meditation, breathing exercise, raw food, and fasting cannot be fully learned, in the precise sense of that term. For the person seeking truly to *respect* the human body, these practices must be *contemplated*. By doing so, you turn the conceptual knowledge of your body into a rich experience.

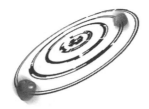

Chapter 6

Dead or Alive: Do We Know the Difference?

Go up to an average American man. Ask him, "What is life?" He'll tell you it's watching football in his Barcalounger with a beer and a bowl of barbecue corn chips. Ah, well — it keeps him out of the pool halls ... Here, however, I'm asking a straighter, more serious question, and one much more worthy of your reflection.

Life and non-life are intermingled throughout the entire universe. We believe that we have no trouble distinguishing living from non-living things. Consider an eagle nesting in her rocky aerie. The eagle is alive, animate. The rock is not, so it must be dead. The very question of what is alive and what is not seems absurd. The answer seems obvious. Yet it's not all that easy to define. There is, we believe, a sharp dividing line between living and nonliving systems. But scientists cannot seem to find it. No single, simple defining quality distinguishes the living from the nonliving.

The mystery of life's origin has puzzled philosophers, theologians, and scientists since thought began. Even with all the progress in molecular biology, scientists still can't decide exactly what it is that separates a living organism from nonliving things. Science has been battling with the enigma: How can life arise from non-life? In fact, science isn't yet able to define "life" or "non-life." All the definitions so far ventured are limiting and flawed.

We know there is a radical difference between what is living and what is nonliving. So what is it? When is a piece of matter said to be alive? What is it that distinguishes living organisms from non-living things? Dylan Thomas described the living organism as "The force that through the green fuse drives the flower."

Aristotle considered the essential quality of living organisms to be the internal ability to initiate independent action. "For nature is in the same genus as potency; for it is a principle of movement — not, however, in something else but the thing itself."

One obvious feature of life is the ability to grow — a blade of grass springing up through a sidewalk crack, a tree taking root in a gutter. This ability to move against external forces is a fundamental property of life, a resource that is lost when life is lost. Somehow, as long as an organism remains alive, it is able to resist external forces and perform actions to benefit the whole organism. Even inanimate objects can perform such actions; the difference is that their movements are predictable.

Imagine throwing a stuffed bird and a live one into the air simultaneously. Both birds lift into the air, all right. But could you predict their actions? There are no surprises with the stuffed bird. All we have to do is take into consideration the height from which it was thrown, its mass, force applied, direction of travel, air resistance, etc. Given these, we can predict, with great accuracy, where the stuffed bird will land. The dead bird cannot direct its actions. Its behavior is predictable, entirely deterministic. Not so with the living bird. No formula can tell you where the live bird will end up. It may fly high up in the branches of a tree, land on a rooftop, return to its nest, or go off in pursuit of food. The possibilities are endless.

Dead matter is passive, inert, responding predictably when external force is applied — the carcass plunges to the ground under the pull of gravity. But living creatures have literal lives of their own. They can do as they please, limited only by the boundaries of terrain and their own physicality. Even bacteria do their own thing in a limited way. They seem to have freedom of choice. Life offers an infinite choice of possibilities that cease only when death occurs. A living organism has a kind of intelligence of its own. It "knows" what to do. Matter is alive when it goes on about its own business, moving, striving, exchanging material with its environment and so forth. Not only does living matter interact with its environment, but it is capable of doing so much longer than we would expect of an inanimate piece of matter in similar circumstances.

Ilya Prigogine conjectures that order and organization can actually arise "spontaneously" out of disorder and chaos through a process of "self-organization." Living and dead entities are collections of molecules. In a living organism, molecules are put together in much more complicated patterns than the molecules in non-living things. Physicists observe *periodic crystals*. These are very complicated objects. They fascinate scientists with the most complex material structures observed in inanimate objects. But no matter how strikingly beautiful and complex these crystals are, they do not hold a candle to the *aperiodic crystal* present in living organisms. Periodic crystals become modest and homely when compared to the intricate organization of living tissue.

The most essential part of a living cell — the chromosome — looks like an *aperiodic crystal*. Chromosome molecules are "aperiodic solids." These molecules represent the highest degree of well-ordered atomic association we know of — much higher than the ordinary periodic crystal. In the living organism, each single group of atoms exists only in one copy.

Erwin Schrodinger in his famous book *What Is Life?* explains it this way: "The difference in structure is of the same kind as that between an ordinary wallpaper in which the same pattern is repeated again and again in regular periodicity and a masterpiece of embroidery, say a Raphael tapestry, which shows no dull repetition, but an elaborate, coherent, meaningful design traced by the great master."

In other words, aperiodic crystals, which make up the very fabric of life, are infinitely more sophisticated than most complex patterns observed in inanimate matter. All processes in an organism's life cycle exhibit an admirable regularity and orderliness, unmatched by inanimate matter. The arrangement of all the atoms along DNA chains is anything but random. In DNA we see atoms and subassemblies of atoms intricately organized in a highly specific way. Here, precisely in such organization, lies the difference between a moth, a manatee, and a man.

The higher temperature itself speeds up the chemical reactions involved in living. Heat increases the commotion among molecules — that is to say, increases the entropy. This is exactly what happens when you cook once-living food. When you heat it, you destroy the neat, permanent arrangement of the atoms or molecules and turn the arrangement into chaos. If you don't like thinking of cooked food as *dead*, think about it as *chaotic* or *jumbled,* or *plain ugly.*

Life, as a sharply defined concept, disappears when dissection reaches the level of the individual cell. Now we no longer have an answer. Is a chromosome alive? What about a gene? DNA? A ribosome, or a protein, or an enzyme?

Trying to peer into life by looking deeper and deeper, we lose life itself.

No matter how sophisticated technology becomes; no matter how deeply scientists penetrate into nature searching for its ultimate building blocks, life disappears before their very eyes. The main lesson here is that life cannot be understood in terms of parts.

As incredible as it might seem, living organisms are made of exactly the same elementary particles as inanimate objects. What constitutes a living cell is no different from chemical components of the inanimate. The whole *is* larger than its parts. Life seems to emerge only at higher levels of organization. There must be a border between the quantum and the classical world. The border must lie somewhere above the level of electrons and protons but below the level of a whole cell.

There is no such thing as a living molecule — only a system of molecular processes that, taken collectively, may be considered alive. To find this life, we must look inside living cells. But here is a problem that can only be appreciated by quantum mechanics. To examine the cell's interior structures with a powerful electron microscope, the cell would first have to be frozen, sliced, dried and, inevitably, killed. We cannot examine a living cell *in action.* You can't perform an autopsy on a living human being. Not, at least, without some protest from the living human being. And not without killing him. Likewise with a rutabaga — the protest may be slight, but the cells must die in order for their inner workings to be examined.

The living cell is the most complex system of its size known to humankind. Its host of specialized molecules, unique to living material, are themselves already enormously complex. Nanotechnology — building structures and devices measured on a scale of billionths of a meter — promises to revolutionize our lives. As we admire the achievements of micro-engineering, breathtaking in their implications, let us keep in mind that the living organism is already full of nanomachines — living cells.

Scientists construct nanoscale microelectronic devices. Living cells are already working at these levels without any help from science. A living cell is a nanoscale device. Interpreting life by the ordinary laws of physics is very difficult. The complexity of the living cell is astonishing. It operates with the exact precision of a great laboratory, yet on the tiniest scale. The innermost workings of a single cell are immensely complicated and strikingly sophisticated. Each cell "knows" what its specified function is and it stays in its designated place. Each atom individually is unthinking. Yet somehow, collectively, these unthinking atoms get it together and produce a life of exquisite complexity. Think in terms of bees and ants in our macro world. The individual ant or bee doesn't "think" in our sense of the word. Yet they build structures and societies of marvelous complexity.

Cells communicate with each other for the benefit of the organism they belong to, and they do so with meticulous precision. In the process of carrying out their duties, each has errands to run, meetings to attend. Everything they do is important in the overall well-being of the living organism. Communication takes place at every level. Molecules must travel across the cell to meet others at *just* the right place and time in order to carry out their roles properly. Somehow, these unthinking atoms get it together and collectively form a living entity. How does this colony of cells come into a being all on its own? How does a single cell, which can only push and pull its immediate neighbors, cooperate to form and sustain something as ingenious as a living organism?

No law known to physics can explain what compels a colony of atoms to follow a prescribed blueprint. The critical difference between a collection of cells and a living organism is the ability of an organism to act in a synchronized manner for the benefit of the body as a whole. At the moment of death, organization ceases. A dead body still hosts plenty of live cells, but live cells do not make life in the same way that neglected instruments piled in the band room will not make music of their own accord.

Variety and complexity are essential characteristics of life. In familiar inorganic substances, such as air or water, a typical molecule will consist of two or three atoms bound together by electrical forces. In contrast, a molecule of a living thing, like a molecule of DNA, may contain many millions of atoms. All the chemical reactions and biological processes in a living system follow a controlled program operated from an information center. The aim of this reaction program is not only the self-reproduction of all components of the system, but the duplication of the program itself.

Quantum physics sees the difference between living matter and dead matter in internal intelligence revealed through the organization of information. And the assembling is done by following blueprints, programs. These instructions are part of life itself. There is a nonmaterial "something" inside living organisms, something unique and, literally, vital to their operation. Some call it a *life force.* Quantum physics prefers to call it *information.* The secret of life comes from its informational properties. A living organism is a complex information-processing system.

Life is distinguished from dead matter by a network of organized information. At death, the *information* which has kept the creature *alive* gets cut off. Atoms of a once-living organism stop functioning together and regress to their natural state of chaos (which we recognize as death).

If you don't like saying that cooked food is *dead,* how about *comatose?* In fact, it is equivalent to an unconscious human being — the information web is completely lost.

" … Intelligence is more important than the actual matter of the body, since without it, that matter would be *undirected, formless,* and *chaotic.* Intelligence makes the difference between a house designed by an architect and a pile of bricks." — Deepak Chopra, *Quantum Healing*

There is constant quantum dialogue between the living organism and the environment. When you pick a fruit or cut off a stem, the dialogue is still there. In plants, death does not happen instantaneously when part of the plant is removed from its original position or state. When we consume plant food, the raw plants begin to communicate with our own body. That aspect of living food shows how limiting it is to think about food only as a source of proteins, carbohydrates, fats, minerals, vitamins, and water necessary to support life.

Food is also information. Just as we do not die immediately when cut off from our food supply, plants (greens, fruits, vegetables) are not dead when we pick them from the garden. They show great diversity in the way they ripen and how long they will maintain a semblance of life before becoming either withered or rotten.

What animates living organisms? These are networks of instructions, directions with feedback. Your body is an information system. Your cells are constantly talking to each other through different kinds of messenger molecules. Some of the more familiar ones are neurotransmitters and hormones.

"When we eat a head of lettuce, every leaf expresses the beauty and complexity of the cosmic intelligence that formed it, and so we are partaking of cosmic intelligence by ingesting it directly. The same for each perfect grain of rice, each generous fruit. At the biological level, we are preying on them, but at the level of intelligence and consciousness, we are collaborating with them in a sacred rite, for the intelligence that

organized their form and function also organized ours."
— B.K.S. Iyengar, *Light on Life, The Yoga Journey to Wholeness*

Recent scientific research about food and nutrition has focused on phytonutrients (also called phytochemicals). These natural compounds in plant foods communicate directly with our body chemistry to assure our health. When phytonutrients enter your body, they join your own network of messenger molecules. This discovery has brought a new significance to the very word *food*. There are thousands of different phytonutrients. Now, nutritional scientists research them for their abilities to prevent cancer and protect against forms of heart disease, arthritis, and other degenerative disease.

When are we going to learn that dissecting life only moves us further away from discovering the sanctity of life? Unfortunately, the grand importance of the raw-foods-only lifestyle still remains overlooked, even though it remains the most logical and attractive direction for research.

Quantum physics reveals that the raw plant food on the atomic level is vastly intelligent, highly organized, and intricately beautiful. And this is the only food that will be able to communicate with your body to assure your health and longevity.

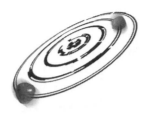

Chapter 7

Nutritional Science and Green Pudding,

or

"It Isn't Easy Being Green"

I'm a great fan of Victoria Boutenko, author of the remarkable book *Green For Life*. I am deeply indebted to her for introducing me to a marvelous culinary delight: green smoothies. During my visit with her, I made my own variation by mixing a ripe mango and a leaf of Swiss chard (stem removed) in a Vita-Mix, with no water added. Victoria said she loved it but said it looked less like a smoothie and more like "green pudding." You can't argue with Victoria's expertise: Green Pudding it is!

Traveling the country giving raw food presentations, I originally used a *tahini* drink called "Better Than Chocolate Mousse" — see the recipe in chapter 34. My husband Nick helps me at these events. Lately he's been in charge of making and serving the Green Pudding. The day I decided to switch to Green Pudding, Nick smirked: *Who's gonna drink this green* — he searched for a word — *stuff?* It came as a big surprise to Nick, when he actually served Green Pudding for the first time, that people were delighted with the emerald mix, even asking for seconds. They were ready for my message and they were converted. From one event to another, north to south, east to west, my Green Pudding was a smashing success. With all this success, though, we started to take things for granted. Until one day, it all changed.

The Symposium for Mid-South Nutritionists and Dieticians invited me to speak at their conference. These were licensed professionals. We came well prepared, wanting to give our best presentation ever. Nick, as usual, served our Green Pudding. The audience members began to eat. During a break in my presentation, Nick approached me and whispered, "They're making faces! They don't like it!" His own face contorted in complete bewilderment. Seeing my disappointment, he joked, "Since they don't want to eat it, maybe I should turn the cup upside down and say it's for external use only?"

These are people educated *scientifically* to know the importance of eating greens. Combining fruits with greens in a smoothie is a great innovation — it creates such a palatable, even pleasurable, way of getting this wonder food down. I thought this group would be really excited. But Kermit the Frog is right: It isn't easy being green. Nick was right, too. Not only was there no enthusiasm, but the resentment in the air was so thick that, if processed in my Vita-Mix, it would have burned up the motor. After the lecture, a woman from the audience came up to me and said: "You are so fortunate that you can say what you did. If I were to say it, I'd lose my license."

What on earth was I saying? *Eat more fruits, vegetables, nuts, and seeds in their unprocessed, unheated form! There are more nutrients in green plants than in pills!* In my arguments I used common sense. I told interesting anecdotes of healing and recovery from serious illnesses. Mostly, however, I delivered a straight appeal for a "go with nature" principle.

I have given hundreds of presentations to different groups of people, but never before have I felt so alienated. I was intruding on their profession — I felt like a plumber making a presentation to a convention of obstetricians.

After it was over, I felt as green as my pudding. I thought to myself, nutritionists or not, I would not let this happen again. I've discovered an awkward truth: there are so many people who want to hear my message that I simply do not have the time and energy for those who are not ready for it.

For me the burning question was: *Why* are they not ready? As always, if there's something I don't understand, I'll explore it. I went to the university library to get a self-taught crash course in nutritional science. Once there, I faced literally shelves upon shelves of books related to this subject. As I tried to figure out how to narrow my search, I occupied myself counting books with the word *protein* in the title. I gave up at 87 — there is a limit to how high even a mathematician is willing to count.

Nutrition is the science of nourishment. The main objective of nutritional science has to be to make us all healthier and make us live longer. Pythagoras knew this. He ate only twice a day, and then very little. He was never sick, and was full of vigor, and handsome even in his "old" age! How did Pythagoras manage to do this without knowing any of the science in the books I faced? Thinking of Pythagoras gave me hope. Good! With my unusual food regimen, among all this research I had begun to feel like a freak. Yet, with this massive body of research, we are still sick. The more new solutions we find, the more new diseases surface.

I wanted to learn what kinds of research methods are used in nutritional studies. What courses did students have to take to qualify as nutritionists? I finally bought two textbooks on the research courses involved — one an under-graduate text, the other on the graduate level. Never mind that it cost four hundred bucks for the pair! I did find out how the research was approached. But mostly I found out what *wasn't* considered. Quantum physics, which I believed more and more to be the key to understanding nutrition, was nowhere to be found in the research curriculum.

It amazes me how many nutritionists I meet risk losing their licenses by promoting total body healing through raw foods and holistic methods. I question the validity of how nutritional science is taught.

Nutritional science is not under attack here. The error lies in the discipline's desire to apply classical laws where they are not always applicable. My prescription: All nutritional majors should be required to take a course in Quantum physics. Please don't think I am belittling nutritional science. (Or getting back at them for not eating my pudding!) The new physics does that job for me. In fact, it humbles all scientific methods.

Nutritional science is still based on a classical Newtonian view of matter and energy, even though a "post-mechanistic" view of the universe is spreading across a broad front — in cosmology, chemistry, new physics, quantum mechanics and particle physics, in the information sciences and, more reluctantly, in biology.

Mathematician and scientist Rene Descartes created the method of analytic thinking — the method of breaking up complex phenomena into pieces in order to understand the behavior of the whole from the properties of its parts. The material universe, including living things, was for Descartes a "machine" which could be understood completely by analyzing its smallest parts.

Ilya Prigogine, in his book *Order Out of Chaos: Man's New Dialogue with Nature,* says: "One of the most highly developed skills in contemporary western civilization is dissection: the split-up of problems into their smallest possible components. We are good at it. So good, we often forget to put the pieces back together again."

Is it possible to discover what drives an almond to become a tree? Suppose a scientist — a botanist, let's say — looks inside an almond seed, trying to discover how it works. After his inquisitive dissection of the almond's insides, the seed will never produce an almond tree. So whatever information he learned, if any, it is not about a real almond at all. The whole almond he wanted to explore, if set in fertile soil, would have grown into a tree. But now, instead of an almond, our scientist is left with two things: One ... some scientific data that's probably in pretty good shape. Two ... the remains of what used to be an almond, probably in pretty bad shape. The data might grow, given more investigation. The remaining ruined almond never will.

Most biologists attempt to explain the great mysteries of whole living things by breaking them down into microscopic parts. The universal method of science is dissection — splitting up problems into their smallest possible components. This trend of thought is, in fact, quite strong even today. Nutritional scientists try to understand food in terms of its "basic building blocks." Their theories are based firmly on experiment, and they call this method "The Scientific Method" — as if it were the *only* scientific method. In so doing, they ignore the complex interactions between their small area of research and the rest of creation. Imagine Martians judging the entirety of humankind by a single weekend visit to Las Vegas.

Scientists focus on *one* particular thing at a time. They separate it, isolate it, and remove it from the flow of life. But once that thing is removed from its context, taken out of the living framework within which it exists, it is no longer what they thought it was. Nor does it have much resemblance to its original form. The separation is *un*natural, so the results are false. No matter how much you dissect it, you will never reveal the absolute meaning.

Science, being highly specialized, tends, in the way it examines and considers things, to separate, to examine, to break the links of network connections and still learn nothing of value. Individual results are useless when taken out of context of the bigger picture. Science, with its emphasis on the analytical mind, focuses on elements and completely overlooks the totality. A linear, static mode of cognition is applied to an infinite network of changing realities.

Remove a cell from living matter, and it becomes impossible to study the cell's properties. Those properties depend on the cell's position as a component and on the coupling of these components which, together, give rise to the many interactions characteristic of life.

The arrangement of atoms in the most vital parts of an organism, as well as the interplay of their arrangement, differs substantially from the arrangements of atoms which physicists and chemists study in their experimental and theoretical research.

Experimental scientists generally take into account only laws formulated by experiments on dead matter and on isolated molecules devoid of life. They deduce laws based on the evidence discovered in their laboratories. But nature doesn't work according to the settings scientists want to use in approximating life. Layers of complexity will be superimposed over the relative simplicity of laboratory experiments.

You cannot measure nature with finite tests and instruments. These reveal only linear, simplified expressions of reality. Conventional scientific research in itself is basically a dead end because nothing can be definitively proven. Answers lead only to more questions, not to ultimate answers.

"We shall see but a little way if we are required to understand what we see. How few things can a man measure with the tape of his understanding! How many greater things might he be seeing in the meanwhile?" — Henry David Thoreau

Scientific methods are about measuring and taking apart in an attempt to discover the whole of nature. Says Heisenberg, "What we observe is not nature itself, but nature exposed to our method of questioning." Our method influences what we observe. According to Heisenberg, when we speak about nature, we speak at the same time a great deal about ourselves.

In order to measure an object, the scientific observer decides how he is going to set up an experiment and exactly what measurements to take. This plan of action will determine, to some extent, the properties of the object observed. But the properties can change during these experiments; if scientists conducted their measurements on pieces of macroscopic equipment and then another researcher came along and modified the experimental arrangement, the properties of the observed object would, in turn, change.

However successfully one sets up an experiment to research nutritional needs, that experiment would still be in some sense incorrect. We can never be sure that today's description of the nutritional needs of the human body is correct. However certain we may feel that our present picture describes how the human body *actually is,* there is always a possibility that some new and better way of looking at things, unimaginable to us now, will be discovered in the future. Generally, the deeper science moves into the smaller world, the more general our approximation of the truth becomes. Our "truth" constitutes a mere approximate model. The deeper we look, the less we see the whole picture.

Consider this. About a century ago, the United States Department of Agriculture (USDA) developed a procedure for measuring food energy which remains in use today. The gross energy value of a food is measured by completely burning the dried food in a calorimeter. The heat released through combustion is what is measured. Are you thinking what I'm thinking? — not just cooking, but burning! In order to learn about food, we must *burn* our food?! Talk about science giving only approximate knowledge! No wonder nutritional science remains unexcited about 100 percent raw food consumption. (Imagine burning money to find out what it's worth!)

Nutritionists talk about the protective properties of vitamin C, vitamin E, beta-carotene, phytochemicals, folate, and potassium, for example. And they look at how each of these nutrients individually affects diseases. Here is where the forest is lost in the trees.

"Isolated material particles are abstractions, their properties being definable and observable only through their interaction with other systems." — Niels Bohr

---

At the macroscopic level, nutrients are not distinct entities, but are inseparably linked not only to the parent plant (which is obvious) and to the rest of the environment. The properties of nutrients can only be understood in terms of their interactions with the individual body and its environment. Nature, at the atomic level, is not a mechanical universe composed of fundamental building blocks. Rather, it is best viewed as a network of relations such that, ultimately, there are no parts at all in this interconnected web. Everything is influenced by everything, because, deep down, everything is an intermingling of energy.

Nutritional science goes by unrestricted inquiry into natural products and foodstuffs. The point is: Our efforts to take things apart disrupt the natural product, no matter how careful we are.

It seems that we learned everything about lipids, carbohydrates, proteins, and so on, but failed to see the whole plant that represents all of it, and much more.

"If you look at nutrition only on a level of calories and macronutrients, vitamins, protein, carbohydrates, — meaning only on a level of biochemistry, you look at only one billionth of what you eat." — Christian Opitz, German nutritional biochemist

---

To say that there are six classes of nutrients that the body needs — carbohydrates, lipids, proteins, vitamins, minerals, and water — is like saying the USA consists of 50 states. It's true — but there is so much more, an infinite number of facts are omitted.

Because scientists name the entities they find and study — carbohydrates, lipids and proteins, for example — they believe they understand them. Examining *parts* of a living thing in isolation effectively kills the living entity. The act of separation is the equivalent of killing it. Every new discovery is not bringing us one step forward in understanding what life is, but, in fact, it is taking us miles away from grasping reality. It reveals that life is more complex than scientists think. Why not acknowledge our ignorance? And go along with nature.

Nutritional science research is based on the conviction that whatever one observed as being out there, really was out there. I sound like the *X-Files*: The truth is out there. It is. The problem is finding it and knowing what you have found. The particle has properties totally dependent on the observer. What we observe appears to depend upon what we choose to observe. Or, as the saying goes: What you know depends on where you stand. In a way, we see what we want to see.

Traditional researchers pride themselves on their objectivity. Yet genuine objectivity does not exist. So they knead their data — subconsciously, at least — to make it fit with their preconceptions. They start the experiment to prove some conclusion ... and so they prove it, unless it is obviously negated by the experiment.

Research by experiment is very subjective. You get what you are looking for. That is what quantum physics is saying. But concentrate on one particular issue or feature, and you bring it into your world. Research is more often than not driven by human factors: political agendas, media pressure, personal prejudices and the vested interests of the one who is paying for the research. Scientists are real people, with feet of clay, and their conclusions are often clouded by the desire to prove expected or desired results.

When we conduct an experiment, we disrupt the natural order. In the subatomic world, an examination requires that light be cast upon what we are trying to observe. It is this trespassing that creates tiny disturbances in what we observe. In other words, our observation affects quantum objects. In the simple act of observation we are intruding into that reality. To observe a thing is to interact with it physically. Think of switching on a light and watching the night critters scurry for the dark.

I don't seek to undermine conventional science's ability to give us the truth, the whole truth, and nothing but the truth. Quantum physics does that job for me! As we have learned in the previous chapter, the structure of living matter operates in a manner which cannot be reduced to the ordinary laws of physics and chemistry.

"We don't know a millionth of one percent about anything," Thomas Edison said. Quantum physics says we know less than that. The more we learn, the less we know. If quantum mechanics sounds like conceptual quicksand, it is. Einstein experienced the same shock when he first came in contact with the new reality of atomic physics. He wrote in his autobiography:

> "All my attempts to adapt the theoretical foundation of physics to this [new type of] knowledge failed completely. It was as if the ground had been pulled out from under one, with no firm foundation to be seen anywhere, upon which one could have built." — Thomas Edison

Modern science is making a shift from "absolute" truth to approximate descriptions. Descartes' paradigm is been replaced by the recognition that all scientific concepts and theories are limited and approximate. They can never provide any complete and definitive understanding. Scientists do not deal with truth per se. They deal with limited and approximate descriptions of reality, simply because a precise correspondence between the description and the described phenomena cannot be achieved.

There is no absolute truth in science. Whatever scientists discover is only an approximate description of the way they understand things at that moment. These approximate descriptions are improved, but never perfected. *All* knowledge is approximate. We must be satisfied with an approximate understanding of nature.

This is not to say that approximate knowledge isn't useful. In fact, it can be lifesaving for some individuals whose problems (like deficiencies and toxicity) have reached macro proportions. That is what acute symptoms are — disturbances of the body that have grown far beyond the subatomic level. This detailed, but isolated, island of knowledge deserves praise for arresting symptoms and alleviating suffering. However, a different approach is needed for achieving superior health and addressing aging, and this approach is happening on the quantum level.

Quantum theory exposes the fact that the essence of material creation is interconnectedness. It shows that we cannot render the world into independent smallest possible units. As we penetrate deeper and deeper into the fabric of life, we find that it is made of particles. But these are not the "basic building blocks" Democritus and Newton envisioned. They are merely symbols — representations which can be useful from a practical point of view, but a far cry from what is "really out there."

Often researchers forget to put things back together, getting lost in the fragments and failing to see the whole picture. But if we were to just passively observe, as the Greeks suggest, we would learn nature's secrets. They believe the mere act of touching disrupts what *is* and we learn nothing. In other words, we should go along with nature.

The idea of participation instead of observation through dissection has been formulated in modern physics only recently. But, it is just such participation as this that is now needed in the new approach to creating and maintaining health. By passively observing, as the Greeks suggest, we would learn that the food chain begins with green vegetation of one kind or another. On land, these are green herbs and edible greens. In the sea, plant life largely includes the one-celled green plants called algae. These individually microscopic plants are so numerous that they outnumber all multi-cellular life taken together.

Green plants are very special living organisms. Unlike humans, animals and fungi, plants do not consume any organic matter. Green plants cannot grow in complete darkness because they need sunlight, direct or indirect. All raw food of vegetable origin starts out as a growing plant and is turned into carbohydrates by your body. Carbohydrates are concentrated sunlight. By eating greens, we recover the sun's energy that was captured in the plants through photosynthesis. So instead of dissecting plants in search of new nutrients, why don't we pro-actively participate in getting the nutrients? Consuming a green smoothie will be a giant step in the right direction. Then just marvel at what it does for our health and appearance!

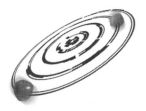

Chapter 8
Less Calories,
More Years

CBS News correspondent Mika Brzezinski did a segment on our Memphis raw food support group. She visited me at home, as part of the program, to discuss my nutritional lifestyle. We served Mika and her crew green pudding. She was genuinely surprised that something so green tasted so good. Ever since, I've secretly hoped that we "grabbed her," and that she's moving toward becoming "one of us."

A few months later she did another segment, "Looking to Live a Long, Healthy Life?" featuring Cordell, a 47-year-old who follows the CR diet. Twice a day, he enjoys a bowl of "blueberries, nuts, and apple peels." For lunch, he has a huge salad made up of the right kinds of fresh greens and vegetables. His largest meal is dinner, with his family, This could be another salad, broccoli, asparagus, and salmon. The main idea of the news segment was: The followers of the "120-Year Diet" believe they'll live a lot longer by eating a lot less.

The segment also featured Dr. Luigi Fontana, who among others doctors conducting long-term studies of CR, believes that Cordell's life expectancy will probably be longer than that of the average American. CR devotees are convinced that the diet protects them from major diseases. Dr. John Holloszy, principal investigator, agrees. "There's no chance of them getting type II diabetes, they have very low blood pressure, and the risk of them developing cancer is markedly decreased." Mika reports: "His doctors say Cordell has the blood pressure of a child, the cholesterol of a teenager, and his risk of heart disease is close to zero."

A number of experiments, including those at the National Institute on Aging in Baltimore, suggest that a calculated restriction of daily calories forestalls aging and is beneficial in maintaining good health. Calorie restriction has been tested in a variety of species such as rats, mice, fish, flies, worms, yeast, and now Rhesus monkeys.

Calorie restriction researchers believe that the CR animals are reducing their metabolic rate in response to a lack of food. In turn, this reduced metabolic rate is responsible for longevity. It extends the life span and retards age-related chronic diseases.

Nothing causes more confusion than the term *metabolic rate*. The phrase "speed up your metabolism" has become the slogan for the fitness industry. Because exercise increases the metabolic rate, the fitness industry concludes that such an increase should be pursued for health and longevity.

It is true that the metabolism slows down with aging and is consistently slow in overweight people. It is also true that muscle burns more energy than fat. So it does appear that speeding up the metabolic rate *should* be the way to achieve health and longevity. Should we then conclude that a low metabolism is synonymous with poor health? Not exactly.

Strenuous training increases the metabolic rate greatly. But athletes and record breakers are not known for their longevity or their physicality in later life. Dr. Douglas Graham, in his book *The 80/10/10 Diet,* brings up one analogy with a car that I find interesting. We all know that a car which gets more mileage per gallon is, by definition, more efficient. Similarly, your body works more efficiently if you can run on less fuel. People who eat a lot of food and do not gain weight are fast metabolizers. Their bodies are less effective in their use of nutrients.

Animals on the CR diet show that slowing down the metabolism will greatly increase the life span. So what do we do — look for the way to *increase* or to *reduce* our metabolic rate for optimum health? It seems a dilemma. There is no simplistic answer.

We cannot simply or absolutely say which is better — slowing the metabolic rate or increasing it — without considering other factors. When a person is full of toxins, his metabolic rate is going to be slow, causing the body to utilize food ineffectively. In this case, raising the metabolic rate by exercise, for example, is a good thing. Now, if a person is beyond the cleansing phase and is healthy, the goal should be to *lower* the metabolic rate by *reducing* calories.

The metabolism works like fire. Real fire uses oxygen to turn organic molecules of burning wood, coal, or paper into carbon dioxide, water vapor, and heat, which is energy. Our metabolism uses oxygen to turn the organic molecules of food we digest into the carbon dioxide, water, and energy we need. But there's a difference. Our body has a strong measure of control over its metabolism. By contrast, a piece of coal, wood, or paper has no control over the fire consuming it. During metabolic processes, there is a slow energy release. All fires, controlled or not, wild or deliberately set, are damaging. Our internal fire, our metabolism, inevitably also causes damage. We call that damage disease and aging.

Slower heart rates, slight drops in body temperature, decreases in nervous energy all are signs of reduced metabolic rate. Less food will spare organs and will encourage longevity, as experiments on CR animals have proven again and again.

The metabolism is the breakdown of nutrients. It's not just about burning up the food we eat, but about how the various nutrients from that food are utilized to produce energy. As James L. Groff and Sareen S. Gropper state in their *Advanced Nutrition and Human Metabolism:*

> "The extent to which different organs are involved in carbohydrate and fat metabolism varies within the feed–fast cycles that underlie the eating habits of human being. Food consumption often occurs at a level 100 times greater than the basic requirement, allowing us to survive from meal to meal without nibbling continuously. Excess calories are stored as glycogen and fat, and these can be used as needed."
> — James L. Groff and Sareen S. Gropper, *Advanced Nutrition and Human Metabolism*

In the beginning, humans lived on raw foods. No one quite knows how long it was before fire was used to cook the foods that early man gathered or killed. Early civilization lived in a consistent state of feast or famine. During winter, drought, or other natural deprivations, food sources could become nonexistent. Humans survived owing to a built-in mechanism which allowed them to store internal energy sources in times of plenty to be ready for times of deprivation. What humans are not designed to survive is eating, eating, and eating every day. To compound the problem, we no longer extend ourselves physically to get these meals. (Walking to the refrigerator door does not count as aerobic exercise, and closing the dishwasher door is not "weightlifting.")

A century ago, even with their physical demands, people ate much less than they do now. These days in America alone, adults consume 500 more calories every day, on average, than they did in the 1930s. What's more, we are no longer walking behind the plow to use those calories.

Christopher Newgard, director of the Sarah W. Stedman Nutrition and Metabolism Center at Duke University Medical School, explains that the reason behind being overweight is what he calls the "feast and feast economy." With a characteristically slow metabolism, not only does an overweight person burn fat less efficiently, but now all the unused calories get converted to fat for storage — all in preparation for a famine that never comes.

Now, with Quantum Eating, that needed "famine" does come! This is "famine," of course, only in a limited sense — the deprivation is only short-term, and carries none of the negative connotations or consequences we would usually associate with the word *famine*. When the body is free of mucus and toxins, every morsel of food is absorbed and we can live on very little sustenance — so long, that is, as what we do eat is wholesome and nutritious. In fact, one of the signs that the body is very healthy is that you *can* run on very little food.

Our bodies are built to store fat. Quantum Eating capitalizes on the body's fat storing ability. If humankind once survived without food for days on end, you will be perfectly all right for 16 hours. I hear you saying: *I do not want to store fat.* Sorry — that's how the body works. But because Quantum Eating uses low-fat raw foods and regular daily dry fasting, this fat will effectively not show up at all. On Quantum Eating, you use *all* calories you get from food. There are no extras to be converted into stored fat.

CR is the only non-genetic intervention which has been shown to extend lifespan and to retard the development of degenerative conditions. The effect of CR on lifespan has been studied in rodents for more than 60 years.

You might ask: Are there any other ways of retarding biological aging or extending lifespan besides CR? None known to science at this time. "Many interventions, such as human growth hormone and other hormone "replacement" therapies, as well as nutritional supplements and a variety of drugs, are claimed by some people to be "anti-aging" therapies. These notions are often plausible-sounding on their surface, and are attractive because of their simplicity and ease of implementation. However as of this writing, there is no reliable evidence to support the notion that anything besides CR is capable of retarding biological aging or extending maximum lifespan in adult mammals.[1]

No one doubts the enormous potential of CR for humans. Gerontologists already know CR works. This is not what they are after now. The general research strategy, according to Brian M. Delaney and Lisa Walford's *The Longevity Diet,* is this: "A researcher first selects one of the many differences between CR animals and normally fed animals. Let's say it is a hormone or particular unknown gene that is expressed at a higher or lower level in CR animals. Now by manipulating the targeted hormone or gene they will try to elicit this one change in normally fed animals. Then, the researcher hopes to see that the alteration of one factor in normally fed animals can elicit the CR effect. Another strategy is to suppress the positive change in CR animals and see if this nullifies the CR effect."

The belief that there is a magic "aging button" in the form of a hormone or gene in the human body is still alive and well. Researchers do not even give credit for the positive effects of increased quality and reduced quantity in minimized food intake.

Many gerontologists still insist that it is already too difficult for people to restrict their calories to the recommended levels to lose weight and curb obesity without asking them to restrict their intake by 60 to 70 percent to ward off aging.

---

1. *A website devoted to CR:* http://www.calorierestriction.org

Said *New Scientist* magazine: "The whole idea of CR is about as attractive to us as poking ourselves in the eye with a sharp stick. Hence our quest for a molecular end-run around CR."

But what social force is *really* operating here? I suggest that it is not an enormous reluctance on the part of people to follow CR. Rather, it is an enormous reluctance on the part of scientists to let the population achieve anti-aging goals without medical science interfering.

Scientists are fixed on what they consider the unacceptable difficulty of what they call the "semi-starvation diet." Trying to demean CR as a practice, scientists emphasize the discomfort of chronic hunger pangs. Among the words used: *torment* and *restraint.* Is cutting back on calories really scarier than having your stomach stapled? Not to me — I'd rather go hungry. Of course, the point of this book is that, if you practice Quantum Eating, you will not be hungry. As adaptable as the human body is, why on earth would anyone assume that CR will cause "chronic" hunger pangs? As far as I know, researchers have never systematically asked people on the raw food lifestyle whether we experience these symptoms or how long they last.

The "eat less" message is at the root of much controversy in nutritional practices. It directly conflicts with the food industry's demands that people eat more of their products. Thus, food companies work hard to oppose and undermine the "eat less" message. Each separate guideline has its own lengthy history of lobbying pressures.

The gerontologist's dream is to develop a drug which will produce a biochemical clone of the aging retardation process involved in caloric restriction. Do they simply suggest lowering calories? No! Eating is still sacred! Eating *as much as you want* is the ultimate target of every study. Consider the language of diet supplement advertisements: *Eat all you want! ... Never go hungry!* Like the diet-supplement industry, gerontologists are looking for drugs which will bypass the body's sensors and activate the body's effectors directly, allowing us to eat as much as we want while reaping the benefits of CR.

The scientific community believes it is possible to determine the mechanism or mechanisms and find chemical compounds that *induce* the effects of CR. The ultimate goal and overweening dream of CR researchers is the development of a "CR mimetic" — a drug which mimics the effects of CR without the need to cut calorie intake. Ah, the elusive miracle pill! But no drug, hormone, or supplement has yet been documented as an effective CR mimetic in mammals. And, make no mistake, we humans are mammals.

They claim that future benefits to public health will more likely come from identifying biological mechanisms that are responsible for the effect, "rather than encouraging the adoption of diets that almost nobody wants to follow." The critical word is *almost*. Besides how could the drug companies charge you for not eating or the scientists make millions by patenting the miracle pill?

Even researchers directly involved with CR do not collectively follow the diet as a lifestyle. Most talk about what their research will do to further the future technology, "to lay bare the secrets of aging and pave the way to the rapid development of sweeping new treatments for aging."[2] *Prescription* treatments of course.

Gerontologists strive to find out the root causes of aging. They are convinced that their research will lead them to the technology needed for genetic interventions for aging. They hope to speed up the pace of drug intervention for forestalling and reversing aging and for the development of other bodily invasions to preserve youth.

Aubrey de Grey, Ph.D., is a controversial biomedical gerontologist from Cambridge, England. He argues that the

---

2. *"Aging Revealed!" by Gregory M. Fahy, Ph.D.* Life Extension Magazine *November 1999*

fundamental knowledge necessary to develop effective anti-aging medicine exists today. De Grey believes that there are seven broad categories of molecular and cellular difference between older and younger people that we need to fix in order to gain 20 years of life extension. He calls these the "seven deadly sins," or as De Grey puts it, "the set of accumulated side effects from metabolism that eventually kills us."

The Unfortunate Seven

1. A chromosome is a very long DNA molecule with associated proteins that carry portions of the hereditary information of an organism. Abnormal changes in DNA or to proteins which bind to DNA are the first dreadful problem. These very mutations can lead to cancer.

2. Mitochondria are the energy factories in cells that convert nutrients to energy. Degradation or mutations in our mitochondria may accelerate aging.

3. Our cells are constantly breaking down proteins and other molecules that are no longer useful. This process produces intracellular junk. Everything that can't be digested simply accumulates as trash inside our cells. So accumulation of chemically inert but bulky "junk" in our lysosomes is the another age causing factor. Atherosclerosis, macular degeneration, and all kinds of neurodegenerative diseases (such as Alzheimer's disease) are associated with this toxic buildup.

4. The next observed problem in the deadly deterioration called aging is harmful junk protein that also accumulates outside of our cells, in extracellular space. The amyloid plaque seen in the brains of Alzheimer's patients is one example.

5. Some of the cells in our bodies cannot be replaced, or can only be replaced very slowly — more slowly than they die. Post-mitotic tissues are tissues which have stopped dividing after adulthood. So the fifth problem is

a decline in the number of cells in certain tissues. For example, this decrease in cell number causes degeneration of the heart. It is also the cause of Parkinson's disease and impairs the immune system.

6. Cell senescence is a phenomenon where the cells are no longer able to divide. So the sixth problem of aging is an accumulation of unwanted cells of certain types. They do not die, but they start doing some crazy things, like secreting proteins that could be harmful. Immune senescence and type II diabetes are caused by this condition.

7. Cells are held together by special linking proteins. Random cross-links occur between long-lived extracellular proteins. Extracellular crosslinks become a big problem associated with aging. When too many cross-links form between cells in a tissue, the tissue can lose its elasticity and cause problems such as arterioscerosis.

In case you didn't notice, as we age, *everything* becomes a problem! These seven sins weigh heavily upon the body and make you old. Aubrey de Grey has proposed seven strategies to reverse the damage we call aging. According to his *Strategies for Engineered Negligible Senescence,* scientists can use various growth factors to stimulate cell division. Senescent cells can be removed by activating the immune system against them, or they can be destroyed by introducing "suicide genes" which only kill senescent cells. For the prevention of mitochondrial and chromosome mutations, he plans to use gene therapy. He believes that protein cross-linking can be reversed by drugs that break the links. Extracellular garbage can be eliminated by vaccination that gets immune cells to "eat" the garbage. For intracellular junk, he hopes to introduce new enzymes that can degrade the junk (lipofuscin) that our own natural enzymes cannot degrade.

It seem that a whole medical crew will have to work full time to get the junk out and the repairs completed on all my

70 trillion cells. (And I thought having my teeth cleaned twice a year was too much!) There has to be another way, or I am simply not their candidate.

These problems, as well as the proposed solutions, are monumental. And if the human body behaves as it usually does, the deeper the science goes, the more complicated it becomes. Ignorance drives science. If scientists saw all the complexity at the beginning, they would be too discouraged even to try. That is why I am no longer a scientist in the conventional sense.

I am reminded of ancient maps before the discovery of the Americas that said simply, beyond a certain point, "here there be dragons." I choose the way of humility. I trust my body's instincts to decide what needs to be done. It is certainly more competent. If the CR diet pardons most of the deadly sins, that is the way I choose.

Life Enhancement magazine (August 2006) interviewed Drs. Richard Weindruch and Tomas Prolla, leading figures in CR research. They shared the findings of their research on genes expression in CR monkeys versus control subjects. Gene expression is the process by which a gene's DNA sequence is converted into the biologically active proteins of the cell.

Aging results in a dramatic increase in the activity of genes that have to do with stress responses, including oxidative stress and responses that have to do with DNA damage. In CR monkeys, various types of damage to DNA were greatly reduced. Caloric restriction, which one would think might act by inducing DNA repair, actually results in a lower level of DNA repair enzymes. The repair enzymes are made in response to DNA damage. The restricted mice apparently have lower endogenous DNA damage, so they don't need to synthesize repair enzymes as much as the controls do. There you are — the first sin is ameliorated.

Mitochondrial dysfunction and other problems in energy metabolism were quite strongly diminished by caloric restriction, absolving you of the second sin. The CR diet reduces toxic buildup within the cells, pardoning your third sin.

The post-mitotic tissues, such as brain, skeletal muscle and cardiac tissues, share the characteristics of using high amounts of oxygen for their ATP production. These organs are the major targets for aging. In calorically restricted mice, the level of damaged proteins is much lower. The decline in expression of genes that are involved in refolding damaged proteins is observed. Protein turnover is activated in muscle by caloric restriction, whereas, in normal aging it seems to be going down. Thus the fifth sin is expiated.

Limiting the dietary intake of monkeys slows the age-related decline in the immune system. Specifically, CR delays the phenomenon known as T-cell senescence, at least partially forgiving the sixth sin.

Glucose is a sugar that cells use for energy. Glucose is always present in the bloodstream. Every cell takes it as needed from all over the body. Glucose can also cause collateral damage as it circulates through the body. According to the glycemic theory of aging, circulating glucose leads to the pathological changes which occur as we age: cross links, browning reaction, and free radical damage.

Picture collagen as a cable of three coiled strands. It provides the foundation for your arteries, veins, lungs, and skin. It forms the cartilage that cushions our joints. Its flexibility ensures that tendons and ligaments twist and bend without breaking. When too much glucose is floating around, it attaches to collagen and forms bridges, or crosslinks, within each collagen molecule as well as between molecules. When calorie intake is restricted, it reduces the glucose level circulating in the blood, which in turn affects crosslinks forming. The seventh sin is thus avoided.

Browning is a central process of aging. The anti-aging effect of caloric restriction might be partially explained by a reduced browning rate. Free radicals cause "oxidative stress" that in turn damages cell membranes, causing inflammation. CR lowers free radical production.

Quantum Eating *is* CR, so it may slow aging simply by retarding the damage caused by high blood glucose levels. On the Quantum Eating regimen, your stomach is empty and glucose levels are low. Your body learns to use glucose very efficiently, turning it into higher energy despite the lower levels. Stretching your daily non-eating time reduces the negative effect to a minimum. This effect may cause the body to age more slowly than normal.

Calorie-restriction diets cause research animals to live longer and healthier lives, but they are not made immortal. They die anyway. Some biomarkers change with aging but remain unaffected by calorie restriction. CR researchers have found that 30 percent of the changes that happen with aging are not affected by a caloric restriction diet. One example of such a stable marker is serum amyloid. It is known that amyloid deposits form in several tissues of mice and in humans as they age, unaffected by caloric restriction. Gerontologists do not know why. Amyloid is part of the junk accumulating in extra cellular space. So, CR does not give complete clearance from the fourth sin. We might still do penance for this one. Six out of seven is not bad!

Scientists and researchers who attend anti-aging conferences are not pictures of health — most are not even health oriented. They are too dedicated to the belief that anti-aging science will relieve them of the effects of old age in the very near future. They do not choose meals at a health food store but head off on a gastronomic binge. As one attendant reports: "Later that evening, in traditional French style, we feasted for hours on goose liver pâté, duck, steak, rich pastries, and large quantities of wine. Clearly, it is easier to advocate an abstemious lifestyle than it is to adhere to one."[3] Grey himself was observed drinking too much beer.

Gerontologists are among the biggest believers in anti-aging potions. Some gerontologists eat massive amounts of melatonin each day. Others take Resveratrol. As at this writing, Resveratrol is the leading anti-aging drug. It contains a natural poluphenoic compound found primarily in grape skins and red wine.

I want you to pay special attention to the words *dehydration* and *nutrient deprivation*. Could it be that our own bodies develop something similar to deal with environmental stress?

Do not rush to the pharmacy to get this drug. The secret to anti-aging is to develop the same response within your body. This is the research that interests me. But who on earth is going to fund it? Who is going to spend money to prove scientifically that an individual can succeed in anti-aging lifestyle on his own, and does not need to buy anything at the pharmacy?

Whether prolonged CR increases the humans lifespan remains uncertain because it has been untested, scientifically, in the sense that no double-blind, placebo-controlled long-term study has been conducted on human beings. While we're at it, how about some scientific research, some double-blind studies, to determine whether CR practitioners actually even *know* they're not eating? For me, it's no longer as deliberate a program as it once was. I no longer struggle. The regimen has simply become natural.

There are several thousand people who are already practicing the CR diet. Most of them appear quite thin, and some comment that they fantasize about food all the time. This is, I suggest, is because they practice CR eating *cooked* food. I can see how this could feel like constant deprivation. I can see how it can lead to dismal moods and emaciated bodies.

---

3. The Quest for Immortality *by Jay Olshansky.*

CR on the raw food diet produces glowing health and a joyful disposition. You will have no hunger pangs or feelings of weakness, but instead a youthful bliss and teenage energy. How could this have been overlooked? I wrote a long letter to the National Institute of Aging requesting to speak to CR scientists eager to share my experience. The response was short and succinct: *The NIA staff involved in caloric restriction is unable to meet with you.*

"Unable"? Perhaps they were at lunch. A steak sandwich, perhaps, at their local steakhouse.

One thing is for certain: You cannot see it if you are not looking — or don't even want to look. To this particular scientific institution, I can only say: You are on your own!

And so are we.

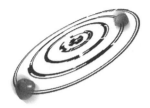

Chapter 9

Dry Fasting as a Remedy for Dry Prunes

Almost 100 years ago Arnold Ehret stated, "The less you drink, the more aggressively the fast works."

Several years ago, a friend of mine was visiting. She made a batch of dehydrated mango strips from a box of ripe mangoes we got from the market. After tasting just one, my sweet tooth activated with a vengeance and I couldn't stop eating them until my teeth started to hurt. One particular tooth was crowned and already traumatized. I know that the sugar I ate in such abundance in my childhood and young adult life was responsible for my numerous fillings and several crowns. I used to get at least two cavities every year. In Russia, painkillers were only used when a tooth was pulled. Never novocaine for a mere filling! I suffered a lot a pain in the dentist's office.

After moving to 100 percent raw food, my cavities stopped and my gum health improved dramatically. But eating so many dry mango strips that particular day did a number on my tooth and an abscess developed. I knew exactly what was coming. My tooth would have to be removed. I was terrified. Losing a tooth is always heart-wrenching, but to lose a tooth where it would show felt like it would be life-wrecking.

I was desperate. I started reading everything I could find on the Internet about abscessed teeth, looking for a remedy. I checked fasting in hopes it might help. At that time, I was already fasting one day a week. Somehow I felt my body was so accustomed to water fasting that even a prolonged water fast would not produce the result I desired.

After several hours' surfing, I came across a posting by someone who saved his tooth by doing a *dry* fast. Dry fasting is known as the Schroth procedure. It was named after 18th century German farmer and naturopath, Johannes Schroth, who used it to cure many illnesses after noticing that his cart-horse ate only dry bran when it had strained a joint. In Russia, it became known mostly due to dry-fasting proponent Porphiry Ivanov, who advised fasting for health and vigor for 42 hours once a week, and who fasted without water for one week and even longer.

I knew doctors are not even allowed to advise dry fasting in the United States. But I was ready to try anything and certainly was no stranger to going against medical advice. I started a dry fast that very evening. It wasn't hard. In fact, it was easier than I thought. By 4 P.M., the next day, the swelling was greatly reduced. By the next morning, it looked as if nothing had ever happened. That is when I knew dry fasting was very special. From then on, when I fasted once per week, it was always a dry fast.

I began to read everything I could find about dry fasting. English-language material was scarce. On the internet I found references about dry fasting made by authors David Wolf, Joe Alexander, and Russian-born author Valery Mamonov. The last-named also has a chapter on dry fasting in his book *Control for Life Extension.*

Dr. Doug Gram called dry fasting "an EXTREMELY dangerous practice and was 100 percent opposed to it." But how can something we are doing every single night be so "extremely" dangerous? For many people sleep is a forced fasting. English language is most precise when it calls the first meal "breakfast" — breaking our night fast. We wake up every morning with all the signs of fasting: bad breath, aftertaste in the mouth, and our tongue is covered in that egregious white fur. In fact, we live as long as we do owing to this nightly dry fast. It keeps us alive.

On the other hand, leading raw food promoter David Wolfe wrote:

"I am one of the few health professionals who promotes dry fasting. Most natural hygienists and fasting promoters consider dry fasting too "extreme" or "dangerous." It is neither, especially when done as I recommend for 24 or 36 hours. My experiences and those of others prove its tremendous value. Test and you shall be convinced."

Since I myself had just experienced a recovery close to a miracle, I wanted to learn more. Resources in Russian provided fascinating reading material. (Aren't you glad I'm Russian!)

Dry fasting is the total absence of food and water consumption. It has been extensively researched in Russia. I found several books in Russian about dry fasting. The general idea was that absolute or dry fasting proves *exceptionally* beneficial to both your health and your appearance.

Oleg Vinogradov, author of the Russian book *Dry Fasting* is convinced that dry fasting eats up not only your diseases and your physical aging, but your wrinkles as well. He writes: "If in your seventies you look your age, you are not using your body's full potential. If in your seventies you look 50, you are using only part of your body's potential and you are over-indulging in food. If in your seventies, you look as though you are 30, you are still eating too much. It is only when you look seventeen when you are seventy that you have found you own path to optimum health. In the end, it all comes down to keeping the balance between eating and non-eating."

That was enough to keep me reading! Reading on, I found numerous stories of miraculous recoveries from dry fasting.

Siberian medical doctor Sergey Filonov, (*www.filonov.net*) hosts retreats for people to undergo a supervised dry fasting. No food, no water is allowed. Even *contact* with water is not advised. During dry fasting, the body is placed under rigid constrictions. Now the body not only has to salvage nutrients but water as well. Everything sick and foreign will be broken down and used up. All diseased tissues get split up and removed from the body in a very short period of time.

Dehydration causes competition between healthy cells and pathological organisms for water. It is a real survival-of-the-fittest scenario. Inflammation cannot survive without water. A wet environment is ideal for the proliferation of pathological bacteria, viruses, and worms — water shortage is as devastating as fire for them. All dead or dying tissues will be expelled from the body. A water fast does the same thing but takes a *much* longer period of time to accomplish the goal.

What is inflammation? Tissues are swollen with water where infection is having a party. Pathological bacteria and microbes love wet terrain. Dry fasting eliminates inflammation the same way a swamp gets rid of mosquitoes and other insects when it dries up. Microbes are annihilated immediately. The shortage of water is a cleansing drought that is disastrous to the body's enemies. It is pernicious for pathological bacteria.

Most people in the United States never even heard of dry fasting, and if they have, they are apprehensive. I believe it is because the idea of eight glasses of water per day has been entrenched in human contemporary conscience. And we are scared to death of dehydration.

Medical professionals advise drinking eight to ten glasses of water per day. This is good advice for people who eat cooked food. Cooked foods introduce toxins into the body, and when we dehydrate the concentration of toxins increases. Water dilutes toxins. And the more toxins you have, the more you need to dilute them. The opposite is also true. The fewer toxins you have in your body, the less water you need.

Normal levels of hydration however, can only be achieved with raw foods. It is a common opinion that drinking water prevents dehydration. The truth is that no amount of plain water intake can replace the loss of vital body electrolytes. Only water containing electrolytes (i.e. sodium, potassium, etc.) and not plain water can prevent dehydration. And this form of water is present abundantly in juicy fruits and vegetables.

A dried prune never returns to being a ripe fresh plum even when it is re-hydrated. When I hear the insistent health message *Hydrate, hydrate, hydrate,* I cannot help but see this image in my mind's eye.

What is wrong with a re-hydrated prune? Why, it doesn't even resemble the fresh ripe fruit it once was. It is not a whole product any longer. The body responds to water in just the same way. It remains a plumped-up prune. That is why eating cooked food and filling yourself with eight glasses of water will not make you look fresh and youthful.

The average human body is 70 percent water. In a mother's womb, a fetus is 99 percent water. When a baby is born, it is 90 percent water. Just as we begin dying the moment we are born, we also begin to dry up. As an adult we are 70 percent; in old age we slip to only 50 percent. Is it any wonder we begin to look desiccated like a prune?

Masaru Emoto, author of the book *The Hidden Messages in Water,* studied the energy of human consciousness and verbalization on the formation of ice crystals. He discovered that water is the medium for transforming energy. Water has the extraordinary capacity to copy and memorize information. Emoto writes: "So how can people live happy and healthy lives? The answer is to purify the water that makes up 70 percent of your body." So how do we purify the water that constitutes our body? Simply drinking any water is not going to alter the balance.

I am always asked *what* water is the best. My unhesitating answer: the water that comes packaged in fruits and vegetables. People are usually shocked when they learn that I do not drink plain water at all. Am I dehydrated? Not at all. I have two cups of fresh-squeezed vegetable juice every morning and two cups of green smoothie for my second meal. And I might have half a watermelon or ten tangerines in between when they are in season. With raw food, my body is getting the most biologically intelligent water.

Quantum physics teaches us that every living thing is distinguished by vast exchanges of information. Water cannot be removed and added back, as in cooking, without destroying networks of information in the living matter. It cannot sustain a high level of regulation within its environment. Self-organization is lost.

Remember that from a physical perspective we are mostly water. Water inside cells, in the *cytoplasm* particularly, is not quite liquid. Much of water is tightly bound to big bulky proteins. What little free water there is resembles jelly, not Poland Springs. It bears more similarity to the insides of a juicy fruit than what we commonly think of as water. It is highly structured: not solid, but not quite water either.

A river is pristine and clear only when it is flowing. Stale water produces decay and deterioration. The body also has stale dead water. Only dry fasting can filter out stagnated water.

Valery Mamonov writes: "During a water fast, all the toxic deposits are flushed out with the water we drink. This water must first be processed, which requires the body's energy, in order to penetrate the cell membranes. In dry fasting, there is no water intake and the water that is present in urine, feces, and sweat is metabolic water as an end product of carbohydrates, fat, and protein metabolism. The wastes from inside the cells are flushed out with that metabolic water, which makes the elimination process easier."

Doctor Sergey Filonov, from the Altai area in Siberia, has been supervising people on dry fasting for fifteen years and has helped hundreds of people. Even though there is not enough medical research done, from his experience with himself and observing others, he insists that dry fasting is the most effective method of healing nature can offer us.

During dry fasting the body begins to resemble the camel. This miracle animal can walk through the desert for a long periods of time without water. A camel's hump stores fat, not water. Water is stored in the animal's bloodstream. Our "hump," says Dr. Filonov is an excess of fat, sick tissues and plague deposits in our arteries. He claims that during a dry fast the body will synthesize water from the atmosphere: Oxygen is taken from air and hydrogen from living tissue.

On his website there is a long list of degenerative diseases which can be helped by dry fasting, including gynecological disorders, musculoskeletal dysfunctions, respiratory tract diseases, circulatory system diseases, neurological pathological conditions, digestive system disorders, skin problems and urological problems. The list of degenerative troubles that can be positively affected by dry fasting — a list very similar to those helped by water fasting — are listed on the website: *www.fastingbydesign.com.*

There are also contraindications to dry fasting, just as there are contraindications to a water fast. It needs to be approached cautiously. It is necessary to improve the individual's overall health before dry fasting becomes an option. Anyone who is very young, very old, very weak, or very sick needs to improve their diet and do some cleansing before attempting a rigorous dry fast. Critically ill people should not go on a fast at all. Also, people who are grossly underweight or pregnant, people with unstable blood sugar issues, advanced cancer, active tuberculosis, active hepatitis, thrombosis, or cirrhosis of the liver should not fast.

During a dry fast, we not only do not eat, we do not drink either. The healthy body can survive 14 days of dry fasting. The sick body can die on the first day, because of the amount of toxins released into the bloodstream.

Dry fasting seems to be a most powerful tool for cleansing all body systems. The body is placed in dire survival conditions, and it expels filth and excess and pathological tissues. The Russian doctors who supervised people through dry fasting insist that it is three times more effective than water fasting.

The common cold and flu can be quickly cured with dry fasting. Folk medicine prescribes drinking lots of liquids, such as herbal teas. Valery Mamonov writes: "However, abstaining from all drinking and eating works even better. In the case of the common cold and flu, with mucus being expelled from the body by a runny nose, the mucus is burned more rapidly and we recover quickly if we decrease our water intake."

Members of my family know the moment they feel any symptom of a cold coming on that my prescription will be to stop eating and drinking for 24 to 36 hours. I cannot say they like it, but it does stop the flu in its tracks.

A famous Russian naturopath, G.P. Malakhov, in his Russian book *Manual on Fasting,* testifies that dry fasting also helps to get rid of kidney stones. Kidney cells normally clean the blood that passes through them, but when a dry fast is undertaken they can also clean themselves with the metabolic water that flushes out the deposited salts and stones.

Dry fasting dramatically improves skin condition. Your skin is an organ of elimination. Skin not only pushes impurities out, it will absorb moisture from the air as well. Usually moisture is getting out, now it is coming in. All skin ducts will be cleaned. Dry fasting drastically facilitates the skin's functioning — the skin simply never works to its full capacity when we drink water.

One of the testimonials people who have gone through therapeutic dry fasting would give is that they will begin looking so much younger that their friends will not recognize them. However, as they resume their regular eating, within several months they return to their former selves.

Russian advocates of dry fasting, however, do not advise 100 percent raw foods. The reason is probably that in Russia it is almost impossible to get fresh fruits and vegetables during most of the year. Kefir is usually recommended to break the fast. They emphasize that dry fasting is a hard physiological test.

People promoting raw foods do not eat before noon and often have their largest meal (even if it is a large bowl of salad) as dinner at 7 P.M.

While others advocate two meals, or even one meal per day, it is always at the end of the day. The advice is: while undergoing the purification process, one should gradually adjust to two vegetarian meals a day, so as to later change to one meal a day. Conventional practice says to initially give up breakfast, and later lunch. Finally what is left is one meal at the end the day.

I reasoned thus: There have been people who eat 100 percent raw, there have been people who eat only one or two meals per day, and there have been people who occasionally perform dry fasts. All of those practices were highly beneficial — I already knew this firsthand. But something was still missing: either permanency, enjoyment or visible anti-aging effectiveness. That lead me to the idea that I should do dry fasting every single day. No, I was not trying to live on air, I decided to extend my nightly dry fast to several hours longer. Before too long I was neither eating nor drinking after 2 P.M., practicing 16 to 18 hours of dry fasting every day.

The longest I ever performed a dry fast was three days. The last two days were progressively harder. The last day, frankly, felt unbearable. So I started to think how could I combine the benefits of dry fasting without the agony. I was already not eating in the evening. So I combined all three ideas together and boom: it was magic. I woke up feeling ecstatic.

Quantum Eating combines the miracle of raw foods, the benefits of dry fasting and respect for the subtleties of the body's circadian rhythms. And you get an additional bonus: Not only is there is no deprivation, but the experience is euphoric. You will feel heavenly.

Dry fasting is an excellent detoxification tool for cleansing the body. But to provide visible anti-aging benefits, it must be done daily for a relatively short period of time to make it safe and practical as well as easy to follow. For good health, we need a balance of cleansing and nourishing. Both cleansing and nourishing require healthy organs. During the digestive process, the body separates the good from the bad, assimilating what is nourishing and eliminating the waste. Fasting is a method to promote the cleansing of old waste. Fasting resets the digestion process for better assimilation, and improves nourishment. Dry fasting and raw foods is a perfect marriage between cleansing and nourishment.

You must become an experienced water-faster before moving to dry fasting. Water fasting is the most widespread method of fasting in clinical practices. During the first days of a water fast, hunger, cravings, headaches, weakness, day-time drowsiness, restless sleep, and occasionally, sickness and vomiting are common. Occasionally a sucking pain in the stomach, feelings of discomfort, and intestinal peristalsis are part of the initial fast. Usually, the first experience of fasting is the most difficult. However, when the body is cleansed during several years on raw foods, none of these conditions will be experienced.

Oleg Vinogradov, in his Russian book *Dry Fasting,* describes how he broke his fast with commercial tomato juice and nearly ruined his health. His body was very vulnerable after a 10-day fast and the toxins in processed food poisoned him. Do not ever attempt fasting unless you educate yourself first and gain experience through short fasts. Not only are short fasts very beneficial, but they perform the even more important role of giving you firsthand experience which can be not only health saving, but even life saving.

In Russia, both types of therapeutic fasting are practiced: water therapeutic fasting, absolute (dry) therapeutic fasting and their different combinations. Dry fasting produces cleansing. However, if the body is too toxic, dry fasting can bring serious consequences. Organs of elimination (kidney, liver, lungs) cannot cope with the volume of toxins leaving the body. A weak organ that is overburdened may shut down. Often an initial liver and colon cleansing is required as preparation.

Just as with everything else, unless you know what you are doing and are ready to take full responsibility, you should never attempt it. Dry fasting can kill a person who is full of toxins, and yet it is a very powerful anti-aging remedy for a person who is already clean and free of degenerative problems. When you attempt Quantum Eating, which includes a short daily dry fast after being on raw food for several years, the risk is minimal, but the anti-aging benefits are striking.

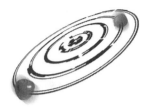

Chapter 10

Not All Waters Are Created Equal

Russian folklore fairly brims with fairy tales that include "living water" and "dead water" motifs. Live water obviously resurrects, but it is dead water, contrary to its name, that will make whole again a hero who has been cut to pieces by evil trolls. In fairy tales, it is often a beautiful maiden who uses the combination of these life-generating waters to bring her beloved back to life. She will sprinkle dead water onto the mutilated body to heal the wounds, then apply live water to restore life.

Certain Russian health practitioners believe that only a dry fast can remove dead water from the human body. Is there any dead water in the human body? Yes, it is called D_2O (or deuterium oxide). This time the term "dead water" lives up to its name. This water is harmful and poisonous to everyone's system. According to some gerontologists, dead water is responsible for our aging and degenerative diseases. In scientific papers, D_2O is called *heavy water*.

Deuterium can replace the normal hydrogen in water molecules to form heavy water (D_2O), which is about 10.6 percent denser than normal water (H_2O). The peculiar property of this naturally occurring deuterium oxide, or heavy water, is that it has a tendency to accumulate in the fat deposits of the body.

D_2O and H_2O are almost undistinguishable by taste alone. However, you cannot sprout seeds in D_2O, and you can actually die of thirst while drinking this water straight. Deuterium oxide causes the metabolism to operate at abnormal rates: It either drastically accelerates or dampens the chemistry of cell metabolism. Both situations are detrimental for the human body.

Can you avoid heavy water absorption? No way! Your body consumes heavy water in the ratio of 1 drop for every 6000 drops of ordinary water. Two-thirds of the moisture absorbed by the body is through the skin. Every time you drink water, take a shower, or simply absorb water from the air, you are building your accumulation of heavy water.

Heavy water has been found to be extremely harmful to living organisms in many ways. For one, it impairs cell division, hindering or damaging the cells in the process. Normally, cells are carrying out regular metabolic activities such as translating proteins into energy. Periodically, the cell undergoes mitosis (cell division) and two daughter cells develop.

Normally, the DNA of each cell contains hydrogen, which actually gives DNA its double helix shape. If deuterium oxide is present in a cell, deuterium atoms gradually replace the hydrogen atoms, forming much stronger bonds between the deuterium atoms. Now the DNA molecules are more rigid. The more rigid the cell membranes, the harder it will be for cells to divide. Thus, heavy water actually inhibits cellular division in the healthy cells.

Another way in which heavy water damages the body is by contributing to irregular cell growth such as cancers and tumors, and slower cell division, stunting new cells' growth causing accelerated aging. Cancer cells are left to mutate unhindered. D_2O inhibits the body's immune system, making it less able to deal with the malignancy.

Experiments on mice have shown that the metabolic rate depends on the concentration of deuterium oxide in their bodies. Heavy water at concentrations up to 20 percent accelerates aging by abnormally speeding metabolic rate, and when its concentration goes above 20 percent leads to death through a sudden drop in the metabolic rate.

One interesting review article, "The Turnover of Body Water as an Indicator of Health,"[1] summarizes the results of the research done on body water turnover. The replacement of body water that was lost in a given period of time in different individuals was studied, as was how this criterion is related to health and slowing aging.

The authors propose that the water turnover in the human body may be used as an indicator of overall health. The idea of drinking eight to ten glasses of water apparently follows the same logic. Until at least fifteen, children show a higher body water turnover than adults, most studies show. Your daily water turnover decreases with age. In people of the same age, those who exercise exhibit a higher rate of water turnover than sedentary people.

This article also quotes research that concludes that in tropical climate water turnover in individuals is 50 to 100 percent greater due to increased water loss from heat and the intense perspiration that is the body's response to it. Were there a direct correlation between water turnover and health, then people in the tropics would be healthier and live longer, but this is not necessarily the case.

If the same principle applied to people who exercise regularly, they would live much longer. They don't. A Harvard Alumni Study showed that exercise added only two years to the average lifespan. Athletes, who probably have

---

1. *Hideki Shimamoto and Shuichi Komiya "The Turnover of Body Water as an Indicator of Health."* Journal of PHYSIOLOGICAL ANTHROPOLOGY and Applied Human Science *Vol. 19; 207-212 (2000)*

the highest water turnover, are not known for longevity — quite the opposite. Exercise increases *mobility*, but not longevity. Exercise definitely improves the quality of life, but seems to add little to the lifespan. The irony is that the time we add through exercise is probably about the same as the total time we spent actually exercising.

Exercise does a great deal to keep body in shape, but almost nothing to keep the face youthful. It seems unfair, but often people who do not exercise have a better looking complexion, owing to fat and retained water padding, than those who do exercise. The common prescription that we should drink eight glasses of water daily to improve health and longevity is an oversimplification. I am a habitual exerciser myself and believe that regular physical activity is an essential part of having a vital and youthful body.

However, something about the idea of drinking a lot of water is not working. Something is amiss. The body definitely needs water. Not, however, from bottles and faucets, but rather from the vessels nature hands us.

Dr. Doug Graham, in The *80/10/10 Diet*, writes:

"Some animals, especially the grazers, are notorious for drinking huge quantities of water. The anthropoid apes, however (biologically, humans are classed as anthropoid apes) are rarely observed to drink water, but they can do it if necessary. Their tongues are not designed to lap water the way carnivores do, so they have to suck water if they must drink."

Anthropoids are very creative when they are thirsty: dipping a furry extremity into water, rubbing it over wet leaves, slurping up water from their fur or from the hollow of a leaf. Luckily for them, they are not instructed to get eight glasses of water or it would become a real challenge. All of their water needs are supplied by eating juicy ripe fruits.

Water is a vital component of any healthy diet ... This is a mantra repeated over and over without question as to its validity. Just because the human body's dry weight is made up of protein, many assume we should stuff our bodies with protein rich foods. Just because we are mostly water, we are told to guzzle copious amounts of water. The laws of nature are not that simple. What is often obvious to a lay person can be overlooked by scientific minds simply because some narrow aspect of their research becomes their entire focus.

While writing this chapter, I lectured in Havana, Georgia. During the presentation, I mentioned that I would be 50 on my next birthday. A lady from the audience came up to me afterwards. "Are you sure you're not 25?" I have heard similar comments many times. Being human, I am pleased, but I am beyond being flattered, because I know it has nothing to do with me personally. I use such testimonials only as a tool to strengthen my message: There is nothing special about me, but everything is special about raw foods and the body's miraculous God-given ability to rejuvenate.

I have achieved great results using a combination of raw foods and extending the night dry fast to at least 15 to 16 hours. I do not drink free water, sometimes for many months and even years. All of my water comes from fruits and vegetables. So I am doing absolutely the opposite (and not for the first time!) of what nutritional and medical science teaches us to do.

When a person's body contains a quantity of toxins, water definitely helps to dilute them and helps the kidneys filter them out. Simply drinking eight glasses of water, however, will not remove heavy water from the body.

Let's see why a short, dry fast can be so effective. Total body water in a healthy individual has two major components — intracellular fluid and extracellular fluid, distributed in the proportion 40 percent to 60 percent. It is believed that all chemical reactions take place in intracellular fluids, in other words, inside 70 trillion cells or on the surface boundaries. Water, as a main fluid medium, is present in all cells except fat cells. Carbon dioxide and other metabolic wastes leave the cells and enter the fluid in the spaces between the cells. There, these materials are mixed and transported by the blood throughout the body, delivering nutrients to the cells and carrying away waste products.

During dry fasting, temporary dehydration thickens the blood. A difference in the osmotic pressure between blood and extracellular fluid is created. Under these circumstances, active water diffuses from the extra cellular fluids into the blood. At the same time, foreign substances are extracted from the cells and forced into the extracellular fluid to be carried away by blood plasma. As the water gets moved, it carries away toxins and promotes cleansing. It cleans away cellular waste and heavy water. The reverse osmosis created by dehydration may be needed to remove dense molecules of D_2O.

Heavy water present in the body accumulates in fatty deposits. It is not subject to the usual tissue replacement turnover. In fact, liver fat often contains two to three times as much deuterium as do other fat deposits. During fasting periods, the body will use up fat deposits and trapped D_2O will be released and removed from the body. Some experts believe that dry fasting is the only way to get rid of deuterium buildup.

Eating results in the formation of metabolic water. By definition, metabolic water is the water produced by living cells as a by-product of oxidative metabolism. The end result of the complete oxidation of glucose is carbon dioxide, water, and energy. During dry fasting, when you do not drink free water, the body depends on the water produced by the oxidation of food you have eaten before.

The Quantum Eating lifestyle calls for a short dry fast of 12 to 16 hours. When you do eat, you consume only raw, "living" foods. The abundant metabolic water produced will safeguard against dehydration during the times you take no food or liquid. This metabolic water is enough to compensate for any moisture loss at optimal body temperature.

Fat is the most efficient source of metabolic water. Fat yields 107g of water for every 100g of fat oxidized, compared, for example, to the 60g of metabolic water from the oxidation of the same amount of carbohydrate. Studies on animals and humans show that the amount of fat burned by the body is influenced by the degree of dehydration present.

Dehydration may therefore be an important determinant of fat metabolism in humans. The scientists' conclusion: Dehydration may stimulate a preference for high-fat foods that lead to obesity. But another conclusion might be just as worthy of consideration: A short term dehydration might be beneficial for burning more fat. However, for now the prevailing opinion in science is that the effects of starvation and dehydration on lipid metabolism have not been clear. Of course, fasting is not starvation, but scoffers like to use the disparaging term "starvation" even when talking about short, deliberate abstinence from food and water. The irony is: Scarcely anyone in western culture "starves." We suffer largely from *over*-eating, not under-eating

Dry fasting practitioners have testified that the more overweight a person is, the easier it is to perform a dry fast and more likely the pounds are to stay off, when compared to a water fast. This is in complete accordance with the fact that, during a dry fast, the body is using up metabolic water produced by burning fats and the information it stored gets lost. By resetting the metabolism, a fasting person, so to speak, has a better chance at getting a healthy start.

On the other hand, the fewer fat deposits a person has, the harder a dry fast becomes. Thus a dry fast should not be undertaken by underweight individuals. If you are too thin, consider water fasting as described in the book *Miracle of Fasting* by Paul Bragg. You will be particularly interested in Chapter 24: How to Gain Weight by Fasting. Water fasting is often able to slow a fast metabolism back to normal. Because eating ample amounts of food is never a healthy solution to gaining weight, I believe you can still benefit from Quantum Eating, but in this case by setting the curfew time to 5 P.M. instead of 2 P.M.

Some nutritional scientists have begun to question the long-held recommendation of drinking 64 ounces of water daily, suggesting instead that you should drink only when you are thirsty. I believe from my own experience and the testimonials of others that if you eat enough fruits and vegetables, you will never be thirsty.

The obsession with "hydration" has given birth to an entire industry of water bottles, drinking water filters, and energy drinks. But according to the Institute of Medicine, most people actually do get plenty of fluids. Their verdict: Drink when thirsty, and, instead of gulping water, reduce salt intake. I think they are getting closer to seeing the whole picture. On the raw food lifestyle, we (ideally) do not get any salt, so we are rarely thirsty. Should we conclude that we shouldn't be drinking so much free water?

The main idea behind all weight loss programs is, the faster your metabolism, the slower your propensity to gain weight. The increase of the metabolic rate can be beneficial only for those who eat cooked foods. After being on raw foods, completing the detoxification process, and achieving your optimal weight, your goal should be reducing your metabolic rate. The last thing you want is to lose more weight. This book is about a youth-preserving lifestyle, not about losing weight. Your ideal weight should be reached during the transition to the raw food lifestyle that I detailed in my first two books.

So I'm warning you ... Don't go around telling people there's this crazy woman urging us not to drink water. That is not what I am telling you. What I am telling you is that when you are turning onto the super health highway, you are on your own. There is little research done on healthy people. It is up to you to learn everything about how a healthy body operates and make a decision about what is good for your body right now.

If you do drink water, there are several factors to consider. Water from pure springs, lakes, or wells introduces a lot of inorganic minerals into your body that, in time, will form cement-like deposits in your joints, gallbladder and kidneys, and clog your arteries. Most bottled water is simply tap water run through filters or special treatments. Bottled water may also contain carcinogens that leach from plastic containers.

Distilled water should be a viable alternative. But there is evidence that it is basically "dead" water because distilling causes it to lose its structure. There are also claims that it can leach small amounts of calcium and other minerals from the body. However, turning dead water into living water is only a matter of exposing it to sunlight for several hours, or adding a few drops of fresh-squeezed juice. You can even do it by adding some crushed blades of grass. I hope you see in this general recommendation one more proof: the miracle is in raw foods! If even a drop can restore water, why not restore yourself with a whole glass of fresh juice or green smoothie?

The rejuvenation and cleansing effect of dry fasting is two to three times more effective than a water fast. In case histories, incidents of dry fasting for three, four, and five days are not unusual. Several naturopaths who have supervised clients' fasting believe that dry fasting of such lengths can help the body to cure almost every degenerative disease, including cancer and AIDS.

I do not recommend that you *ever* fast longer than for 24 hours. In fact, I believe you will achieve the best anti-aging results by using fasting's marginal benefits *daily* — and only for 16 to 18 hours at a time. Regularity in fasting is of much more importance than duration for your youth-preserving lifestyle.

Don't expect fairy-tale results overnight. Kiss all the frogs you like, and none will turn into princes. Dry fasting may not awaken your fairy tale prince from the dead, but 16 to 18 hours of dry fasting daily will help keep your internal maiden from premature aging.

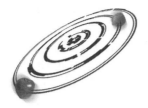

Chapter 11
Salt and Water: Myths and Legends

Kidney specialist John Daugirdas, M.D., in his book *The QUD Diet: Eating Well Every Other Day,* introduces a new diet that consists mostly of eating every other day. Seeing the connection with Quantum Eating, I became interested. Our metabolic rate is greatly affected by how much food we eat. When the body is deprived of food for several days, survival and starvation mechanisms kick in and fuel is burned more efficiently. The body learns to get by with less. Your body goes into survival mode by slowing down the rate at which you burn food for energy — it reduces your metabolism and uses *everything*. Since eating is inherently destructive, you should welcome this as the biggest blessing! At the same time, most dieters know that food cravings turn this efficiency into a curse. When you do resume eating at your former level, cravings will come with a vengeance and you will gain all the weight back.

Diets don't work. Why? On almost any diet, you'll lose a few pounds quickly — most of this as excess water — but with time it usually gets harder and harder to continue losing weight. When you reach a plateau, you cannot continue eating the same amount of food. You must start eating less. However, eating less on a cooked food diet is hard to do. You experience a continuous feeling of hunger or deprivation. Eventually you get discouraged and fall (or jump) off the diet wagon. You return to eating as you did before. Only now, your body has lowered its metabolism as well, and you not only rapidly regain all of the weight but now you gain more. Experienced dieters all know this boomerang effect.

Biologically, our bodies store short-term energy reserves in the form of glycogen. If our glycogen reservoirs are full, any excess of food goes to long-term storage in body fat. By fasting 16 hours, the body dips into glycogen storage. When you eat, you refill glycogen reserves. Your hunger is a phantom sensation that is called forth by the siren call of cooked food. The constant feeling of deprivation that it creates does not allow you to reduce your food intake.

John Daugirdas' solution to short-circuiting the starvation mode is to keep the non-eating period to no more than 24 hours. On non-eating days, he recommends taking supplements. On the day you eat, he allows you to eat anything and everything you want, once again observing the sacred law of stuffing your face. Daugirdas suggests that his diet is meant for healthy people who need to lose only 25 pounds or less. This makes the diet a temporary solution for losing weight, but not a permanent lifestyle designed to keep you young and healthy. Even though there are many things I do not like about the QUD Diet, the author has a valid argument. Eating every other day temporarily activates the body's survival-starvation mode, can be very beneficial for a healthy person. If you practice Quantum Eating, you do not eat for 12 to 16 hours and the body has a brilliant mechanism to accommodate this routine.

Hunger is equated with a drop in the blood sugar level. One day at my yoga class, a lady felt lightheaded and had to lie down. The instructor asked whether she had eaten that morning. The woman admitted that she hadn't, and the instructor concluded that her blood sugar was low. This is the common assumption taught by health professionals. I thought to myself: If she had only known I had not been eating or drinking for 18 hours and I had none of the symptoms associated with low blood sugar. The healthy body has compensatory mechanisms that keep up the level of sugar in the blood during a fast. When you have mastered Quantum Eating, you will have no such negative symptoms.

Daugirdas gives another explanation for the weakness and dizziness associated with non-eating. Most people take in a great deal of salt each day. If we eat too much salt, it is the kidneys' job to eliminate it. Over your lifetime, the kidneys adjust to this higher salt level, and program themselves to excrete through urination the salt (sodium) your body doesn't need. When a person first begins to fast, it normally takes the kidneys a couple of days to adjust to the lower salt intake. On the first day of a fast, your kidneys continue to excrete a large amount of sodium. When the salt content begins to lower, the volume of water and blood in your body begins to decrease. This lowered blood volume can lead to dizziness and weakness.

To avoid these unpleasant sensations, Daugirdas suggests taking extra salt on the days off to keep body salt and water content more stable. He wants you take extra salt on days off so your sodium level will be relatively constant because sodium fluctuations can lead to weakness. I don't get it — why not reduce salt on the days when you do eat, instead of adding salt on the days you do not eat?

What amazes me is that the author does not distinguish between salt (NaCl) and sodium (Na). Naturally, he knows the difference. But his text seems to equate them. I have not touched sodium chloride in years, but I make sure I get plenty of sodium through my food. For example, I always have four stalks of celery in my morning juice. Celery is abundant in sodium, as are all the other fruits and vegetables I eat daily.

Another book examining the topic of salt and water is *Your Body's Many Cries For Water* by F. Batmanghelidj, M.D. This is a well documented, passionate work, one you'll find eminently readable. The author methodically makes a case that chronic cellular dehydration is the cause of most degenerative diseases. He successfully treated 3000 peptic ulcer sufferers with water alone. I almost dashed for a glass of water, but I knew I would find the flaw in his logic. Near the book's end I did find the flaw when I read: "The Salt Free Diet is utterly stupid."

Batmanghelidj further writes: "After a few days of taking six or eight or ten glasses of water a day, you should begin to think of adding some salt to your diet. It you begin to feel muscle cramps at night, remember you are becoming salt-deficient. Cramps in unexercised muscles most often mean salt shortage in the body." Of course, he has a solution to the problem of cramps: You should add a half teaspoon of sea salt for every two quarts of water you drink.

Then the author warns that if your ankles swell, do not panic. This is a reaction due to the fact that your kidneys are not working properly, causing you to retain liquid. Now you should reduce your salt intake and increase your water intake for several days until the swelling disappears. Has anyone else zoned out by now? Trying to remain healthy should not be that complicated. Who wants to spend their time monitoring their ankles as though they were on life support? You do not offset damage by taking alternate corrective measures — you shouldn't be causing the damage in the first place.

I can see how the information in this book may be absolutely life-saving for a person on the cooked food diet, but it is almost irrelevant to a person on raw foods. Pure water is excellent, but the water in juicy fruits and raw vegetables is better. Drinking ten glasses of water is unnecessary and can be too much of a good thing if you drink fresh squeezed juices, eat one to two pounds of juicy fruits and enjoy green smoothies daily.

Now "if you do not eat properly," you need a lot of water. If you drink a lot of water, you need to take extra salt, not sodium (this is in the fruits and vegetables that you are not eating, remember!). When you take extra salt, your body becomes unbalanced. You need all those supplements to compensate for all those fruits and vegetables you haven't been eating. And we have come full circle, back where we started. You need everything that is in raw foods — water and all the nutrients. You can get them separately and make your life complicated, or you will fail and get sick and old just like everybody. And I can assure you: you are never going to get *everything!*

So Batmanghelidj recommends adding extra salt (NaCl), especially if you do not eat enough fruits and vegetables — "if you do not eat properly" as he phrases it. You are *not* going to get this option from me. My books are a tribute to raw foods. They hold the key to an anti-aging lifestyle that assures superior health. You will get no compromise here.

Nutritional science typically makes little distinction between raw and cooked produce, but our eyes do. Cooking removes water from food. Look what happens to perky vegetables and greens after cooking. Even surrounded by water they look shrunken, spongy, and dull, as though the life has gone out of them — which, in an important sense, it has.

Cooked food does contain water, but it also harbors the dehydrating agents and toxins that cooking produces. The body now needs more water to dissolve these toxins and eliminate them from the body.

Blood becomes concentrated after food consumption. It definitely becomes more concentrated as a result of eating cooked food. When the blood becomes condensed, it draws water from the cells around it and we become permanently dehydrated.

Consuming salt provides the body with unbalanced sodium. This sodium has no business arriving in the body on its own. It must be accompanied by a myriad of other nutrients. Otherwise, sodium is detrimental to the body and the main cause of permanent dehydration, which is just another name for aging.

I was hoping that Batmanghelidj, in his recent book *You're not Sick, You're Thirsty!* would make a distinction between salt and sodium, but he doesn't. He writes: "Salt is a vital substance for the survival of all living creatures, particular by humans, and especially people with asthma, allergies, and autoimmune disease." It is not salt, but sodium that is a "vital substance for the survival of all living creatures." In the complete absence of fruits and vegetables, salt might be life-saving. But why on earth, in America in the midst of year-round abundance of fruits and vegetables, would doctors advice taking salt, as if not having fresh produce and not wanting to eat it were the same thing?

Here is the paradigm shift in understanding that we need: The sodium provided by celery is life-giving, while the sodium provided by sodium chloride is life-taking. Read my first book, *Your Right to Be Beautiful*. There, I devote a whole chapter to explaining this difference and how table salt is the worst source of sodium for your body.

Most people see a swollen face in the mirror in the morning. If you consume no salt, you will see less swelling. To my way of thinking, this morning slimness is another sign that abstinence is beneficial, not detrimental.

According to nutritional science, sodium and potassium together regulate the water content of the body. It is too complicated for the individual to figure out how much of what supplement to use. Let the body do it — your body knows best. Just feed it what it is meant to eat.

Few westerners consume too little sodium. Even fewer get enough water eating cooked food. What we need to do is get the right amounts the right way. *Natural* is the order of the day. Your body has an extraordinary capacity to regulate itself, to get things right on its own. Free your body. Let it use nature's gifts, and let them do their work. By eating raw foods you can let the body regulate the blessings and curses of water and sodium. It will do a much better job than you ever can!

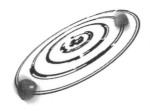

Chapter 12

Our Living Clock: Body Rhythms

"Happy families are all alike — every unhappy family is unhappy in its own way."

Thus begins Tolstoy's masterpiece, *Anna Karenina*. To paraphrase: Healthy people are all alike — every sick person is sick in his own way. Diseases are many, but health is singular. As we strive toward our pinnacle of health, and as we struggle with issues in health, each of us will be doing it in our own way. But the closer we get to optimum health, the more alike we become.

I met a man in Santa Monica who has been on the raw food lifestyle for about nineteen years. He was glowing with health, positively exuding a bright, vibrant energy. He never feels hungry or thirsty, he told me. I wanted to hug him — this, you see, is exactly how I feel most of the time. Individuality is the key that unlocks the door to the changes each of us must make to achieve our health. But as we get closer to our optimum health, the same program will work for most of us. The best example of this truth: our body's internal clock.

Observing the natural world reveals the presence of daily, monthly and annual rhythms — sometimes, rhythms of astonishing precision. Plants open and close their flowers at the same hour each day. Bears hibernate through the winter, awakening to changes in temperature and moisture. Biological clocks rule all life — from bacteria to plants, fish to reptiles, small mammals to human beings. Time is embedded in our genes. The reason for this dominance of clocks is obvious: We live on a planet of rhythms. Our planet revolves around its sun once every 365¼ days, with its axis tilted at 23 degrees — hence the rhythms of summer, fall, winter, spring, and summer again. We live on a planet that rotates once every 24 hours, exposed daily to periods of daylight and dark.

A trial study treating cancer patients in France, Italy, Belgium, and Canada found that patients given drugs at an optimum time in their day cycle of cell growth had far fewer side effects.[1] After studying these results, researchers have begun to realize that these natural rhythms also apply to other medical conditions, with implications for all kinds of treatments. This research has initiated a new field of medical research, called *chronotherapy,* which administers drug treatments to work "in harmony with the body's natural time rhythms."

To some, it may seem rather pretentious to discuss the notion of "harmony" in reference to drug treatments, but there is a lesson here that cannot be ignored. Since our physiology alters between day and night, it is hardly surprising that the actions of drugs vary depending on the time of the day they are administered. If the medical implications of popping pills according to the biological clock are so profound,

_1._ Independent on Sunday, *February 2000.*

it's an exciting but entirely sensible step to imagine how you might improve your health if you apply the same respect for good timing to your eating and sleeping practices.

Ticking away underneath your outward self, beneath your overt behavior, is your own personal clock. Your biological clock functions very well in preparing you and your individual body parts for the next periodic event facing you — a time of activity, or a mealtime, or sleep. Most of what goes on in our bodies, all our physiological and biochemical processes, are rhythmic, showing strong differences depending on the time of the day or night. Our bodies have a built-in 24-hour cycle called the *circadian rhythm*.[1] The term was coined by chronobiologist Franz Halberg in 1959. The human body has over 100 identified circadian rhythms.

We humans spend about a third of our lives asleep. Sleeping is the most obvious (but not the only) process regulated by our biological clock. There is a daily rhythm in heartbeat, heart rate, blood pressure, kidney function, the generation of new cells, body temperature, the production of many hormones, and even your pain threshold. The amount of glucose circulating in one's blood is highest in the morning and lowest in the afternoon. The liver metabolizes sugars, lipids and proteins at different rates over the course of the day.

"Scientists have not isolated how the brain clocks time but they know that a major factor is its reliance on outside influences — called "zeitgebers" (ZITE-ga-berz) — that keep it on a 24-hour schedule. The major zeitgeber is daylight, which enters through the retina and signals the brain to get going as we awaken. Other zeitgebers are sleeping and eating. Zeitgebers send clocked signals to your brain to keep you on schedule. Every area of your body relies on circadian

1. *The English* circadian *derives from the Latin* circa *("about") and* dies *("a day").*

rhythms." — Jay Dunlap, Department of Biochemistry, Dartmouth Medical School

Night and day count as the most important rhythmic cycle among all our natural cadences. Some people think of themselves as "night owls" or "night people." Whether dancing till three at the latest club or simply sitting home reading or worshiping the great god of late-night TV, these folks invariably claim *I'm not a morning person.* Someone else, though, is up at oh-dark-thirty, out for a jog, and finished the morning paper while others are yawning. These are, by their own description, "morning people," sometimes, "larks." The idea here is that individuals are somehow *inherently* oriented toward remaining awake at night, or "programmed" from birth to get up early. But the notion of "night people" is pure fiction. Human physiology renders us quite incapable of surviving without daylight and sun exposure. We're not bats, rats, or muledeer — our sight and hearing are not acute enough to allow us to function well in the dark.

Is there *no* truth to the notion of the "night person"? Of course there is. There *are* people who come habitually to function this way. But the habit is learned behavior. Consider the college student, for example, who develops the practice of studying into the wee hours on weekdays, partying till similar hours on weekends, largely because friends do it. The notion of the *night owl* is a social construct, often formed in late adolescence and the early twenties during high school and college. Graduation, a job, and parenthood then typically take an individual into a lifestyle and a set of social constraints which practically rule out the very possibility of staying up till three and sleeping in till ten. The night owls become larks out of necessity. There will be some complaining but largely the exigencies of life and livelihood prevail. Towards the retirement years, "night owls" rhythms move to become even more larkish.

An experiment was performed on some 47 British sailors considered either larks (introverts) or owls (extroverts). See the partying dynamic at work? Participants' oral temperatures were taken at regular intervals over a two-day period and averaged in order to identify patterns. The average for both groups was 97.9°F, but peaks and valleys showed some variation. The internal rhythms of the larks showed that they started warming up earlier in the day, then peaked and faded sooner than the owls. Body rhythms were all constant within that framework.

You are healthiest when you live in harmony with your rhythms. Besides the obvious rhythm of sleeping and waking-night and day, circadian rhythms monitor every bodily function from dividing cells to releasing hormones that enhance mental and physical performance. All activities are essential to our well-being whether they peak during waking or sleeping.

Another important cycle — and the one over which you have the most control — is eating. Studies are beginning to show that *when* you eat may be as important to long-term health as *what* you eat. However, very little research has been done toward optimizing eating times to accord with the changing physiology and biochemistry of the body.

Newborn babies cry for food about every ninety minutes. From their second to third month of life, most demand food only four to five times a day. From their fourth to sixth months, they are trained to the adult pattern of three meals a day. Contemporary society is geared toward three meals a day with snacks in between. This pattern is so strongly imprinted in our psyches that even people in time-isolation studies will experience hunger pangs three times a day within hours of the times normally set aside for meals.

Normal body temperature is said to be 98.6°F, but not for everyone. This reading is only an average. Body temperature ranges from about 96°F to about 100°F over a 24-hour period. For someone who sleeps nights and gets up at about 7 A.M., it is lowest between 4 A.M. to 5 A.M. If you habitually wake up at four, your body temperature starts rising before the normal wake-up time. It will plateau in the early afternoon, dipping a fraction of a degree in mid-afternoon, then climb slightly, reaching its high at about 7 A.M. Every day, before you wake up, your body temperature and blood pressure rise, your heart beats faster, and numerous glands squirt out pulses of cortisol and other hormones you'll need to get going.

Your body performs entirely different chores at night during sleep than it does during waking hours. At night your organs perform a tune-up on the complex engine of the human body, detoxifying, repairing and restoring you internally. This maintenance program is the reason we sleep — the body does not have the energy to keep the brain at a conscious level while it diverts its attention to healing.

Every night, before you go to sleep, your temperature, heart rate, and blood pressure fall, and the body produces a nighttime hormone — melatonin. This hormone tells us it is night, directing us to get ready for sleep. Both day- and night-active species secrete melatonin mainly in the dark.

"Everything is rhythmic unless proved otherwise."
— British chronobiologist Josephine Arendt.

Human Growth Hormone, also known as *somatotropin,* is one of many endocrine hormones. What makes GH special that the body can produce large amounts of GH right into old age. It is the most abundant hormone secreted by the pituitary gland. Just like estrogen, progesterone, testosterone, melanin and DHEA, Human Growth Hormone production declines as we age. However, this hormone is superior to all the other hormones because when it is replaced it supposedly not only prevents further biological aging, but reverses its signs and symptoms. Growth hormone levels go up when insulin levels go down, about four hours after a meal. James Jamieson and Dr. L. E. Dorman, experts on hormone replacement therapies in the book *Growth Hormone: Reversing Human Aging Naturally* state: "It is at this point that the fat burning potential of GH tends to be at its daytime peak. But remember, the largest burst of GH is released during the early hours of sleep — hence, our evening eating habits are crucial to maximizing this nighttime secretion. By avoiding food during the last four hours before bedtime we may enhance circadian growth hormone release, and fat burning potential."

The practitioners of Oriental healing arts believe that there are twelve major energy meridians in your body. They run from the top of your head, through your fingers, and down to your toes. Meridians are channels that carry subtle energy through the body. There has been progressively more research into discovering the parallels between these traditional "meridians" and the veracity of acupuncture. Orthopedic surgeon Dr. Robert Becker has researched the body's electromagnetic fields, even going so far as to design a device to measure electrodes by rolling it over the body. The final results recorded in his book *Body Electrical* indicate that electrical charges consistently parallel the Chinese meridian points.

Circadian rhythms are connected with the ancient Chinese belief in meridians, our energy pathways. The meridians are used in acupuncture as the *healing gates*. Each meridian is most active for a two-hour block of time every 24 hours. The circadian rhythms coupled with meridians schedule their daily activity something like this (see following page).

1:00 – 3:00 A.M.	Liver meridian
3:00 – 5:00 A.M.	Lung meridian
5:00 – 7:00 A.M.	Colon meridian
7:00 – 9:00 A.M.	Stomach meridian
9:00 – 11:00 A.M.	Spleen/pancreas meridian
11:00 – 1:00 P.M.	Heart meridian
1:00 – 3:00 P.M.	Small intestine meridian
3:00 – 5:00 P.M.	Bladder meridian
5:00 – 7:00 P.M.	Kidney meridian
7:00 – 9:00 P.M.	Pericardium or circulation meridian
9:00 – 11:00 P.M.	Thyroid/thymus meridian
11:00 – 1:00 P.M.	Gallbladder meridian

The liver meridian — read just "the liver," if you'd prefer — is the most active from about 1:00 A.M. till 3:00 A.M. The liver is the key organ in toxin elimination. It filters the blood, and is very active at night when we are sleeping. "When man moves, blood moves; when man is still, blood returns to the liver," states the *Yellow Emperor's Classic.*

The time frame of the liver's greatest activity is the essential reason why it is unhealthy to eat our main meal late at night. Most food eaten in an evening meal will be stored as fat and may lead to obesity. The liver rebuilds the body during the night. Within the context of the daily circadian rhythm, we note that the liver has a biphasic rhythm, with the assimilatory phase beginning at 1 A.M. and reaching its maximum at 3 A.M. It is more beneficial to consume no food during this time. Abstinence gives this hard-working organ the chance to do its job. When the liver is overloaded, we tend to wake up in the middle of the night — usually between the hours of 1:00 A.M. and 3:00 A.M.

The stomach meridian is active between 7:00 A.M. and 9:00 A.M. in the morning. Shouldn't that tell us that the best time to eat is in the morning? Your living clock has prepared your stomach to receive food at that time. Your stomach empties 50 percent faster after breakfast than after dinner. Since hunger and other digestive rhythms slow down in the evening, the healthy body doesn't need or expect food in the afternoon and processes it more slowly. This works to your advantage, keeping you from hunger pangs for the rest of the day.

The spleen/pancreas meridian is active between 9:00 A.M. and 11:00 A.M., just after breakfast. It is the pancreas that completes the job of breaking down protein, carbohydrates, and fats using its digestive juices combined with juices from the intestines. It manages enzyme production for digestion and metabolism. It secretes hormones that affect blood sugar levels. The pancreas produces chemicals that neutralize stomach acids that pass from the stomach into the small intestine by using substances in pancreatic juice. You want the pancreas to be active when you have just eaten, since pancreatic failure in the production of enzymes causes food to digest poorly.

Another inducement to having breakfast during this time window is that the spleen can readily transform food into energy. Western science agrees with Chinese medicine that individuals who consume the majority of their calories in the morning have more energy and are able to maintain their optimum weight more easily, whereas those who consume the majority of their calories in the evening tend to be sluggish and gain weight.

The heart meridian is the most active between 11:00 A.M. and 1:00 P.M. "Chief of the Vital Organs," the heart regulates other organs by controlling blood circulation. The heart is a muscle slightly larger than your clenched fist. It works as a pump to send oxygen-rich blood throughout your body.

Blood contains oxygen and nutrients needed by every cell in your body. How hard your heart has to work is strongly connected with digestion. Therefore in Chinese medicine the heart is paired with the small intestine, which separates by-products of digestion, and absorbs nutrients which are sent to the heart for circulation throughout the body. More strokes and heart attacks occur in the morning than at any other time of day. Blood clots form most frequently about 8 A.M. Blood pressure also rises in the morning and stays elevated until late afternoon. Then it drops off, hitting its lowest point during the night. Experts believe morning changes in your body may be responsible for cardiovascular problems. I am confident that late meals the afternoon or night before are responsible for this. Not eating at night will alleviate the burden on your heart.

The small intestine meridian is the most active between 1:00 P.M. and 3:00 P.M. The small intestine is the part of the gastrointestinal tract between the stomach and colon. It is the portal for absorption of virtually all nutrients into the blood. The small intestine is also the place where the most chemical digestion takes place. Once within the small intestine, macromolecular food aggregates are exposed to pancreatic enzymes and bile which break everything into molecules capable or almost capable of being absorbed. In the small intestine, proteins are changed into amino acids, fats into fatty acids, and carbohydrates into sugars. What could be a better time for your second and last meal of the day?

The kidneys meridian is the most active between 5:00 P.M. and 7:00 P.M. The period of highest activity coincides with the traditional western dinner hour. The logical question to ask: Since this is an organ of elimination, shouldn't it now be *cleansing* instead of dealing with a heavy meal? The kidneys are the body's most important reservoir of essential energy.

They convert excess waste and water to urine, which is then stored in the bladder. All life processes are closely related to the kidneys. If the kidneys are strong, growth and maturation will be vigorous, leading to a healthy body. Conversely, if the kidneys are weak, you will age more quickly, becoming susceptible to various diseases of the old and infirm. The first sign of the weakening of the Kidney Meridian is fatiguing easily. You may feel pain or weakness in the knees and lower back. Your brain function will decrease, resulting in poor memory. Other symptoms include a darkening complexion, hypertension, dry mouth and throat, and shortness of breath.

The amount of urine we pass is less at night than during the day. This is *not* because people do not drink or eat while sleeping. Interestingly enough, rhythms in urine volume persist even when people are kept in bed all day and made to fast, or were fed identical small meals at short intervals all through the day and night. This shows that the kidneys' output is rhythmic. The same is true for all excretory organs. There are times of the day when they purge more toxins and we must free them from other chores, like dealing with food, to do their job.

The five organs of elimination and detoxification are the colon (large intestine), kidneys, liver, lungs, and skin. Four of these are our main concern here. All four are active either at night or during the latter part of the day. These are the organs of elimination. They should be cleansing the body and restoring our energy instead of dealing with a heavy meal. When these organs are active, you should not be eating at all, so that you allow these organs to perform to their utmost the job of elimination.

Nutritional science teaches that food consumed in the evening prompts an increase in the unhealthy low-density type of cholesterol, and a decrease in the protective high-density type. Moreover, the body stores carbohydrates in liver and muscle tissues in the evening more extensively than during the day. In the morning, the body converts these stored carbohydrates into sugar to use as an energy source. I believe the best time to eat your breakfast is between 7 A.M. and 9 A.M. Your second meal should come between 1 P.M. and 3 P.M. when your stomach, spleen/pancreas, heart and small intestine meridians are most active.

Knowing your rhythms helps you coordinate your body to achieve maximum performance. We must respect our internal clock and eat at approximately the same time each day. People who eat regularly usually have regular sleep habits — another important facet of circadian rhythms. But to eat regularly is only one aspect of eating patterns.

For most adults, breakfast is the smallest meal of the day, with lunch and dinner progressively larger. It should be the other way around. After 5 P.M., it takes more food to make us feel satiated than it did earlier in the day. This is a key reason we eat more in the evening. Ask any dieter: What time of the day is the hardest? Typically in western societies, we eat the most in the evening. People who stick to a diet for most of the day often lose their resolve in the evening. Overweight people report more intense feelings of hunger in the evening than do people of normal weight. They also consume a larger proportion of their total daily calorie intake then. Breaking this pattern is crucial to achieving health and ideal weight.

While you sleep, your muscles and brain consume less energy. The body is engaged in repair, healing, and detoxification, and your body maintains a high level of sugar in the blood. This sustained sweetness of your blood at night is your body's way of delivering the sun's energy to your liver and all the other organs. When you are healthy and do not eat in the evening, your body is able to keep a uniform blood sugar level between midday and 6:00 A.M. by converting glycogen to glucose, even though you are not eating anything.

In the mid-1970s at the University of Minnesota, weight control studies showed that people who ate only one 2000-calorie meal a day for a week lost weight when they ate their meal in the morning. They gained weight when they ate the same meal in the evening. In one research study, normal-weight volunteers ate meals chosen from canned goods and military rations. They lost weight on the breakfast schedule. The volunteers who ate on a dinner schedule maintained the same weight or gained a little. If you want to lose weight, eat early in the day. If you want to gain, eat later in the latter part of the day. But in either event, *never* eat at night, two to four hours before going to bed. In my Quantum Eating system, you set that curfew earlier and earlier until you reach 3 P.M.

Body rhythms, however, are a two-way street. By changing your meal schedule, you can actually shift your body's rhythms. High-fiber fruits and vegetables are more filling than cooked foods. Your brain waits to say "time to stop" until about twenty minutes after a stream of signals starts arriving from your stomach. You'll get the message whether you eat a lot or a little. To help resist the urge to snack in the evening when you are dieting, turn off the kitchen lights. This will signal your body that it is time to stop eating. If you do eat in the evening, choose fruits or a green smoothie.

If you ingest, inhale, or absorb more toxins than your elimination and detoxification systems can handle, you will become ill from the toxic buildup. If you eat raw foods but you disrupt your elimination organs with excess food while they should be performing toxic clean-up, you are accumulating an excess of toxins. The excretory rhythms should not be violated on a day-in and day-out basis.

Many raw food people skip breakfast. I think this is a mistake. The reason stated is that *we have to earn our breakfast*. What is there to earn? In the morning, after dry-fasting overnight, we *need* energy. For healthier eating, the standard pattern of progressively larger meals from morning to evening needs to be reversed, putting the emphasis on breakfast and gradually eliminating any meal after 2 P.M. or if you can train your body not to eat after 1 P.M. for larks or 3 P.M. for owls.

Rhythm and *discipline* are the keys to all healing and rejuvenation. The body processes food more slowly later in the day because our rhythms are not based on absorbing late meals but rather on rejuvenating the body. All of your day's total food intake should be consumed within a span of eight hours, preferably during the daytime, between 7 A.M. and 3 P.M. Eating must stop six hours before going to sleep. This way, you achieve 16 full hours of fasting. This regime will assure that your body gets its cleansing function entirely done every single day. This is essential for health and youthfulness.

But won't this make you feel hungry later in the day? When you begin this regime — or if you begin the regime too abruptly — the answer is Yes. A little, at least. But equally (as Quantum Eaters, raw-food enthusiasts, vegetarians, and even good, experienced dieters in the "ordinary food" world will tell you), that hunger quickly begins to carry with it a sense of vitality, mental energy, and clearer thinking. What's more, much of what we *call* hunger is not really hunger at all, in the true, physiological sense. It's a merely a psychological hunger that arises from the accumulated weight of our individual and cultural past eating habits. Rarely indeed do we in the burger- and doughnut-fuelled affluent western world experience genuine hunger at all. Such "hunger" as you may feel as you first adapt to your new timed eating discipline quickly dissipates. I have not been hungry in the evening for some time now, precisely because I have not eaten after 2 P.M. for several years.

Quantum Eating capitalizes on the implications of time cycles in the body. Since we are all on basically the same clock, give or take minor individual variations, what works for one individual will work for everyone. You can go all night without eating easily. To adopt Quantum Eating, all you have to do is extend the duration of your nightly fasting. If we want to change our eating habits by reducing the number of meals, this has to be done gradually. The process might take a year or more. Your body will need time to adapt to a new schedule. You can be perfectly fine on just two meals per day. The idea is to get the last meal as early in the day as possible, beginning, say, at 6 P.M. Then 5:30, 5:00, and so on, finally combining your third with your second meal.

I was very interested to learn that Buddhist monks and nuns do not eat after noon. Buddhism goes back to a single founder, Siddhartha Gautama, the so-called 'historic' Buddha. He lived in India in the middle of the sixth century BC, during the extraordinary period that saw the birth of so many spiritual and philosophical geniuses — Confucius and Lao Tzu in China, Zarathustra in Persia, Phythagoras and Heraclitus in Greece.

I was puzzled: Why is Buddha himself typically depicted as fat? How could he become so huge on so little food? If you've had the same question, here is one explanation that I found. These are not images of Buddha (Shakyamuni) at all. Images of a fat "Jolly Buddha" or "Laughing Buddha" are actually depictions of Jambhuvala, the guardian king of prosperity, *Mi Fo*. Buddha is sometimes represented as fat because this portliness has become a universal symbol of wealth and prosperity in a world where deprivation can mean starvation. But that obesity is best understood as symbolic, not as a literal picture of or prescription for health.

Buddhist religious communities typically practice a tradition of two meals daily. Their last meal is around noon, though some may have a light broth later in the day. The Kitagiri Sutta of the Majhima Nikaya explains the practice:

"Once when the Buddha was touring in the region of Kasi together with a large Sangha of monks, he addressed them saying: 'I, monks, do not eat a meal in the evening. Not eating a meal in the evening, I, monks, am aware of good health and of being without illness and of buoyancy and strength and living in comfort. Come, do you, too, monks, not eat a meal in the evening. Not eating a meal in the evening, you, too, monks, will be aware of good health ... and living in comfort."

In such a conclave, monks or nuns who eat after noon are guilty of Paccittiya. They must confess their transgression to another member of their community. This penance reinforces duty and self-intent without resorting to outright punishment. You may find a similar practice useful as you work on developing the discipline of moving your eating to earlier times in the day. If you don't happen to be Buddhist, you'll avoid all the trouble with spelling exotic names for methods and practices — you can simply call your method the "buddy system." Your "buddy" doesn't even have to be a Quantum Eater — just a friend who recognizes the worth of what you're trying to do, and who's willing to be a sounding board, an ear for your confessions of small eating sins, and a source of applause for your day-by-day successes.

Emulate one ingredient, however, of this Buddhist practice — forgiveness. Let it be a Christian, a Hindu, a Muslim, or an agnostic forgiveness, if you like. The fact of the forgiveness matters more than its flavor. You'll need time to shift your food timing away from what the culture commands and toward what your body's natural rhythms dictate. The degree of forgiveness you'll need may vary with your starting point. If you're already a dedicated raw foods afi-cionado, your main issue will be timing. If you're a vegetarian who eats both cooked and raw vegetables, you'll have a couple of kinds of "sins" to catch and correct, timing being one. While most of my readers have progressed at least this far, some are starting still farther back.

Whether your sin be a culinary orgy at Luigi's Pizza Parlor or, more likely for most of my readers, just a bowl of big salad downed as you watched the ten o'clock news, forgive it. Confess it, forgive it, and move on. Beating yourself up serves *no* purpose. Quite the contrary, it's demotivating. Each day dawns with a brand new date. If this is day 2, or day 200 — congratulations! If you slipped yesterday, then thank yourself (or thank God) for your climbing back on the wagon this morning. Today, eat a little earlier, and thank yourself for it. Feel the good effects. Move forward in small, conscious, deliberate, and *disciplined* steps. And one day we will hug each other as you will tell me: "I almost never feel hungry or thirsty."

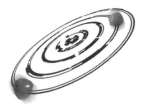

Chapter 13

2 P.M. Curfew

Curfew? say my uninitiated friends. *You've got to be kid-ding! First I have to eat all this raw food, and now I can't leave the house after two in the afternoon!* You initi-ates can chuckle. You newbies — relax. Read on ...

My husband Nick used to seduce me with food. "How can you go around the country telling people that they are supposed to eat less?" he would say. "You are taking away one of life's biggest pleasures!"

This is a huge misconception. One of the biggest pleas-ures, when you're attuned to it, is when your stomach is empty but you are not hungry. Once you have been released from the bondage of food, a euphoria will envelop you. So my answer is: Why would I trade my perpetual bliss for a short-lived gastronomical pleasure?

A calorie-restricted diet does not have to be difficult or unpleasant. Detractors like to say, "A longer life, not worth living," which itself promotes the idea that eating is our greatest pleasure. People always talk about the pleasure of eating, especially the pleasure of dining on rich, fatty foods. We treat this intense pleasure of excess as something delightful. But it is not real pleasure — it is penance! I don't think of myself as an ascetic. Rather, I simply say that everyone else is indulging in a food perversion.

Food gives only crumbs of pleasure. Not eating can be exuberantly satisfying. If you cultivate the joy of non-eating, the energy within you, connected to that never-ending source of energy, the sun, you will not perish; you will gain a joyous, radiant feeling as though you are in love and want to hug the whole world. You can go all day without food and not even notice it. Less food is not the same as fasting, when detox symptoms kick in. I am talking about a state in which you are effortlessly nourished by energy and you "forget" to eat. You are divinely in touch with a clarity of feeling that there is nourishment beyond just food. You stand inspired with an abundance of joy and vitality. This is how I feel when I do not eat after 2 P.M.

A primary concern of people is where to eat, what to eat, and with whom to eat — never why we eat. What is food?

Common experience shows that items considered to be good food, even delicacies in one culture, are considered by others unfit for human consumption. Cow lips (hair, teeth and all) are a local delicacy in Madagascar, but they give nightmares even to non-vegans in the West. Greasy pork rinds turn up noses in Seattle; in Memphis, they're a food group. Nutrition experts never dwell on the answer to the question of just what food is. They accept the notion that food is simply the stuff people eat.

According to Webster's, food is "material consisting of carbohydrates, fat, proteins and supplementary substances (minerals, vitamins, et al) that is taken or absorbed into the body of an animal in order to sustain growth, repair vital processes, and furnish energy for all activity of the organism." This definition is flawed. Even during a fast, these functions are going on. Even the unfed body still produces new cells, and without any food.

But this definition powerfully illustrates how much common beliefs about food are part of who we are. Marooned for weeks on an uninhabited desert island, some people manage to refrain from cannibalism, while others in society refuse to give up hamburgers to avoid early demise from a heart attack. People would rather die than violate the clean-your-plate norms of our culture. Without paying attention to the cumulative effect food has on the body, people choose food according to comfort, entertainment, and pleasure.

Food definitely brings pleasure. Most people report feeling more cheerful and less stressed during mealtimes. Appropriate centers in the brain are stimulated by some chemical components that react like drugs. While eating, your subconscious is on an endless search for this particular reaction, that special food that will give you definitive satisfaction. The ultimate gastronomical experience is alluring, but never attainable.

What eating can never deliver, non-eating will. With Quantum Eating, your stomach is empty and you are not hungry. Satisfaction is no longer dependent on food consumption. You experience tremendous joy, and feelings of sublime ecstasy come over you. The realization strikes you that this feeling is what you have looked for all your life.

The pleasure you derive from cooked foods is passive. The enjoyment of raw foods and of Quantum Eating in particular is active, caused by psychological attention to the goodness it is bringing to your body. So growth occurs as a result of invested psychological energy. Growth in health, in spirituality, in body awareness.

Isn't food essential in order to survive in this world? How much food does one need? Enough, I submit — and not an ounce more! For different people, the amount will vary greatly. The small amount that will kill one individual because of the detox symptoms it will initiate will make another live a non-aging life. Our goal should be to eat as little as possible without creating a nutritional deficiency. Therefore, you should not attempt a full program of Quantum Eating until you have completely cleaned your body of toxins and all degenerative conditions.

Metabolism is derived from a Greek word meaning "change" or "exchange." Energy which maintains life comes from what an organism absorbs from its surroundings. The fact that one dies when deprived of food is the main reason our culture assumes that it is mainly food which gives us energy. Other processes, like breathing and direct assimilation through the skin, are completely overlooked.

Food consumption is actually the main reason we *lose* energy. After food is consumed, the process of digestion begins, which slows down our system, depleting our overall energy. The mere activity of digestion exhausts us. Consider one inescapable fact of life, which I'm going to express rather bluntly: No matter what we eat, it will ultimately be transformed into poop. Toxins and waste are continuously coming out, even from raw foods.

Yes, you lose energy even if you eat an all-raw, living food diet. No matter the amount, you are still losing energy. Raw food greatly improves your health and appearance — the evidence is overwhelming. But to achieve long-term anti-aging results, I believe that reducing your calories is essential. Keep in mind: it is fasting that makes us look and feel better.

"When you fast, the Light will illuminate you." — Gandhi

Each time you eat more than your body needs, you put extra stress on the body. Excessive eating is a dispensed violence you perform against your body. The more we eat, the hungrier we become. The more we drink, the thirstier we become. Nowadays food, instead of being the means to an end (living), becomes an end in itself. Treat food as a means to life, rather than life's ultimate goal. Eating itself is inherently destructive. Go "Raw and Low" (raw in nutrients and low in calories) and you will be on the threshold of bliss. Experience release from the bondage of compulsive eating and freedom from hunger.

It appears that we cultivate greater life-sustaining energy through smaller amounts of food. In fact, the healthy body's daily requirements of vitamins and minerals are less than a thimbleful — a very small amount compared to what we're accustomed to believe. After a certain time, the body can accommodate little or no eating for some time. Sounds futuristic? Quantum physics supports my claim entirely.

The descriptions that are commonly applied to quantum physics are: *absurd ... bizarre ... mind-boggling ... incredible ... beyond belief!* Is it any wonder the same adjectives come to mind when we think about not eating or very little eating? I understand that introducing Quantum Eating to a food obsessed society is like introducing a round-world reality to a flat-world civilization. Let's break through the barriers of conditioned norms and open to a world of greater possibility when it comes to eating. After all, this is *Quantum* Eating!

A living organism consists of tissues, which are built of molecules. And molecules are built of atoms. Atoms consist of electrons and protons, which in turn are built of smaller components. Eventually, we reach a point where matter, as such, effectively ceases to exist. At this point, we have only something called the vibration of energy. At the most elementary level of matter, the world is nothing but swirls of energy.

Here is the main assertion quantum physics makes: All existence, at the subatomic level, can be described equally well as either solid particles (like tiny balls) or waves (like undulations on the surface of water disturbed by a paddle). If that isn't confusing enough, quantum physics goes on to tell us that neither description is really accurate on its own. Quantum physics insists that both the wave and the particle aspects of being must be considered as we try grasp the nature of things. From the quantum perspective, the stuff we're made of, as well as the food that we eat, is essentially behaving as waves and particles simultaneously. It is up to us what we want to explore at any one time — the particle or the wave — but we cannot do both.

In physics, if we expose the particle aspect of the wave-particle duality, we destroy the wave aspect. Vice-versa, if we expose the wave aspect of the wave-particle duality, then we destroy the particle aspect. We must therefore contend with two different experiments — one revealing the wave feature, the other revealing the particle feature. The results of the experiment depend on the nature of the whole experimental setup. According to quantum physics, the more we impose one concept on a physical "object," the more the other concept becomes uncertain. This is Werner Heisenberg's *Uncertainty Principle.* (Werner never knew what he wanted for lunch, either.) By concentrating only on the *matter* aspect of food, we completely overlook the energy aspect. This means that the more we insist we should eat to live, the more important food becomes and the less capable the body becomes of taking in energy as nourishment. If you are stuffing your body with the *physical* aspect of food only, then you're neglecting the energy aspect.

Strange? It gets even better. Quantum physics insists there is no defined border where what we perceive as matter ends and nothingness begins. On the subatomic level, sunlight and plants are all the same. In *The Matter Myth, Dramatic Discoveries That Challenge Our Understanding of Physical Reality,* Paul Davies and John

Gribbin supply a good analogy. Does it look to you as if we have gained something from nothing? The Great Roman philosopher Lucretius said, "Nothing can come out of nothing." Physicist and cosmologist Alan Guth contradicts this, saying: "It is often said that there is no such thing as a free lunch; the Universe, however, is the ultimate free lunch."

I will give you an example from my own life. I do Bikram yoga every day. It is a very intense 90-minute practice in a hot room. It is estimated that during one class a person burns up to 850 calories. But on many days all the food I eat in a single day equals that many calories. On some occasions I take two Bikram classes per day, without changing my eating pattern. Where is the energy coming from?

It is a complete misconception that food consumption is the sole or even the only essential ingredient in our vitality. In fact, the *less* we eat, the *more* energy we absorb directly from sunlight. We already receive some energy directly from the sun and some from the food we eat. The less toxic the body is, the more open and receptive are these pathways to receiving still more energy.

The life energy we speak of is known by many different names: Sanskrit calls it *prana* (light). In China, it is called *Chi* and in Japan *Ki*. All the matter in the universe, including the human body, is comprised of these swirls of vibrating energy. When you practice Quantum Eating, a higher level of nourishment becomes activated. You begin to realize there is a vast realm of nourishment beyond food, that food is only a tiny aspect of that *prana* feeding. Some suggest that the nearest traditional concept of *prana* in the West is the Holy Spirit of Christianity, a sacred power that is both immanent and transcendent. *Prana* is also often called wind, vital air.

Your body will adapt to whatever you impose upon it, so long as you do this gradually. Just as there are always consequences to pay for abuse, there can also be rewards to gain. Gradually, the body will need less and less food while consciously demanding sustenance from the all-pervading cosmic supply. Could it be that which transforms the energy directly into matter is dormant while we eat more than we need? By moving to two meals per day in the first part of the day, you will unlock the mechanism in your body that will lead to absorbing energy from the environment. Weird? Quantum physics insists that we are already doing it.

The body has amazing abilities of adaptation. But adaptation takes time. Approach any drastic change like the 2 P.M. curfew with caution and common sense. Do not force yourself to start eating this little all at once, it will be impossible and you will fail. Allow yourself to take gradual steps. Giving your body time to adapt to this healthy new environment, it becomes not only possible but also extremely enjoyable. Even on 100 percent raw foods, you still must keep upgrading and refining your diet.

In my books, I sometimes say *raw food diet* and sometimes I say *raw food lifestyle*. So which is it? Diet? Or lifestyle? Of course, it's both! During transitioning, it is definitely a diet. Dieting has a temporary element built in; it is something passing, something to endure. The element of deprivation is very strong, so it is a struggle. That is why diets do not work, why they are hard. But the raw food diet is the only diet that has the potential to become a lifestyle. Quantum Eating can be developed into a lifestyle. It can grow into a lifestyle if you persist. It will become a lifestyle when you begin *enjoying* it.

I enjoy my raw food very much, but I actually relish the second part, the not-eating part of the day much more. No I am not going to give up food entirely. I'm already goofy enough — any additional goofiness would be gilding the lily.

But I do want to try to adopt the practice of Buddhist monks and nuns to stop eating after noon. Provided, that is, that I do not have to be sequestered in a monastery.

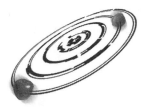

Chapter 14
Quantum Eating Made Easy

"Everyone I've ever known who ate every other day or less was healthier, stronger, and more intelligent and loving than people who eat every day." — Leonard Orr, *Breaking the Death Habit, The Science of Everlasting Life*

People often ask me: How can you eat raw and eat so little? Is it hard? Let me give you an analogy. Assume you are a chocoholic. You will remain a chocoholic only as long as your body does not make you really sick when you eat it. The moment your body develops severe allergic reactions to your chocolate consumption, you will know better than to eat it again. In fact, you will make every effort to be sure there's no chocolate in any dish you eat ever again.

Pleasure and pain are very powerful motivators in everything we do. So how can I live now without ever eating cooked food? I am neither a saint nor am I a fanatic. The answer actually is entirely mundane: Cooked food makes me sick. The wrong quantity and quality of food will make me miserable.

I feel like I have overeaten when I eat anything after two in the afternoon. Overeating can happen at different points of satiety, but it always feels *gross*. For me now, even a small bowl of salad after 2 P.M. feels like overeating — I feel stuffed after eating these vegetables, when before I would have eaten half a chocolate cake. When I move to lighter food consumption, I undoubtedly begin to feel and look better.

The problem with many other people is that junk food does not make them sick immediately, though it may be killing them one bite at a time. You have to cleanse your body to the point that it will not *let* you eat unhealthy foods. How do you improve your chances to make it on the 100 percent raw food diet? Cleanse your body with sound practices: juice fasts, water fasts, and colon hydrotherapies, and each time reduce your calorie intake accordingly.

You can actually train your body to stop craving food after 3 o'clock, 2 o'clock or even 1 o'clock in the afternoon. One day we were traveling. I felt hungry around two, but there was nowhere to stop along that stretch of road, so I waited for us to reach our destination, thinking: I'll make an exception and eat later. But when we stopped about four and I was ready for my second meal, I felt no hunger. I ate anyway and felt heavy and stuffed later. Now, if I miss my usual mealtime, I eat nothing until the next day. You can actually learn to enjoy not eating, just as you enjoy eating — only more so.

Most of us know that the hardest thing is to keep the stomach flat. A distended stomach is a universal affliction. For so many among us, stomachs are overstretched, giving us that unattractive (and unhealthy) overhang. Nothing could be more obvious: We eat too much. When you do not eat after early or mid-afternoon, the stomach is sucked up during the rest of the day and remains so for a prolonged time time during the night. An empty stomach creates a situation where pressure inside is less than outside, pulling the stomach in. Because this happens every night, over time the stomach will retain its flatness, even without your doing a hundred crunches. Before and after my pregnancy, I never exercised. After my son's birth, I was left with a bulging lower abdomen. No amount of exercise seemed to reduce it. Raw foods helped dramatically, but only on the Quantum Eating regime I am beginning to win the battle of the bulge completely.

Raw food eating will make you feel *present* within your body. You will know when oils and dehydrated food will eventually have to be left behind. They were needed only as a raft to cross from the cooked to the non-cooked banks. It is time to move on.

Your body will signal you that it is ready to adopt Quantum Eating. For example, if you have a bowel movement in the middle of the night, your body is telling you that you are eating too much and too late in the evening. Time to raise the bar. If the urge to urinate awakens you, it is also an indication that you are consuming food too late. Your sleep will improve dramatically as you adjust the time of your last meal. You should never wake up in the middle of the night to go to the bathroom.

I read that in another era, French beauties always knew not to keep the colon full and would use an enema every night to achieve a beautiful complexion. I would never recommend doing this, no matter how tempting. Regular enemas can be habit-forming and will eventually have bad consequences on the function of your digestion system.

An interesting thing happened to me several years into Quantum Eating. Like most people, I had a bowel movement every morning when I woke up. But as a result of not eating for 18 hours (after 2 P.M.), my bowel-emptying time moved to 5 P.M., three hours after my last meal. At night my digestive system is basically free from waste products collected through the day. After this change, I noticed a profound improvement in my complexion. It happened only when the last meal was something very light, like a green smoothie. Even if you have another bowel movement in the morning, this late day bowel evacuation will greatly improve your energy level and your looks and will give you a euphoric sensation upon awakening. Everyone's body is different, so keep experimenting with different foods and amounts for your last meal to achieve the results you want. Even now it does not happen to me every day. I am still learning.

> "People can tell a measure of their health by their bowel movement. Nothing is so overrated as sex and so underrated as a good bowel movement." — Ted Loftness, MD, an internist in Litchfield, Minnesota.

Forgive me, please, for talking so much about bowel movements. Indelicate as the subject may be, we do need to know what is going in our bodies, and elimination is a big part of it. I once gave a speech at my Toastmasters club and, as you have already guessed, I spoke about raw foods and their effect on the human digestive and elimination system. My evaluator commented, "It takes guts to talk about the bowel movement with such ease." I thought to myself: *All it takes is one healthy gut!* When the foul smell and hard time in the bathroom goes as a result of the raw food diet, the foul attitude toward the body's excretions goes as well.

When you eat cooked food, you spend a lot of time in a kitchen either preparing meals or devouring them. On the raw food lifestyle, it is the bathroom that becomes your favorite place in the house. During the transitional period, as your digestive system cleanses itself, you will delight in the fact that you evacuate more than you consume and as you progress to the Quantum Eating regimen, you will like going to the bathroom because you *know* that elimination is much more important than eating.

At the same time, if you are attempting to stop eating and drinking after, say, 5 P.M. and you have a hard stool the next morning, it means you are not ready. In this case, drink some water in the evening and make your "curfew" later in the day.

The raw food lifestyle is as much art as it is science. At some point the concepts and ideas you have learned must yield to your own firsthand experience. Your body must be treated with diplomacy. Never allow your impatience for results to push your body into doing something it is not ready to do. Even though everyone can benefit from not eating at night, raising the dinner-time bar must be done gradually.

The secret to success on the Quantum Eating regimen is to concentrate on changing your lifestyle at whatever pace your body can accept change. You proceed experimentally, attentively, relying upon the responses you receive from your body. Move gingerly. Watch for any signs the body is giving you, and adjust your eating accordingly. Changing your diet abruptly can be dangerous, but so can be any act of living.

It is my opinion that eating at night contributes to aging — even on a 100 percent raw food regimen. As you are trying to master Quantum Eating, you will want to stop eating by, say, 5 P.M. But your body or mind may try to sabotage you by demanding food. Your mind will think, even insist: It is time to eat. Before you know it, your body is marching dutifully into the kitchen. This also can happen the other way around. Your stomach growls and signals the mind to find some food. Before you know it, your feet are heading toward the refrigerator or pantry. Indeed, we sometimes become quite Pavlovian about this. Only half tongue-in-cheek do I say to TV football fans: You know those moments ... Commercial — grab a beer. Half time

— into the kitchen for a gigantic dagwood sandwich. Even practiced vegetarians and raw-fooders may well still be subject to external cues that prompt arbitrary, superfluous eating.

Resist that first impulse to get up and go for food. If you are still in the transitioning phase and you are experiencing detox symptoms, direct your attention to the discomfort. Mentally embrace it. Welcome it. Any discomfort you have associated with not eating — such as stomach growling, dizziness, even nausea — accept these without judging or reacting to them as undesirable and trying to eliminate them by giving in to eating. Unpleasant as these detox symptoms might be, these bodily sensations can be used to teach you something about yourself. Your detox symptoms are not only changing your physical body, they are also teaching you to accept your body unconditionally. Resistance is the source of all discomfort. You will discover that it is possible to relax even when you feel physical discomfort.

After your body is cleansed of toxins, the unpleasant physical symptoms will go away. Quantum Eating frees your body from enslavement to food, and helps you enter the freedom of little eating. It brings liberation from incessant eating. But your body is only part of the equation. Your body will accept Quantum Eating months, even years, before your mind is thoroughly re-trained to live with little food.

Realize that it is not always your body that tells you to eat — it is often your mind. It is offering food as a panacea to other problems that are unresolved in your life. You respond to outside stimuli — when you receive bad news (or even good news), when you are nervous, when you are excited, when others are about to eat, but almost never to actual hunger. By offering food as a solution to any new thought, we actually limit the range of feelings we allow ourselves to experience. Restlessness and nervousness are mistaken for hunger. If you have a reason, it is all right to be sad or to be anxious — this is part of the normal process of living. What is *not* all right is feeding every passing emotion instead of accepting it or trying to resolve the underlying source. Ask yourself a question: Is it *genuine* hunger I feel?

We eat compulsively because we are barely in touch with our body, unaware of how it is really feeling. To be aware is to be able to focus on the present moment. The moment the thought of how much you want to eat comes, acknowledge it and treat it like a random thought, such as wanting to go to the Bahamas, or you may be up and chewing before you know it. You are not even aware that you decided to stop what you were doing and start eating because of a random impulse. Chaperone your thoughts. Don't allow your mind to pull you into actions that compromise your healthy food choices. Observe the impulse to go to the kitchen or the food thought that enters your mind. Listen to the monologue in your head. Understand how much of it is simply moaning and groaning, and how much is expressing gratitude, love, and hope.

When the strong urge to eat comes from your mind, lie down on your back in a comfortable position and concentrate on breathing. Allow the images and thoughts of food that flood your mind to dissipate. If your attention strays back to food, just observe it and escort it back to the breathing. Feel the rising and falling of your belly as you inhale and exhale. Discipline your mind as you would an unruly child — firmly and with loving kindness. When your mind tells you to go and grab something to eat, smile, shake your head, and say *No* — firmly.

Each time your attention wanders, bring your mind back, make it acknowledge your non-eating comfort. Take a few moments to feel your body nurtured and safe, feel the pleasure of non-eating. Enjoy it! Observe, on exhaling, how your stomach can go deeper into your frame. Enjoy the emptiness, the lightness in the stomach, and the feeling of exhilaration that comes from within.

A newly acquired elasticity of tendons, ligaments, and muscles will increase flexibility and vitality beyond your ordinary range of movement. Also, when falling asleep, there will be a few moments (lasting only a fraction of a second), when you will experience occasional sensations that feel as though a surge of energy has bolted through your body. You will begin to actually feel the body rearranging its faculties and functions to accommodate raw food and smaller food quantities. You will feel as if remodeling and the rearrangement of furniture is going on inside you. These moments, rare and transitory, cause no distress, but only a feeling of wonder. One of the signs of significant improvement in your health is a sensation of intense pleasure floating through your body, especially at night.

Remember Pavlov ringing his bell for the dogs at mealtimes? The sound began to trigger salivation in the dogs because the bell activated a "bell equals mealtime" mechanism. I chew some kale just after my second and last meal. It has become a habit. Now I believe this taste sends the signal to my brain that eating is over.

Initially, as you begin going to bed with an empty stomach, the sensation of buoyancy might make you so keyed up that it is hard to fall asleep. This is because your body is adjusting. As your body adapts to this lightness, your sleep will become deeper and shorter within several weeks.

After you have practiced Quantum Eating for a while, a sensation of lightness will fill your body. You will want to move, to go outside and run, leap, jump — anything to release the energy percolating through your system as euphoric feeling.

"Energy is eternal delight" — William Blake, English poet and artist

By continuously eating and never purifying the body through non-eating, we deprive ourselves of this exalted state. Drugs can give you this high only temporarily and are ultimately destructive. The fact that you never earned it means that the high will be followed by a low. All addictions are about getting undeserved highs, stealing unearned pleasure. So negative energy rushes in on the heels of this high. And negative consequences will show up uninvited.

While you practice Quantum Eating, enjoyment bubbles from within during each living moment, rather than in a temporary burst of pleasure. You'll feel an extraordinary lightness when you are awake and moving. You earned this state by making yourself super-healthy. This joy is a grand reward for being healthy. This is the high that does not come with a low.

At the beginning of your health-seeking adventure everything is against you. Your body is against you — it gives you detox symptoms. Your mind is against you — it wants to lure you back to old habits. Your friends are against you — they think you are nuts. But as you dive deeper into the lifestyle, the body becomes your biggest ally. Non-eating can actually be captivating. There are no words available to me to describe this sensation — they are not vivid enough to include the reality to which it points as a signpost. Once you have experienced this sense of exhilaration, you will redouble your efforts to attain it again. You will want to intensify and deepen your enjoyment. These feelings are so powerful that, once they have been experienced, they are never forgotten. That is when Quantum Eating becomes effortless.

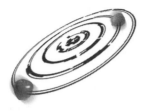

Chapter 15
Eating as a Ritual

At the Optimum Health Institute in Austin, Texas, I met an interesting German lady whom I wanted to get to know better. Our class schedule was so tight we could only talk briefly. I looked forward to lunchtime, hoping for a longer chat. At lunch I held a place for her and, being extra thoughtful, I brought her food along with mine. To my dismay, when she got to the table she picked up her plate, said, "I need to find a quiet place to eat" and simply walked away. My jaw dropped. I felt like a kid whose computer crashed just when he's ready to play a new video game. Despite what I at first thought of as outright rudeness, this woman's actions became a pivotal learning experience for me. I now believe it *is* best to eat alone.

We're socially conditioned to eat together. As Malcolm de Chazal put it, "Women eat while they are talking; men talk while they are eating." There is no better way to describe how our society combines these two diverse functions — eating and talking.

We tend to eat more when other people are around. Every one of us, for example, has at one time or another chowed down like hippo on a plate of canapés or a favorite snack at a Christmas party. We become so completely immersed in conversation that we pay no attention to our eating process. Our mind's energy is so engaged in our thoughts and what we're going to say next that our body becomes like a robot, blindly shoveling food into our mouths without conscious thought. Most people place more focus on talking and thinking, disconnecting from the nourishment component of eating, and from the amazing effect on the body that eating *consciously* has. We are almost never present when we eat. We have to learn to concentrate on eating, concentrate on being fully present in the moment. Most of us do not know how to do this.

From childhood onward, our ability to control what we eat, or whether we eat at all, is the single most basic aspect of life over which we have full power. Since our being ultimately depends on the food we eat, each time we eat we take our life and well-being in our hands. The act of eating is singularly fundamental to experiencing self-awareness. You can transform eating (and not eating) from the most mundane act to a sublime experience.

Thich Nhat Hank says in *The Miracle of Mindfulness*: "Raising your cup of tea to your mouth is a rite. Does the word *rite* seem too solemn? I use that word in order to jolt you into realization of the life-and-death matter of awareness." Of course, a cup of tea is only a symbol here, and the author wants us to carry each act of our daily life in mindfulness, whether it is doing dishes or running errands. But eating is a good place to start.

In the same book the author tells a story about sharing a tangerine with a friend. This friend was very excited about a new project he was eager to begin. So immersed was he in his future that he completely forgot about what he was doing at that very moment — eating a tangerine. He was popping sections of tangerine one after another without ever being present. The author pointed out to his friend (and to all of us) that he should eat one single section of tangerine, not his future plans.

Concentrate *only* on eating *whenever* you are eating. Let this principle become your mantra. The organ involved in eating is the same organ used for talking. Don't use your mouth for both at the same time. Social eating leads to overeating and impaired digestion.

"While I am eating, I am deaf and dumb." — Russian Proverb

Being psychologically present when you eat is the key to liberating yourself from hunger. When you eat and socialize at the same time, your awareness of eating diminishes. You'll quickly feel hungry again. Eating is *personal*. You can allocate other times for family gatherings. Teach children to eat in silence and gratitude, concentrating on the moment. Use books — not spoons — to bring your family together.

We all have a special closed room dedicated to daily evacuation — the toilet. So why not a place for eating? Think about it: We are actually more present in the moment when we defecate than when we eat. We give more concentration to our bowel movements than to our fork movements. Could it get more absurd? We pay more attention to what goes out than in.

Create a special place to eat — preferably a place that connects with nature. A porch, a bench, a swing — being out in nature can be very beneficial in helping one to concentrate. If you can't go outside, set aside a special place that includes flowers, plants, and outdoor light. Be still. Smell your food and savor every bite, with full awareness in that bite.

While working on *Quantum Eating,* I found a book by Maureen Whitehouse — *Soul Full Eating: A (Delicious)*

Path to Higher Consciousness. She writes: "Now if you happen to choose a piece of Devil's Food Cake, eat it with awareness. A little treat now and then needn't plummet you into the depths of hell."

My view is different. When you are eating mostly raw foods, and you allow yourself such slips, your body will rebel. If your body does not punish you, it has not been cleansed enough — and that is nothing to be complacent about. On the other hand, if your body is clean and free of toxins, even if this treat does not "plummet you into the depths of hell," it will make you extremely sick. Since such a so-called "treat" can become torture to a purified system, it should not be encouraged. You can trust me: No amount of mere awareness will help the matter.

In another place Maureen Whitehouse writes: "We can eat anything we want, any time we want, as long as it is indeed furthering our connection to our Divinity." Let me ask you: Where did this "chicken soup" idea get us, health-wise, in the first place? Why should we think that eating helps us establish a connection with the divine? If anything does that, it's fasting — non-eating, the absence of food. When we read about the heroes of the Bible, one thing is mentioned again and again — the forty days' fast.

An ascetic diet is almost always associated with attaining the highest levels of spiritual and moral wisdom. Throughout history Native American shamans, Christian hermit monks, and Indian gurus, among others, have engaged in prolonged forms of fasting in order to master the animal instincts that could block their spiritual development. They aspired to a profound form of spiritual experience. Mastering the denial of food is essential to achieving higher consciousness. I am not saying that one *cannot* be a highly spiritual individual while eating plenty. I am saying that I do not know *how* it is possible. With all my experience and research, my mind refuses to comprehend the idea. I see a full stomach as a tremendous obstacle!

To continue your habitual eating practices, having all the treats you crave, while at the same time relying only upon your mind for your spiritual transformation, is unrealistic. Your body will be confused by the contradictory messages it receives. The mind cannot transform your body while you are in the act of murdering its faculties.

Eating fruits and vegetables in their raw unprocessed form is like taking communion with nature. Eating raw foods offers a redemptive quality by bringing attention to the food you are about to eat, observing it carefully as if seeing it for the first time. You'll not only be satisfied with very little food, but you'll also enjoy the sacred time that is spent mindfully nourishing yourself. You'll find in this process a joy that fills your being with such an enriching high-octane energy that you will eventually realize how little food you actually need. You will eat *less*. You will eat *slower*.

On the Quantum Eating regimen, be sure every bite gets your full attention. Because you know there will be no food in the latter part of your day, you never eat just to get it over with. It's a good thing to stop thinking when you eat. Take your time. *Be there* for every bite. While eating, be *aware* that you are eating. Let go of your busy-ness and your problems while you eat. Pay attention to all of the senses involved in the activity of eating. Pay close attention to every muscle contraction, every jaw movement, every swallow. Be totally present.

When you eat, act as though this is the most important time in your life: here and now. Do not allow your thoughts to drift away. If consuming a juice or a smoothie drink, be mindful. Be present — do not gulp it down. Ascend to the state in which the distinction between the food and you is no longer there. This way eating becomes a wondrous experience. And an amazing thing will happen — the more mindful you become of eating, the more enjoyable non-eating becomes. The non-eating state might become infinitely more joyful than a food feast could ever be.

But this will come later. In the meantime, during the next lunch break at work or at a family gathering, pick up your plate and say: "I need to find a quiet place to eat." On second thought ... don't do it! Others might think you have lost your marbles ... while in fact you have just found them! There will be many times you can be alone, choose them wisely. You do not have to make others feel rejected to preserve your integrity. With enough discipline and time, you can concentrate on your meal without physically removing yourself and calling attention to yourself. Most gatherings have enough conversation going on around you that your mental absence will scarcely be noticed. Be well, be alone, but don't be anti-social.

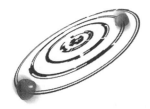

Chapter 16

Health Is a State Where Medicine Loses the Vote

'm Russian. I prize democracy, I treasure the right to vote.

But I'll tell you: If I ran the show, Modern Western Medicine would be denied the right to step into the voting booth in a state named "Health."

The object of the medical science is to devise approximate descriptions or models of aspects of the human body. Basically, this consists of asking a question, suggesting a hypothesis, testing it, and then, on the basis of the results, rejecting or accepting that hypothesis. The ultimate arbiter of correctness is the available empirical evidence.

In mathematics, however, the measure of correctness is proof, as distinct from experimental evidence. For a mathematical conclusion to be accepted as a true, it takes a chain of reasoning statements that demonstrate that the conclusion must *always* follow from the hypotheses. Mathematicians sneer at empirical evidence. It's never good enough for them, because a new piece of evidence may force a conclusion to be modified or rejected outright:

"No amount of experimentation can ever prove me right; a single experiment can prove me wrong." — Albert Einstein

In mathematics, nothing can be proven by experiment — only by deductive reasoning. Research in medical and nutritional science, on the other hand, is done by pattern recognition. Data is collected from experiments and patterns are explored for similarities and differences. Let's say 1,000 people are involved in an experiment. Most of these people, if not all, eat cooked food. Most of these, if not all, are sick to some degree. So, when the scientists collect the data, extrapolate the data, and come up with a suggestion ... that suggestion will be good *for whom?* For people who eat a cooked food diet and who therefore hover perpetually on the edge of illness.

After being on a 100 percent raw food lifestyle for ten years, I noticed that most recommendations coming from medical or nutritional science do not work for me. A few examples ...

In the hospital after my hip replacement surgery, I was drinking three freshly squeezed vegetable juices, loaded with greens, every day. Like many people undergoing surgery, I had been prescribed the drug Coumadin, to prevent blood clotting. I was lying in bed and, having nothing else to do, I began to use deductive reasoning: *There is no way my blood is thick with all this juicing,* I reasoned. *There is no way I need Coumadin.* Most people on a cooked food diet have a condition called Rouleau or "sticky blood." It is caused when red blood corpuscles clump together. The doctor insisted that I at least take aspirin, saying, "If you don't take a blood-thinning drug and you develop a clot, I will be liable." However, the hospital staff does not monitor you when you take aspirin versus Coumadin. I collected all the aspirin and sent them down the toilet. I didn't stay to see whether it made the water any thinner.

A week later, I was released from the hospital. Back home, I continued my research. One book caught my attention: *People's Guide to Deadly Drug Interactions.* I ordered the book. When it arrived, I opened the book randomly and read: "Coumadin can interact with a diet abundant in green leafy vegetables with fatal results."

According to the Journal of the American Medical Association, medical mistakes are the third leading cause of death in the United States. As recorded in the book *Death by Medicine,* a study based on the results of a ten-year survey of government statistics yielded even more dismal figures. The study concluded that iatrogenic illness is actually the leading cause of death in the United States and that adverse reactions to prescription drugs are responsible for more than 300,000 deaths a year.

I no longer get regular check-ups. After two artificial hips, I am uninsurable. But uninsurability is not the only reason I'm not flipping the pages of *Redbook* in the doctor's waiting room. Let's pretend I am going to have a doctor's check-up right now. One of the tests the doctor would order is called a white blood cells differential. A blood sample, drawn from my vein, will reveal a startling abnormality: My white blood count is very low.

The common thinking is that when you hear howling, think hounds, not wolves. When the doctor sees my blood count he will surely think hounds. He will arrive at what will seem a perfectly logical medical conclusion — presuming he were dealing with a patient consuming cooked foods. People on raw food have been diagnosed with AIDS, leukemia, or other cancers because their white blood cell count is low. Blood infiltrated by white cells signals that the body is fighting back, sending its immune cell soldiers into battle against infection. But with most folks on a raw food diet, there's no infection — hence few soldiers. (And those soldiers there are will be milling about the PX at their home base, slurping green smoothies!)

Another experiment was done on a person who has been on 100 percent raw food lifestyle for ten years. His blood differential measured low. Then he was given cooked food for a period of time. His white cells count was checked again and it had skyrocketed! Our bodies treat cooked food as poison.

In the hospital or in the doctor's office, the parameters you'll be compared to are not *normal* — they're more aptly termed just *average*. They're derived by experimenting on people who eat cooked foods. The healthier you become, the more you'll find yourself off the charts!

"The reality is that the tests every patient ... typically undergoes — pressure, pulse, blood chemistry, and x-rays, to say nothing of the more sophisticated (and expensive) imaging technologies — are not simply indices of health but little observation windows looking down on all the things that can go wrong in the human body." — Stephen S. Hall, *Merchants of Immortality, Chasing the Dream of Human Life Extension*

Medications are incompatible with practices like water- and juice-fasting and raw foods, which promote health and longevity. Let me explain by giving a hypothetical example. Mary has been on the raw food lifestyle for several years. She has done a juice and water fast to cleanse her body. Now she can easily go 24 to 32 hours without food, even without water, with no negative reactions. During this period, she is full of energy and has no weight loss.

On the other hand, we have John, who has some serious health issues. He's been treating his symptoms with gradually increased piles of medications for several years. If he doesn't eat or drink for 24 hours, he can easily die because his elimination organs may not be able to deal with all of the toxins released at once.

On the other hand, if Mary, after dry fasting for 32 hours, were given John's medications, John's dosage could kill her. After being on raw foods for several years, her liver is very healthy and not enlarged. It is actually smaller than the livers of people on cooked food diets.

You see why I say that health and medication are mortal enemies and the hospital can be a dangerous battleground for healthy people.

Many books will tell you to check with your doctor before ever attempting a lifestyle change. Up front, I must warn you that if you have been to a doctor for some medical problem in the last few years and regularly take medication, this book is not for you. Leave this book for the future and get my first book or another book about raw foods that can help you deal with degenerative conditions. Even if you had all your tests done on your last medical exam and you were pronounced healthy, that is not good enough for you to begin Quantum Eating. You must be experienced in juice fasts, water fasts, and the raw foods lifestyle, and you must feel very healthy. This is a book about superior health, about an anti-aging lifestyle. You have to have at least 20 to 40 days of fasting experience under your belt before attempting Quantum Eating. These 20 to 40 days do not necessarily have to be consecutive — they can be cumulative. You must, however, feel so good that the idea that you need a doctor's opinion to confirm your health never crosses your mind.

Food intake can affect the absorption of many types of drugs. Usually absorption is reduced on a full stomach. Medications have almost all been designed for people eating three meals per day — and overwhelmingly with cooked meals in mind. For example, the insulin dosage given is linked closely to the estimated amount of carbohydrates taken in. If a patient is being treated for hypertension, it's assumed he'll maintain a fairly constant level of sodium intake every day.

People with diabetes and hypoglycemia don't tolerate fasting well. If they try to get off medications, they must have not just any doctor's supervision, but that of a doctor familiar with the healing powers of raw foods.

Doctors can save your life and they can treat your symptoms. But making yourself healthy and making your life longer is your responsibility. Doctors have as many health problems as their patients. If they knew how to be healthy, don't you think they would heal themselves first? They deal with diseases, so if you have a medical condition that needs special attention, go to a doctor.

My book is about health. I know nothing about diseases. Though I admire the people who know how to help you in life-threatening situations or how to control the genetics of debilitating diseases, I do not apologize for my ignorance of the workings of this disease and that. I do not want to learn about illnesses, do not want to memorize their names, study their symptoms, or learn sophisticated matchmaking between diseases and the drugs that ameliorate them.

All I know is health. All I want to know is health. Only if you believe that responsibility for your health is yours alone and you are ready to take full accountability ... *then* you can greatly benefit from reading this book.

Quantum Eating is not an extreme practice. Alternate-day fasting and one-meal lifestyles have been around for thousands of years in one form or another. You are already fasting for eight hours during the night. It has always been accepted that eating late is bad. Didn't your mother tell you you'd have bad dreams if you ate at bedtime? Add two hours. Many people skip breakfast altogether. Add another four hours. These people already are abstaining from food for 14 hours. Now all you have to do is to add another two hours over the next year.

I use the Coumadin story in my presentations and have included it on my CD. While writing this chapter, I received an email from a lady who attended my lecture. She wrote:

"I let my sister (who has been an ICU nurse for 24 years) listen to your CD and she said that Coumadin has never been given across the board to everyone post-operatively. Now, I'm sure that maybe you had the surgery in Russia or maybe even so long ago that back then it was standard. So, I'm going to hope that you clarify this so that skeptics like my sister don't dismiss the important message of truth you bring."

My hip replacement surgeries were done in the U.S. According to the list on *www.hipsandknees.com* of what to anticipate after surgery, one should expect to be given Coumadin to prevent blood clots from forming. It *is* the most commonly prescribed blood-thinning drug in America. And it is also true that millions are taking this drug world-wide. Yet this is not the point.

Not only do I try my very best to thoroughly verify all the information I present here, I am *living* it. Whether or not Coumadin is the prevailing blood thinning drug being pre-scribed at the time when you are reading this book is irrele-vant. Do not let minor particulars hide the prime point of this book. Bad news: Degeneration is inevitable. Good news: Regeneration is a possibility. Are you going to use this infor-mation for your benefit? Or are you going to wiggle your way out by poking intentional holes in my arguments?

Please don't write and tell me that Quantum Eating is impossible just because *you* cannot do it. It cannot be done? Just watch me — I am doing it! Doctor or not, if you are looking and performing 15 to 20 years younger than your age, I want to know what you are doing. If you honestly have a valid point, I'm all ears. But if you're searching for a counterargument, because Quantum Eating sounds too hard and you're looking for an excuse not to do it, and you are using scientific evidence as your shield, leave me out of it.

If you believe it "cannot be done," then you are right. *You* can't do it. *You* shouldn't attempt it. If you believe you can do it, then you are right, too. This is a good time to think like a scientist, like a real empiricist ... Take the plunge into Quantum Eating. Verify its benefits for yourself. I hear you asking: Is there any scientific evidence? My answer: Try it and become the evidence!

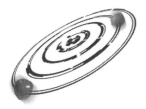

Chapter 17
The Law of Vital Adjustment

Hilton Hotema, in his remarkable book *Man's Higher Consciousness,* written in the mid twentieth century, discussed the body's miraculous ability to adapt. He called it the Law of Vital Adjustment. To explain the little-understood power of adaptation of the living organism to its environment, he offers the example of research done by Claude Bernard. A bird was placed under an airtight bell-glass large enough to allow it to survive for three hours. However, if the initial bird were removed at the end of two hours and another bird put in its place, the second bird died instantly, poisoned by toxic fumes exhaled by the first bird. The first bird, though, would have continued living another hour.

At a Toastmasters meeting, one of our most beloved members — let's call him "Bob" — told us he was battling cancer for the third time. This time it was his lungs. In a voice made hoarse by labored breathing, sounding like the water in old house pipes, Bob gave us an update. He said proudly that this time chemotherapy was not making him as sick as it had before. He was even able to continue working. Taking all this as a good sign, the whole group began cheering and applauding. Bob is a dear friend of mine and I shuddered as a great sadness shot through my heart. The realization hit me that he is still alive for the very reason that he has no health left. Bob is like Bernard's first bird: By suppressing his immune system, Bob, like the bird, is surviving his last hour.

A healthy body fights violently against encroaching poisons, and the quantity of poisons Bob was receiving would have killed a vital, healthy body. Achieving optimum health requires a different approach. The problem must be eradicated. Success depends very much on taking personal responsibility. Unfortunately, sick people would rather go along with the tools and products, methods and prejudices, of modern medicine, delegating all the responsibility to their doctors.

Your body will always guide all physiological processes in such a way as to insure the longest possible survival. This is adaptation. Even a weak body survives longer under adverse conditions that would be scientifically explained simply because it has adapted to these negative forces and learned to survive the consequences of mistreatment.

Your body adapts to the poisons you force feed it. But your body pays a dear price. If the poison is introduced gradually, you will not die instantly of an overdose, but you'll not increase your life span, either. Our bodies must suppress vitality in order to survive present abuses.

A vital body responds with serious violent reactions to chemotherapy as a dangerous poison. It will make an otherwise healthy body "sick as a dog." The patient will not only *be* sick, but *feel* sick. The healthier the body is, the stronger the reaction. However, even that reaction may be minimized because a body containing cancer is not truly healthy.

This is a hard journey. Not everyone is willing to take this route. In fact, very few dare. In the book *How We Die* by Sherwin B. Nuland, the distinguished surgeon writes: "Almost everyone seems to want to take a chance with the slim statistics that oncologists give to patients with advanced disease. Usually they suffer for it, they lay waste their last months for it, and they die anyway, having magnified the burdens they and those who love them must carry to the final moment."

Nuland describes not only the mechanisms of cancer, heart attack, stroke, AIDS, and Alzheimer's disease, but adds also vivid descriptions of the last moments of suffering of real people, because he says that is how most people will die. He set out to show in his book how undignified death is. And I must say he has succeeded: I frankly felt nauseated several times while reading this book. Nevertheless, I believe everyone should read it. Not only does the author dispel the myth of the dignified death, but he delivers a much more valuable service: He shows that despite the technological *hubris* of modern medicine most of the time doctors are helpless and defeated in the face of death. The reader gets the idea: Surround yourself by as much high-tech equipment and as many white coats as you like — death from illness is not going to be pretty.

"Finally, considering the panorama of long-term chronic illnesses of the sort that typically afflict so many elderly people, and seeing the way these constellations of illness leach away the essence of a loved one's vitality and spirit, you begin to realize that the sheer complexity of age-related disease and the process of aging itself threaten to diminish, if not overwhelm, the ultimate promise of any single form of therapy." — Stephen S. Hall, *Merchants of Immortality, Chasing the Dream of Human Life Extension*

The body's adaptive ability is truly astonishing. Its capacity to adjust, to assimilate and to neutralize new poisons that enter the body system, is amazing. For example, if you decide to smoke your very first cigarette today, you will more than likely react to the smoke by coughing, often accompanied by feelings of nausea and a burning sensation in the lungs. Having made the initial decision to allow this toxic air to enter your body, your body immediately and appropriately reacts, signaling to your conscious mind to stop the nonsense and reject the poison. But when you try to smoke again, your body will show less resistance as it brilliantly begins to adapt to the poisons you have chosen to ingest. Adjusting to the new situation, your body begins to alter its functions by allowing the smoke to enter the lungs, even though the body knows the smoke will harm it.

This example shows us that the body is a unique organism with the amazing ability to adapt to new situations in order to survive in spite of the ingestion of poison. When your new acquired beliefs and actions are detrimental to your well-being, the body adjusts, abiding by the new situation and adhering to new programming.

We learn from the behavior of the body that not only can the body accept poison and carcinogens, adjusting its mechanism to facilitate the poison's acceptance, but it also becomes addicted to the chemicals as a result of the poisons. Such body behaviors work on either positive, life-enhancing actions or, conversely, on actions that sabotage the energetic matrix of the body. Our body can adapt to all possible living conditions on Earth, if it is given enough time to allow it to develop in an accommodating way.

The body will adapt itself to high mountain altitudes or sea level, to constant room temperature or to radically different climates, and to an astonishingly varied diet. The exercise of the body's powers of adaptation to these environmental conditions stimulates all its functions. This exercise, this stimulation, is essential to well-being and to maintaining stamina, vigor, powers of endurance, and resistance to fatigue. The same is true of different organs and systems of the body.

After reaching maturity, the body is not supposed to change. The deterioration of the bodily functions and distortions of old age are the body's response to the abuse it is taking from a hostile environment — and, I hasten to add, from *you*. Negative features are forced upon the body and the body fights against these enemies with all its mighty power. It will not admit defeat until the last breath. The aches, pains, and other symptoms that medical science labels disease are actually signs of the body's heroic nature struggling to never give up. Disease is nothing more than the sign of healing of very serious wounds.

Human bodies have the ability to reproduce or change the physiology of any particular muscle group or organ to meet their existing physical needs and demands. The human body is perfectly designed to prolong life by adapting to adverse conditions. But there is a price to pay. The body will alter to meet every new situation. The body that was not supposed to change will change by suppressing vitality. The body will change, trying to accommodate numerous toxins. All organs work together in a focused attempt to survive. When the body is overwhelmed with filth, then lumps, tumors, and cancers appear.

Beauty will be sacrificed first. Beauty will be brought to the altar and tortured for bad habits and environmental hazards. Sallow skin. Spots. Sags. Discolorations. Hair growing in undesirable places. And, most visibly for so many North Americans, an unsightly move from shapely to shapeless as inches build on the belly, the thighs, the buttocks. Love handles become carry-on luggage. Flab — not merely the fat of stored calories, but fat as a by-product of disease — builds relentlessly in individuals, and in our population. (Did you know that standard furniture sizes have significantly increased in the last century? Chair seats are bigger, and not for reasons of mere style.)

Your body has regrouped into survival mode. The body become thicker, larger. Bigger arms, neck, bosom, waist, hips, legs, and buttocks. The disfigurement of old age is the body's way of removing garbage from vital organs. Lacking a convenient landfill, however, we continue carrying this waste about with us, displaying it in ever-larger pants sizes.

That was the bad news. Now here's the good ... the same law that might kill you can actually save you. The same Law of Vital Adjustment will make it possible for you to be very comfortable after following the Quantum Eating regimen for a length of time. As long as you proceed gradually, you can train your body to live on little food and the result will actually *hinder* the aging process.

The body we occupy is pure brilliance, always adapting to the environment and to the lifestyle we hold. It will continue deteriorating unless we listen to its needs and alter our habits to enhance its abilities.

"When you overeat one day, you are hungrier the next. Huge meals stretch your stomach and throw your appetite out of proportion. Conversely, the less you eat the less you want. After you become used to smaller food intake, you may wonder how you have previously eaten so much." — Judith Churchill

---

Go back to basics — or at least, to what vegan raw food eaters would consider basics. Just stop eating meat. Keep faithful to that goal, and three months later you'll find, if you slip or if you deliberately experiment, that meat will sicken you. If you stop drinking milk, within a few months even a morsel of cheese will give you such foul gas that you (and everyone else, I remind you) will know you've made a mistake. After adjusting from three to two meals a day, your body will fight fiercely to return to three meals.

The human body is beautifully designed always to seek equilibrium. When we violate an equilibrium by making a major change, the body, like the pendulum, seeks to swing back into its "natural" position. When we build — as so many of us North Americans have — a sickened equilibrium, the pendulum seeks to return there. An equilibrium based on sound eating, sound hydration, and good breathing, is hard to achieve. Such a lifestyle is a *major* change. Indeed, rightly understood, it's a complex, multi-faceted change affecting many equilibriums simultaneously. The spotted, bulbous, tortured bodies we might see in a western shopping center — public displays of human self-abuse — are actually bundles of simultaneous processes, each striving for equilibrium against the odds of every new order of fries, every cigarette, every over-sugared, creamed-up espresso latte introduced to it.

Every abuse — whether airborne, brought in by food, encouraged by indolence, or even induced by medical science, as in Bob's case — interacts with a complex system of processes seeking to restore equilibrium. Disturb the system enough, and it will even work *against* health, but always towards ensuring the longest survival. Understand the Law of Vital Adjustment, however, learn how your body receives and interacts with each variable in food, water, and air, and you are well on your way to a body — and a life — proceeding ever more surely toward an equilibrium centered on health, vitality, and genuine happiness.

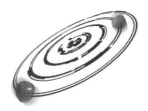

Chapter 18
Oxygen: Dr. Jekyll or Mr. Hyde?

"Man is an obligate aerobe." — Hippocrates

When I married my husband, he had chronic bronchitis, experiencing an acute attack every few months. Nothing we did, through medical means or folk remedies, could cure this recurring condition. One day he excitedly told me that he'd heard a doctor on the radio talking about curing all types of respiratory disorders with what he called "shallow breathing." Many patients who became asthma-free gave testimonials praising this doctor's method. He promoted a pattern of breathing that did not allow the lungs either to fully expand or to fully contract. Airflow was thus restricted and helped asthmatics breathe better. He claimed oxygen was causing their problems. *Oxygen?*

Pure quackery, I thought. I was sure that either Nick had misunderstood something, or the doctor wasn't legitimate. I wasn't about to pursue something that sounded so ridiculous. The matter was forgotten and my husband continued suffering his attacks for years. Only when I went raw and was able to convince him to cut back on lactose did the attacks slow in frequency. A year ago, he finally gave up cheese and they stopped entirely. But I had never forgotten the controversy about oxygen.

While working on this book I came across a fascinating book, *Flood Your Body with Oxygen,* by Ed McCabe, touting the tremendous benefits of proper oxygenation. The author is a journalist who for many years has promoted oxygen awareness, health, and environmental consciousness. He has traveled extensively, interviewing thousands of people who had been helped by Oxygen Therapies, as well as hundreds of doctors who worked with such therapies. Ed McCabe writes: "What are Oxygen Therapies? They are a process of slowly and properly saturating, of *flooding* the body with special 'active' forms of oxygen. Oxygen Therapy is not only one of the oldest therapies, but, as the evidence shows, it is one of the most successful."

We need oxygen to live — of that there's no doubt. Yet there are many microorganisms that are instantly killed if exposed to oxygen. Almost all bacteria, viruses, fungi, parasite, mycoplasmas, and microbes are either strictly anaerobic or at some point anaerobic.

Every breath you take is followed by immediately exhaling waste compounds that your body eliminates constantly. They come out through respiration precisely because they are first combined with oxygen. The main point of this passionately written book is that to eliminate diseases you need to "flood your body with oxygen."

McCabe explains that antioxidants are naturally occurring and found in raw foods. They do not *prevent* oxidation, as their name implies. Instead, they give protection to healthy cells by shielding them like armor. Any cellular life form (such as a bacterium, a virus, a fungus, or any other human pathogen, or weakened, diseased, or dying cells that have no antioxidant coating) will be burned up by oxygen. Oxygen selectively attacks diseased cells because these cells have damaged or non-existing antioxidant protection. Aren't Nature's solutions beautiful and brilliant?

McCabe's book made perfect sense to me. However, while agreeing with the author's explanations and reasons, I could not shake the memory of that other doctor who had stated the absolute opposite almost thirty years before. I remembered that he had cured thousands. I even remembered his name — Dr. Konstantin Pavlovich Buteyko.

I needed an explanation! I called Ed McCabe. He was very courteous and we had a pleasant conversation. To my disappointment, however, he had never heard of Dr. Buteyko and dismissed his claims as absurd. I now felt certain that the doctor I'd heard about almost thirty years ago was exposed as a fraud and long forgotten. But I decided to check the internet just in case.

To my surprise I found a website devoted to his method: (Russian: *www.buteyko.ru* / English: *www.buteyko.com*). I learned that, though the doctor himself died recently, at age 80, he has left behind a very successful institute promoting his "shallow breathing." Published articles claim that as many as 90,000 people have become asthma-free because of Buteyko's system. Bewitched, bothered, and bewildered, I became acutely curious. I had just read one tribute to *more* oxygen and one paean to *less* oxygen. What was going on?

"A great truth is a truth whose opposite is also a truth."
— Thomas Mann

So is oxygen friend or foe? I began to read everything I could find. I realized that scientists were just as confused as I. It seems that oxygen gives life and dispenses death with every breath. Remember truth and its opposite? Quantum physics has no problem with oxygen being both the good guy and the bad guy simultaneously. And neither should we.

But there is another gas that is essential to internal respiration — that is, to the process by which oxygen is transported to body tissues and carbon dioxide is carried away. Carbon dioxide is a waste product of cellular respiration during the production of ATP (energy). The body gets rid of it continuously by exhaling air that is rich in CO_2. Is CO_2 just plain bad? No! As with anything, it is much more complicated than just plain good and bad. In fact, scientists are discovering now that carbon dioxide has many beneficial effects on the body. This carbon dioxide is also the chief regulator of pH levels in the blood, which is essential for survival. It prevents blood from becoming too alkaline or too acidic. It has to be balanced perfectly, because both extremes in pH are life threatening.

The story of how Buteyko made his discovery is interesting. He suffered from a severe form of hypertension. One day, when he breathed rapidly and deeply, it resulted in dizziness, heart discomfort, palpitations, and weakness. When he intentionally slowed his breathing rate and depth, he found immediate relief. After a minute, he felt much better. He concluded that deep breathing was causing his problem. To check his theory, he asked asthmatics with stenocardia (ischemic heart disease) and other ailments to breathe less. The symptoms disappeared at once. When he asked them to breathe deeper, the symptoms resumed.

Wait a minute! When I read this the whole issue snapped into focus. I saw oxygen as not *causing the problem,* but as *aggravating the symptoms.* These are not at all the same thing. Oxygen is a great detoxifier. When oxygen applies its cleansing power to clogged and gummed-up lungs, a person feels worse. As we know, any process of toxic removal makes you feel worse before you feel better. There is no reason in the world why a body afflicted with such a severe disorder should have *no* symptoms, as in the case of Buteyko's test subjects. A sufferer felt better *only* if oxygen were restricted and not allowed to perform its filth-cleansing mission.

This is why even a fairly healthy person may feel faint, dizzy, flushed, or light-headed when doing breathing exercises. This is a result of increased oxygen levels in the body, to which your body may not be accustomed. Should you never do them again? On the contrary! Yoga instructors usually advise to allowing the breath to return to its natural rhythm and to increase your *pranayama* practice and the use of oxygen gradually. *Pranayama* is slow, deep breathing. It is the time-tested art of yogic breathing. Healthy and well-trained people can do breathing exercises without any ill effects.

> "[H]igh vibration people ... display seemingly inexhaustible vitality and stamina, creative power, and/or athletic ability of the highest quality ... What is their secret? How do they live at a superior rate of high vibration? The answer is simple: Such people consume large amounts of oxygen. They breathe deeply and fully, utilizing every square inch of their lung capacity. The more oxygen you can breathe into your lungs, the more energy you will have." — Dr. Paul C. Bragg and Dr. Patricia Bragg, *Super Power Breathing for Super Energy, High Health & Longevity*

If you are not an experienced yoga practitioner, try to begin with the two simple exercises I describe in the next chapter. Regular breathing exercise with resistance will result in slower breathing and gradual extension of breath holding.

By regulating your metabolism, breathing exercises will improve your health and help you achieve your ideal weight. You can actually lose weight simply by doing breathing exercises. Remember the last time you had a back-yard barbecue? If the charcoal did not turn red, what did you do? You blew on it! The more oxygen, the hotter the coals. When you breathe and take in oxygen, fat molecules are combined with additional oxygen atoms, causing oxidation and producing CO_2 and water. Oxidation of fat happens when oxygen reacts with fats, and they get burned as carbon dioxide and water. Through this combustion, energy crucial to cellular work is released from the cleaved (fractured) bonds of the atoms of the fat molecule which, before oxidation, held tightly together.

"Oxygenation through deep breathing boosts the immune system and can rid the body of chronic illnesses."
— Dr. Sheldon Hendler, MD, Medical Researcher Cell Oxygenation, Author of *The Oxygen Breakthrough*

Another way to get more oxygen into your body is with hydrogen peroxide. Hydrogen peroxide is found everywhere in nature because it falls to earth in the form of rainwater. After a good thunderstorm, you get out and it looks as though everything has grown an inch. Everything is alive, green, clean. What's happened? All the vegetation just received a high dose of nature's oxygen and peroxide that aids growth almost visibly. Rain is formed high up in the atmosphere, within an ozone–oxygen-rich atmosphere. The low concentration peroxide formed up there then goes into our groundwater. The roots of plants and trees reach down into the ground water and take up the peroxide. Nature continues this cycle by delivering the cleansing, oxygenating peroxide to us.

Hydrogen peroxide (H_2O_2) is simply a water molecule (H_2O) with an active singlet oxygen (O) attached *(see p. 434)*. That makes it an oxidizer of microbes and toxins when the active singlet oxygen breaks off and turns back into water. Peroxide is a clear, colorless liquid. Its smell is not that detectable, but it does give off a faint bleach-like odor. Almost velvety to the touch, it quickly becomes an irritant when used undiluted. Every cell in your body is manufacturing its own peroxide constantly. Peroxide is necessary for our immune systems. Our body uses hydrogen peroxide to fight infection, parasites, bacteria, viruses and yeast.

One of my readers sent me a list of the many advantages of hydrogen peroxide, from an article by a doctor's wife[1]:

"I would like to tell you of the benefits of that plain little old bottle of 3% peroxide you can get for under $1.00 at any drug store. My husband has been in the medical field for over 36 years, and most doctors don't tell you about peroxide, or they would lose thousands of dollars." The article continues:

1. Fill the little white cap from the bottle and use it as a mouthwash. No more canker sores and your teeth will be whiter without expensive pastes. *[Tonya's note: if you have amalgam fillings you should not do this!]*
2. Let your toothbrushes soak in a cup of "Peroxide" to keep them free of germs.
3. I had fungus on my feet for years — until I sprayed a 50/50 mixture of peroxide and water on them (especially the toes) every night and let dry.
4. Soak any infections or cuts in 3% peroxide for five to ten minutes several times a day. My husband has seen gangrene that would not heal with any medicine, but was healed by soaking in peroxide.
5. Fill a spray bottle with a 50/50 mixture of peroxide and water and keep it in every bathroom to disinfect without harming your septic system like bleach or most other disinfectants will.

---

1. *Excerpted from the* Countryside & Small Stock Journal, *January/February issue, 2006 (used with permission).*

6. Tilt your head back and spray into nostrils with your 50/50 mixture whenever you have a cold, or plugged sinuses. It will bubble and help to kill the bacteria. Hold for a few minutes then blow your nose into a tissue.

7. For natural-looking hair, spray the 50/50 solution on your wet hair after a shower and comb it through. You will not have the peroxide-burnt blonde hair like the hair dye packages, but more natural highlights if your hair is a light brown or dirty blonde. It also lightens gradually so it's not a drastic change.

Folk remedies using hydrogen peroxide go back at least three centuries. Drinking a highly diluted solution kills bacteria, offering a simple remedy for treating many minor infections. However, there is a real danger that an overdose can cause irritation and burning of digestive tract. I do not take peroxide orally. You shouldn't attempt it either, until you educate yourself and know what you are doing. Be sure to read *Flood Your Body with Oxygen* about your options. For me, the best way to get peroxide is to eat fruits and vegetables from plants that consume hydrogen peroxide through their roots and leaves, depositing it into their fruits.

Bathing in a tub full of water and hydrogen peroxide is highly effective. Ed McCabe suggests that the general rule for bathing in peroxide is one pint of 35-percent food-grade hydrogen peroxide into your bath. On the internet, I found a testimonial by one man who claimed his gray hair disappeared after daily baths with hydrogen peroxide. Of course I tried it! It hasn't happened yet. But the experience is invigorating and the improvement in my skin is obvious. The heat of the bathtub water opens the pores in the skin and enables blood vessels below the skin to absorb the peroxide, cleansing them in the process. I love my hydrogen peroxide baths!

Oxygen is good ... oxygen is bad ... Choose either one and you've oversimplified. Choose either one and you're standing on quicksand, scientifically. There is much experimental evidence to support *both* points of view. If you base your position on experimental evidence alone, there will be no end to this debate. Applying deductive reasoning might give us a compromise.

According to Buteyko's website, thousands upon thousands suffering from asthma, hypertension, and other heart diseases have been helped. Here is my own explanation ... his method is obviously working or it would not still be around and still gaining momentum after more than half a century. His method comprises a series of breathing techniques. There is a set of exercises that must be done daily. There are three parts to Buteyko's method of breathing: It is slow ... it is shallow ... and it requires holding your breath. Two of these components — slow breathing and holding your breath — are extremely beneficial and have been used by yogis for centuries.

These two components of Buteyko's method do the healing. What gives his method its symptom-oriented nature is shallow breathing. This allows patients to avoid severe reactions by slowing the healing process. However, people who do not have breathing pathologies are much better off *never* using shallow breathing techniques. Sure enough, I found that critics of the Buteyko method point out this negative side of shallow breathing. They say that, after about six months, the lungs lose their ability to take deep breaths. This gives another indication that breathing should be deep and slow. We should strive to have fewer breaths per minute.

"Deep breathing techniques which increase oxygen to the cell are the most important factors in living a disease free and energetic life ... Remember. Where cells get enough oxygen, cancer will not, cannot occur." — Dr. Otto Warburg, President, Institute of Cell Physiology, Nobel Prize Winner

There is another side to oxygen! Oxygen readily combines with hydrogen. This is the process we call oxidation. You have observed oxidation in action as it affects food. Oxidation turns oils rancid and turns iron into rust. And according to a 'free radical' theory of aging: Oxidation is causing aging and eventually death.

Look at both sides. On the one hand, oxygen gives us the intelligent, handsome Dr. Jekyll. Oxygen's negative side gives us the rather devious Mr. Hyde.

Oxygen is essential and at the same time damaging. If it reacts with the fats or carbohydrates that provide our fuel, we benefit from their energy-releasing breakdown. Oxidation is a chemical reaction that uses oxygen to burn our food and release energy (ATP). Its by-products are called free radicals. This is yet another puzzle in science that is full of self-contradicting experimental results.

The idea is this: Oxygen is essential to keeping you healthy, but at the same time you must strive to take in *less* oxygen in the long term. Confusing? Here is my take on this controversy. Oxygen is absolutely necessary to burn the food we eat. It supplies us with energy, and it is also essential for removing toxins from the body. Here is the catch. While oxygen chases pathogenic microorganisms and other filth out of your body, it is doing you a great service. Oxygen that is burning your food for energy will be doing long term damage — it ages you. Look at it this way: Oxygen is helping you with cleansing for free, but it is charging you hard currency for its job of releasing energy from food.

We're left to ask, then: Is there a way to outsmart this perverse little molecule?

Actually there *is* a way to make the most of oxygen's dual nature. The more we eat, the more oxygen we consume

— and while it is burning up our food, it is burning us up as well, thereby shortening our life span. One way to achieve rejuvenation is to cleanse the body and keep your eating pattern unchanged. Oxygen therapies, in this case, will result in obvious health improvement. But unless you change your diet, they will only keep you afloat. Remember that free radicals are the product of any oxygenation. There is another way to achieve rejuvenation — calorie restriction.

Any wonder the book *Oxygen: The Molecule that Made the World* by Dr. Nick Lane has a chapter titled "Eat! Or You'll Live Forever." In other words the solution is: Eat less! In this way, oxygen will have only limited ability to oxidize you to death, aging you along the way.

The recommendation to gradually increase the length of time you hold your breath through daily breathing exercises serves the same purpose. It trains your body to decrease the number of breaths per minute, which is essential for longevity. Remember that only by getting less oxygen through your lifetime than the next person will you raise your chances of a longer, healthier life.

The more breaths you take in a short period of time, the less oxygen is made available to your bloodstream. Your lungs require a certain amount of time to process the air you inhale. It has been observed through many centuries of yoga practice that the longer the breath can be held after exhalation, the healthier an individual becomes.

To partially neutralize oxygen's nasty aging nature, we should learn to breathe slowly, taking fewer breaths per minute. At the same time, to take full advantage of oxygen's cleansing service, we should take deep breaths.

When you hold your breath on the exhale, it raises the level of carbon dioxide in the body and brain. It also increases the level of nitrogen. Oxygen is delivered more efficiently to the body immediately after holding the breath.

Not eating is beneficial for a short period of time. Not drinking is beneficial for a short period of time. Why should we be surprised that not breathing for short periods of time can be very refreshing to the brain? Of course, what we mean by "a short time" varies. Individual cases have different durations.

I wish the jury weren't still out on this one. I wish the situation were clearer. I wish the empirical evidence were greater in both volume and quality. But that's the nature of Quantum Eating, as it is the nature of all leading-edge science and health practice. The process of discovery remains — for the individual as well as for science as an institution — a permanent part of the picture. The main aim, always, is to discover what works best for you. And my main caution is, whatever range of practices you choose — do keep breathing.

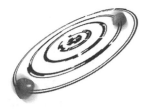

Chapter 19

Breathing Lessons for Health and Beauty

"Those who have mastered the breath experience enjoy spiritual breathing as much if not more than sex because it is a biological experience of God, and it produces physical and emotional satisfaction with every breath." — Leonard Orr, *Breaking the Death Habit: The Science of Everlasting Life*

The Bible begins its description of Creation with the sentence, "God's breath moved upon the waters." Hindus call breath *prana*. The Chinese call it *chi*. God's breath is the energy permeating the universe at all levels. In the Taoist view, the pranic nutrition provided by air through breathing is more vital to health and longevity than that provided by food and water through digestion.

Our culture assumes that food is the only means for nourishing the body and that food is the sole source of energy promoting life. Though we know food in excess can be very harmful, food is still deemed absolutely necessary. In reality, however, there is no way we are getting energy from food alone. There clearly exists another source. Food gives energy and food drains energy. There has to be a happy medium. We receive our energy from air, food, and water.

Human beings can use two systems of nourishment: food and water or pranic nourishment. When you eat food, you are using both systems together, whether or not you know it. When the amount of food decreases gradually, another pathway is activated. The physical body will adapt and adjust to a new regimen or any new situation. New programming will deliver new results. After eating, you begin losing energy. The more a person eats, the more other portals for receiving energy remain shut down. The less food you eat, the more energy you absorb by simply breathing air. By performing breathing exercises daily, you train your lungs to become the main organ for receiving energy and distributing nutrition.

If food does so much to improve your health and appearance, how much more could a simple breathing practice do? You might say: *I already breathe, don't I?* You certainly do, but there's always a better way.

The lungs are not muscles. They cannot inhale or exhale on their own. They are totally dependent on the diaphragm, a large muscle that works like a bellows. The lungs' task is to extract oxygen from a drawn breath and disperse it into the blood stream. Waste, like carbon dioxide, is exhaled. The fact that lungs, unlike the heart, are not a muscle is why you can completely control them through exercise. You are disciplining your diaphragm, not your lungs.

Breathing deeply and holding your breath provides exercise for the diaphragm. Breathing exercises generally increase the volume of air flow, which provides more oxygen and removes carbon dioxide more efficiently. By cutting down the number of breaths required per minute by more than half, diaphragmatic breathing greatly enhances your respiratory efficiency, conserving your heart and preserving vital energy.

Taoism is an English terminology that incorporates a number of interrelated Chinese religions and philosophies maintained through centuries of traditions. Overall it emphasizes the "Three Jewels of the Tao" — love, moderation, humility. Taoism traditionally measures life not by years but by breaths and heartbeats: Slowing the heartbeat and the number of breaths taken over time extends life by the equivalent saved. Paul Bragg writes in *The Miracle of Fasting*: "For over seventy years, I have done extensive research on long-lived people and I find one common denominator amount all of them. They are deep breathers. I have found that the deeper, and therefore fewer, breaths a person takes in one minute, the longer they live, and the rapid breathers are the short-lived people."

Do not underestimate the power of breathing as a part of an anti-aging lifestyle. It is enormous. Food and oxygen are our primary sources of vital energy. Therefore, attention to these bodily functions is fundamental in cultivating health and longevity.

The quantity of oxygen absorbed determines your body's vitality. The faster you breathe, the less efficiently you use oxygen. We breathe faster, now, especially in western cultures, than once we did. As life becomes faster paced, we breathe more quickly, less efficiently. We now average about eighteen breaths per minute. The higher your breathing rate, the faster your body deteriorates from lack of oxygen. Your life span is directly linked to your breathing rate. Similar to lowering the metabolic rate, longevity is aided by slowing your breathing patterns. A breathing rate of once a minute is thought to be the secret of longevity in Indian yogis. Breathing exercises are essential in reducing your breathing rate.

If you are new to breathing exercises, conscious breathing can be overwhelming. At first, you will not only dislike doing these exercises, but will try to talk yourself out of it. Therefore, I give you only two of the most effective and easiest ones for the beginners.

It is almost impossible to empty the lungs entirely — some amount of air will remain even after exhaling. Small pockets inside the lungs will still store stagnant air. Holding your breath is quite beneficial. When you exhale air and don't inhale immediately, stagnant stale air is removed and a supply of fresh air rushes into those pockets when you inhale again. Reduced pressure inside the lungs draws out the stale air. The entire surfaces of the alveoli (air sacs) inside the lungs receive greater amounts of fresh air. As you continue this exercise regularly, you will increase the length of time you can hold your breath as well as number of times you can do the exercise.

While performing your breathing exercises you might feel dizzy. Just rest and keep doing it. You might feel agitated. Just rest. Keep doing it. You might feel as if you are doing nothing. But persist. Be mindful of what you are doing, completely involved with the experience.

1. **Breathing through water.** All you need is a container filled with water and a straw. A regular bottled water container will work fine. Keep the lower end of the straw under about three inches of water. Take a deep breath through your nose. Then slowly exhale through your mouth into the straw, forcing the air into the water. Exhale for at least 15 seconds. Repeat ten times. As your lung capacity increases, you can gradually push the straw deeper to increase the resistance.

2. **Forceful exhale.** While standing, bend your knees slightly, lean over, placing your hands on your knees. Inhale slowly for a count of four. While all your muscles are tight, keep holding your breath for four seconds. Force all the air at once through your mouth making a

"ha" sound. You can help your lungs expel the air by pulling in your belly muscles, forcing your stomach inward toward your spine. When no more air can be pushed out, relax all your muscles as quickly as possible and return to a relaxed position. Repeat ten times. As your lung capacity grows, increase the time you hold your breath to six seconds.

The rhythmic contractions of the abdominal wall during the forceful exhale procedure are highly beneficial. The vigorous contractions not only give a therapeutic massage to the internal organs and the glands, but they also increase oxygenation of abdominal tissues, burning off excess abdominal fat.

Breathing exercises should become an integral part of your daily routine. At first it may seem difficult to go through even a few breathing repetitions. But once it becomes habit, momentum is your friend. The benefits become so obvious that you won't consider abandoning the practice.

"Deep diaphragmatic breathing stimulates the cleansing of the lymph system by creating a vacuum effect which pulls the lymph through the bloodstream. This increases the rate of toxic elimination by as much as 15 times the normal rate." — Dr. J.W. Shields, MD, Lymph, "Lymph Glands, and Homeostasis." Lymphology, v25, n4, Dec. 1992, p. 147

You have to *learn* abdominal breathing. This is also called the "Diaphragmatic Breath" or "Natural Breath." Lying flat on your back with your arms by your sides, palms up, start thinking about what your breathing really is. Inhale, slowly and deeply. Think about it. Your abdomen reacts to your breathing by rising and falling. Feel your breath replenishing your body. Keeping your mouth shut, breathe only through your nose. Now rest one palm or, better, place a heavy book on your stomach and feel it rising and falling as you inhale and exhale. Make yourself aware of the workings of your body as it moves beneath your hand.

The lung meridian is the most active between 3:00 A.M. and 5:00 A.M. It controls *chi,* according to Chinese medicine texts. *Chi* means both "breath" and "energy." Breath *is* energy. Lung weakness can be reflected in the appearance and condition of the skin, which is also a respiratory organ. The lungs and the large intestine are actually internal extensions of the skin. One very effective way to improve the complexion is to do breathing exercises daily.

Some believe that the essential element in air that carries the pranic energy turns out to be the negative ion — a tiny, highly active molecular fragment that carries a negative electrical charge equivalent to that of one electron. Since science does not recognize such concepts as *chi* or *prana,* let us talk about negative ions, which some believe are the same thing.

For any chemical reaction to take place, two molecules must come together and exchange some compatible atoms which are either positively or negatively charged. All of your bodily functions rely on the energy released when molecules in your body couple with molecules of the opposite "charge" caused when food, water, and air enter the body. An ion is any atom that has a positive or a negative charge. A positively charged ion will seek a negatively charged one to join with, and something new is produced. If there are not enough negative ions in the air or in your food, the molecules in your body are left holding a positive charge and are not available for fusing with negative ions to create energy.

Negative ions are invisible molecules that we inhale in abundance in the mountains, near waterfalls, and at beaches. Natural sources of negative ions are sunlight, radiation, moving air, and water. They are created in nature as air molecules are exposed to sunlight, radiation, moving air, and water.

Pollution, smog, chemicals, and the like, are airborne in relatively large ions with a positive charge. They are capable of steamrolling over the good negative ions and flattening out all the good air. Positive ions simply suck all the vitality out of the air. These are the circumstances that cause your local weather man to tell you that local air quality is dangerous, and to avoid long periods spent outdoors.

"Negative ions increase the flow of oxygen to the brain; resulting in higher alertness, decreased drowsiness, and more mental energy." — Pierce J. Howard, director of research at the Center for Applied Cognitive Sciences in Charlotte, N.C. *The Owners Manual for the Brain: Everyday Applications from Mind Brain Research*

Have you experienced exhilarating moods after a thunderstorm, or walking on the beach? The air circulating in the mountains, the country, the forest, and on the beach is said to contain an average ratio of negative to positive ions of about 3 to 1. In cities, the ratio drops drastically to one negative ion for every 300 to 600 positive ions! The vitality of negative ions in the air is greatly reduced by air-conditioning, central heating, and unventilated spaces. Negative ions stand as the vital difference between pure and polluted air. Where else can we find negative ions? One answer: in *organic,* not inorganic, fruits and vegetables. Another reason to go raw!

"[Negative ions] make wider cell nuclei with more volume and enhance our capacity to absorb and utilize oxygen." — Dr. R. Gualaterotti

215

Falling water creates negative ions by splitting otherwise neutral particles of air, releasing electrons. These electrons join with smaller air particles, thus giving them a negative charge.

According to Wikipedia, *feng shui* (pronounced "fung shway") is the ancient Chinese practice of placement and arrangement of space to achieve harmony with the environment. The literal translation is "wind–water." *Feng shui* involves the use of geographical, psychological, phycological, philosophical, mathematical, aesthetic, and astrological concepts in relation to space and energy flow. This discipline, now several thousand years old, has been newly revived to ensure a healthy living environment. Among the chief elements it uses to promote harmony are water fountains, natural sprays, and ferns. All of these items generate negative ions and improve air quality. If you do not have these items in your house, you do have at least one natural ionizer — your shower!

Negative ions are the vitamin of the air. — Dr. E. R. Holiday

---

Daniel P. Reid, in *The Tao of Health, Sex, & Longevity, a Modern Practical Guide to The Ancient Way,* quotes the third century alchemist Ko Hung, who wrote: "From midnight until noon, energy waxes; from noon until midnight, energy wanes. When energy is waning, breathing exercises are of no benefit."

It is best to do breathing exercises early in the morning, according to Western science, which has determined that the concentration of negative ions in the air is the greatest between 3:00 and 6:00 A.M. I get up at 4:00 A.M. to take advantage of these early-rising negative ions.

"At first, one feels little effect, but after practicing breathing exercises regularly for 100 days or so, the efficacy of this method is beyond measure, and its benefits are a hundred

---

times greater than taking any medicine ... The method is actually quite simple, but it must be practiced regularly over a period of time in order to realize its genuine benefits. If you try it for just twenty days, your spirits will improve, the region around your navel will feel warm during practice, your waist and legs will feel light and limber, and your eyes and complexion will grow bright and lustrous. These benefits are permanent for as long as one continues to practice." — Daniel P. Reid, quoting Su Tung-po, a twelfth-century Chinese poet, extolling the virtues of deep breathing

Once your body is cleansed of all the poisonous toxins, your skin can become more of a breathing organ, getting some of its nourishment from the air. If we did not put toxins into the body, we would not have to sleep as much as we do, for the body would not have to repair itself. Toxins create the need for sleep. On the raw food, you will sleep less, and you will *need* to sleep less, because fewer toxins need to exit the body. You will also discover that breathing accomplishes the same thing as sleep does — it re-energizes the body. Breathing refreshes the body very much the way sleep does. Thus by doing breathing exercises, you will discover you need even less sleep. Deep breathing breeds deep, uninterrupted sleep and reduces the time needed to rejuvenate.

Our bodies are mainly composed of the elements of air — hydrogen, oxygen, carbon dioxide, and, of course, water, which in turn is hydrogen and oxygen. Your body already has all of the elements it needs to sustain life simply from the process of breathing good clean air.

If you are sick, fasting will help your body heal. If you are old, fasting will make you more youthful. You can stop eating for a while and gain great health benefits, but your body cannot stop cleansing and removing toxins even for a moment. Elimination is far more important than alimentation (eating). These facts reinforce the notion that most of the food we eat is nothing but waste that will be eliminated through the bowels as feces. What enters the blood does not even remotely resemble the food we have eaten. Only gases and colloid fluid elements will appear in the blood.

The main point of the intriguing book *Breatharianism, Breathe and Live Forever,* by Wiley Brooks and Nancy Foss, is that we do not die of old age. Rather, we eat ourselves to death. Brooks and Foss quote an article by Trubshaw printed in the *Occult Gazette*: "Man's body is electrical, and contains dormant glands and cellular areas which, if stimulated by magnetic forces, would come into action and express powers of a so-called superhuman nature."

The article goes on:

"The degenerative life-shortening practice of eating food for pleasure, forced these aeriferous organs into retirement, as the body slowly adjusted its mechanism to meet the new condition — or perish. And so, instead of dropping dead in his tracks, man dies by degrees, and the dying process is what science calls 'aging.'"

The idea was initially developed by Hilton Hotema in *Man's Higher Consciousness,* first published in 1950. On the book's cover is the statement: "A thousand years hence, the contents of this work will be as up-to-date as at this hour … writings and methods of living based on Cosmic Law are always in order and never become obsolete."

How many authors can declare something like this? I read this book in complete awe. The author was reading my mind. Sixty years ago the author was saying exactly what I felt. Almost every sentence I read, I wished I had said it.

Every person who has been fasting regularly will know this book tells the truth. However, researchers for whom missing a meal is the ultimate crime against the body will never grasp this book and will dismiss it as mumbo jumbo. My editors warned me that I might be stretching my reader's tolerance to the breaking point. This relatively small book stands opposed to all the volumes of nutritional and anti-aging research. Even under this dire prediction, I side with this book. With *Quantum Eating,* I tried to make implementing his ideas more practical and, you will be happy to know, only half as extreme.

Hotema quotes a group of eminent nineteenth century doctors who, after studying the food question from every angle, concluded: *"We eat to live, and we eat to die,"* a belief which coincides with contemporary science's notion that our metabolism keeps us alive, and that it is our metabolism that will eventually carry us to death. Modern science knows that not just eating, but also living, is hazardous to your health. But the clear fact is that eating raw foods is less aging than eating processed food. And eating a smaller quantity of raw foods is less aging than eating a lot.

Breathing fresh air is even less aging. The more nourishment you receive by breathing, the less food you will need. Do your breathing exercises daily and they will become a most vital aid to your success with Quantum Eating.

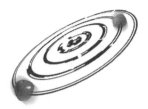

Chapter 20

How Long Should "Beauty Sleep" Last?

Excitedly, one of my readers wrote to me: *You must, simply must, read T. S. Wiley's* Lights Out. *It seems that raw foodists pride themselves on less and less sleep. Fooling with 'circadian rhythms' of the seasons and the sun is only fooling ourselves ...*

I am an insatiable reader. I would never turn my back on a book, especially one that comes with such an enthusiastic recommendation, so I *had to* read this one. In the book, Wiley ventures to prove that obesity, heart disease, diabetes, and cancer are caused not by eating fat or by not exercising, but from stress and sleep deficiency. The author's general recommendation is to sleep 9.5 hours per day.

Interestingly, a few days prior to receiving this email, I read an interview with Bikram Choudhury, the founder of Bikram Yoga. (His series of twenty-six hatha yoga postures is performed in a room heated to 105°F). In the interview, he mentioned he sleeps only two to four hours nightly. The interview included a picture of Bikram, a healthy-looking man who appears to be about forty, though I know he is sixty years old. I've heard numerous stories about how fit and full of energy he is. My instructors like to tell anecdotes about how Bikram begins each teacher training session by stripping to his shorts, revealing skimpy briefs, which he claims are the very ones he wore forty years ago. I was disappointed that there was no picture of T.S. Wiley, the author of *Lights Out,* for comparison. In my area of research, a picture of the author is the ultimate measure of whether or not I will consider the precepts. It is very convincing if the author looks younger and healthier than his or her reported chronological age. A fairer measure might be whether he looks younger than he used to.

Bikram insists that the only real exercise is stretching. This should be done daily. Wiley, on the other hand, writes, "In fact, exercise just might be the last nail in our collective coffins." He believes that exercise deactivates stress responses and should be performed every ten days or so. (I am sure some readers are cartwheeling with joy — exercise in itself, mind you — at the prospect of having to exercise so infrequently.) Why is the experience of these two men so different?

Another book recommended to me: *Take A Nap! Change Your Life: The Scientific Plan to Make You Smarter, Healthier, More Productive,* by Sara C. Mednick. Please pay attention here to the word *scientific*. In fact, this painstaking research was done by a Harvard-trained research scientist. She claims there is "hard scientific evidence that the nap is woven into our DNA." This conclusion was reached through experiments with real people. How many people among these subjects were yogi masters or even raw foodists? I will make an educated guess: *none*. Otherwise, the author would have at least noted a prevailing peculiarity: very little sleep during the 24-hour circadian period.

Mednick begins her book with a rhetorical question:

"Imagine yourself in a perfect world. Your mood is positive. Your brain is operating at maximum. Your body feels healthy, energetic and agile ... In this wonderful land of your imagination, you enjoy a well-balanced diet, get enough exercise, breathe clean air, and spend quality time with friends and family ... So ask yourself, 'If I inhabited such a place, how much would I sleep?'"

Her question is definitely addressed to a cooked-food eater, as the affirming answer she expects is, *A whole lot more than I'm sleeping now.* I do not think so. In fact, I am sure that sleep will be the last thing your perfect, vigorous, and buzzing with vitality body would want to do in this perfect world. Think of young people in love ... napping is the last thing on their minds.

The author then tells us the story of personally discovering the blessing of a midday nap. She was tired, stressed, and "when even the ever-increasing shots of espresso could not keep my eyes from fluttering shut," she "crashed" in her office during the middle of the day. Luckily, a visitor's couch was available. The main idea of the book: Our population is sick and tired and it needs a regular midday nap. If you are sick and tired, this is excellent advice to follow. But what if you are *not?*

If you are reading this book, you probably already enjoy the miraculous results of raw foods. So congratulate yourself: You are already living in "a wonderful land" that others can only dream about. If you are not familiar with what raw foods can do for your health, go back to my first two books. I'll be here waiting while you catch up.

If your body is abused either by cooked foods or stress, it needs more sleep to heal. No one can argue with this life-saving recommendation. The absolute opposite is true if you are healthy. When you practice Quantum Eating, you do not burden your digestive system, and you will need very little sleep.

Books about sleep research usually claim that sleeplessness causes hypertension, which can also lead to strokes. Hypertension is caused by the arteries being occluded with fatty build-up from eating meat, dairy products, and cooked foods. A little sleep does not allow the body to detox and heal itself. In this case, sleep is the remedy, not the cause. This is an example of how screwed up — how's that for a scientific word, dear readers? — scientific conclusions can get when the research is done by experimenting on the general population which is eating cooked food and is afflicted by one or another ailment.

One study of 70,000 women showed that heart attacks increased in those who slept less than seven hours per night. Those who slept five hours had a 40 percent higher rate of coronary artery disease or heart attack. Sounds scary. But this has no relevance to you, because not a single test subject was eating the way you are. The usefulness of this research is zero, so far as you are concerned. When you remove the cause of the illness, you reduce the need for healing time.

Mednick also notes in her research that tested subjects experienced a dip in energy twice during a twenty-four-hour period. One large dip of energy signaled them to go to sleep at night, while another mini-dip hit during the middle of the day, usually after lunch. People on the raw food lifestyle usually do not experience this midday mini-dip. It is extremely rare that I need a midday nap.

Sleep experts brought together an impressive cross section to study sleep patterns across life span, occupation, culture, age, and gender. They are very proud that what they got is a slice of the general population. But all of these subjects share one common curse: cooked food. As a result, they all take the absence of symptoms for actual health. The absence of symptoms is not necessarily health, any more than the absence of darkness is sunlight.

Sleep is like a recovery room. The more you are hurting yourself, the more time you need to spend there to recover. If you do not bang your head against the wall on a daily basis, you will not need to spend a lot of time applying bandages to it.

Am I against a long night's sleep or a nap? Of course not. I just want you to see how irrelevant general recommendations are to you. When you are following the raw food lifestyle you are not general, typical, average, or generic — you are unique and special.

As you transition to the raw foods lifestyle, there will be days when you feel on top of the world and will need very little sleep. However, there will be days when the cleansing has gone deeper and you feel tired and drained of energy. Do not do anything else — just sleep. It is during sleep that the body heals and performs its cleansing chores.

You should never use how long someone else sleeps as a criterion for yourself. You must sleep as much as *your* body tells you to, regardless of what others do. Normally, I sleep about five to six hours. Still, I have days when I sleep eight or nine hours. For example, one day I went for a deep tissue massage. I specifically asked the therapist to work on the scar tissue on my hips. When she was done with me, I felt exhausted. The toxins that had been released from the area that had been operated on so many times made me sick and tired. I took a bath with Epsom salts and barely made it to the bed before falling asleep. I did not awaken fully until twelve hours later. On other occasions when I, being extra zealous, have taken two sessions of Bikram yoga on the same day, I have felt like sleeping in the middle of the day. Muscles in my legs were burning and, as the injuries in my hips were healing, I napped happily for thirty to sixty minutes.

We all get sleepy after a heavy meal. Sleeping and eating are closely connected. After being on the 100 percent raw lifestyle for ten years and experimenting with different raw foods and their amounts, I can say that nothing influences your sleeping needs more than the amount and quality of food you eat. This has long been known. In ancient Greece, Plato and the physician Galen believed that sleep originated from stomach vapors that rise up to the brain during digestion, cutting it off from the rest of the body, causing unconsciousness. The more we eat, the more sleep we need. But the opposite is also true: The less we eat, the less we sleep. Eighty percent of our energy is exerted in digesting and metabolizing foodstuffs. People who fast a great deal sleep little.

Digestion is a hard job for the body, the equivalent of ditch-digging. In fact, this analogy is accurate if you consider that an average person eats 100 tons of food during his or her lifetime. Is it any wonder that food causes the body to need more sleep to recuperate from the burden of processing so much food?

You should never live with sleep deprivation. The classic signs of sleep deprivation are defined as difficulty getting up in the morning, feeling tired throughout the day, lacking energy, and feeling irritable.

How much sleep do you really need? Your body will let you know. Observe how you feel in the morning. The ideal is to wake up feeling refreshed, alert, energized — even euphoric. People in love do not sleep much. No doctor will say this is abnormal. Quantum Eating will make you feel like that most of the time. You are simply not ever sleepy, except five to six hours during the night.

It's an excellent idea to establish a regular schedule for your bedtime and wake-up time. When you have a regular sleep routine, your inner clock can work efficiently so that at bedtime every aspect of your physiology is aligned to help you sleep. When it is time to be awake and alert, all the parts and systems of your body will be supporting your alertness.

Be consistent with your wake time and bedtime. This will assure you a more regular sleep pattern. There are hormonal changes linked to the circadian cycle. As your body temperature drops, levels of *melatonin,* a hormone secreted by the pineal gland, rise, contributing to feelings of sleepiness. Melatonin production prepares the body for sleep by decreasing body temperature, lowering metabolism, and initiating drowsiness. In healthy people with a normal sleep pattern, melatonin levels are lowest during the daytime, increase during the evening, and reach a peak during sleep.

In the early morning, blood levels of *cortisol,* a stress hormone, increase and help prepare your body for action. Work with your body's biological clock and not against it to establish a consistent rhythm of sleep and wakefulness.

If you are accustomed to using a nightlight in your bedroom while you are sleeping, stop. Sleep in complete darkness. You'll find an interesting by-product here — an increased appreciation of your shins and your big toes, two body parts magnificently adapted to helping you find furniture in the dark. Recent research has revealed that any disruptions to your natural body clock, such as being continuously exposed to artificial light or burning candles at night, and especially sleeping with a nightlight on, increase your risk of cancer. In fact, British scientists proposed the idea that a steady increase in childhood leukemia in the UK, Europe, and the United States may be connected to nighttime exposure to light.

I like structure. I believe that having a structured routine for sleeping and eating is essential to succeeding in our raw food lifestyle. Once a habit is developed, we don't have to struggle, decide, and start anew every day, because the momentum of our habit carries us. When you have a regular bedtime and a regular routine before bed, the body will work like a clock giving you times to eat or to sleep or to get up as one cue after another reminds you and prepares you for the next rotation.

I like to take a hot bath before going to bed. I strongly suggest it as part of a daily ritual. The warm water relaxes your muscles. You will feel refreshed and cleansed from the day's concerns. A hot bath will raise your body temperature. Go to bed immediately. As your body cools, you will feel sleepy, just as you naturally feel sleepy when your body cools down at night.

Almost every day I awake at 4:00 in the morning, feeling like a twelve-year-old and ready to go. If I eat after 2 P.M., giving in to social pressures — I have slips like everyone else — I feel miserable, as though I had been mildly poisoned. I toss through the night, and that makes a huge difference in how I feel in the morning. I certainly will not get my blissful awakening.

Where you sleep is also crucial. Numerous commercials will tell you that you need a special bed or pillow — a mattress that won't spill your wine when you jump on it, or a pillow filled with grain. When Victoria Boutenko visited us, she and her husband just rolled out blankets on our living room floor, opened the back door a crack to "get some fresh air" (on a freezing February night!) and slept right there. My guest bedroom was never more useless. The simplicity of what I was witnessing struck me as profound. I decided that I wanted to sleep on the floor.

The first night was uncomfortable. The second was better. By the third, I never wanted to sleep on a bed again. When you sleep on a hard surface, all your ligaments and muscles are stretched. On a soft bed, your body's natural posture is skewed.

You might think that a firm mattress or a board under the sagging mattress works as well for good repose. Not even close. There is nothing like lying on the floor and assuming a "dead body" pose to humble you and bring a feeling of surrender, acceptance, and tranquility. As you begin to move toward sleep you are "dying" to the world, to its craziness, to its demands and crises. No ambitions. No worries. No regrets.

There is one disadvantage, however. It has been a hard task to persuade my husband to get down there with me! It took me ten years to convince him to go 100 percent raw. I hope it will not take that long to get him on the floor. What else will the man have to do for love? He doesn't want to know ...

It is very beneficial for your back to sleep on a hard surface. However, sleeping on the hard surface can give you hip bursitis if you sleep on your side. When I talk about sleeping on the floor, I mean sleeping on your back. You want to sleep on your back to avoid wrinkles, no matter where you sleep. Nothing will leave deeper trenches or pronounced sagging of the face like sleeping in the wrong position. The skin on your face can only recover from this stress for so long. If it is stressed over and over every night, sags and wrinkles will take permanent residence on your face.

Don't tell me that you can't sleep on your back. You can. I had many operations on both hips and for several years, sleeping any way but on my back was simply too painful. I trained myself to sleep on my back. Now I cannot sleep any other way. Your first few nights will be hard. But if you persevere, your body will accommodate you.

While writing this, I decided to test the theory of sleeping nine hours. When I woke up at my usual hour, I made myself fall asleep again. When I finally was up, I felt groggy, in a foul mood and hurting all over. Sleeping nine hours is *not* for me. The simplistic approach of presuming that, if something is good, more will be better, fails again and again when applied to a nonlinear system like the human body.

It was interesting to read in *Physical Immortality,* by Leonard Orr: "I found that missing sleep stimulates suppressed negative emotions to consciousness so that they can be resolved and healed." Is it possible that reduced sleep can even be beneficial? Yogis teach mastering sleep through meditation all night. Bikram talks in his classes about yogis who do not eat much, do not sleep much, and do not age. Even though very few of us will follow yogis to the ultimate extent of their beliefs — becoming reclusive and out of the capricious world — we can certainly draw from their experiences and teachings to enhance our lives.

Excessive daytime sleepiness can be a sign of serious disorder, such as clinical depression. It is interesting that, in medical circles, clinical depression is occasionally treated by keeping the patient awake for twenty-four hours. Why should this be surprising? Eating and no eating, drinking water and no water intake, breathing and holding the breath, now sleep and no sleep. Health and anti-aging mysteries lie in achieving a perfect balance between these opposites in a practiced Quantum Eating lifestyle.

Once again, the main idea is simple ... let your body tell what beauty sleep it needs, and when. Your body knows what's good. And, ultimately, your body knows how to make you beautiful.

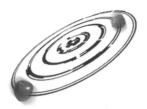

Chapter 21
Getting Warm
by Tempering With Cold

While researching this chapter I came across Victoria Boutenko's article "Tempering the Body with Cold Water," which is a part of the new edition of her *12 Steps to Raw Foods*. I realized that she is much better qualified to write on this topic than I am. After all, she has personal experience of swimming in frozen lakes and rivers at the time when her whole family belonged to the Moscow Polar Bear Club. In *12 Steps to Raw Foods,* Boutenko writes: "After dipping in cold water I feel so good and refreshed that I cannot think of anything else being compatible with this pleasure."

Until recently my only serious experience of cold water tempering was a semi-cold shower at the beach. Absent first-hand knowledge, who would think that dipping into ice cold water could be extremely pleasurable? After reading her article, I was inspired. I saw in this practice a great potential for health and longevity. But only after reading the following sentence in her book did I know I was going to implement cold water into my lifestyle: "During the brief application of cold water, blood vessels in the skin abruptly contract, pushing a large amount of blood inside the organism. This results in the re-activating of the inner capillaries, many of which are typically atrophied by the age of thirty, due to poor circulation and unhealthy lifestyle."

Wow! This coincides with the main idea of this book: When the body is placed in brief adverse situations, it activates the body's powerful survival mechanism. You do not even need to know *how* to utilize it — all you need is to be *willing* to use it.

Vladimir Vasiliev's *The Russian System Guidebook* is based on the training methods used by Russian special forces and talks about tempering the body with iced water.

I hear you moaning! We are combating aging, are we not? I am not suggesting you take three five-gallon buckets of ice water and dump them over your head first thing in the morning. That might be too much for most of us. Still, there is something in cold water tempering that can powerfully affect people on the raw food plan.

At almost every lecture I give, someone in the audience comments, "I have been raw for several months. I feel great, but am always feeling cold." I have to admit, raw foods bring a lot of wonderful sensations, but this is not one of them. During the transitional period, you may feel cold more frequently than before, especially in your feet. I say *might*, because not everyone will go through this stage. It happens mostly to people who are thin and do not have much weight to lose. Guess what! There is a wonderful remedy for the problem — ice cold water. Crazy? Not at all. Victoria quotes a Russian scientific publication:

"Several scientific studies have demonstrated that within fifty seconds after the brief application of extremely cold temperatures, an enormous amount of heat is generated by the transformation of neurons, which is known as the phenomenon of 'instant free heat.' Therefore, despite the initial shock that can be painful, winter swimmers (often called 'Polar Bears') almost immediately experience an amazingly pleasant warmth from head to toe, causing the profound relaxation of the body."

Vladimir Vasiliev explains that a sudden exposure to cold is like a small explosion in your body that raises the temperature inside your body, as if you have a fever. And very much like a fever, this blast will kill most bacteria and viruses, because of the overall body temperature. You can lose weight with cold water tempering. "Fifteen minutes of swimming in 20°C water will force the body to exert 100 calories of heat."[1]

After hearing testimonials that tempering the body with icy water results in an invigorating experience and a special kind of relaxation, is it too great a stretch to accept the possibility I am presenting here — that non-eating can be a very exhilarating experience? Just like swimming in ice cold water, non-eating for sixteen hours might become a hard-to-break habit.

I was almost tempted to join a Polar Bear club. Small problem ... Memphis does not have one, probably because it rarely gets cold enough to freeze anything bigger than a puddle. There is another problem — ice water for my titanium hips would be like having my tongue stuck to a lamp post at a freezing temperature. If you do not have my problems and you live somewhere that has a local club, at least try it. Your effort could create a perfect alignment with your raw food lifestyle: no more cold feet!

If you would rather chill out at home, here are some tips. Begin implementing your cold water procedures gradually. I assume you are already eating plenty of raw foods and do

1. *Baranov A.*, Kidalov V: Healing with Cold, *Kemerovo, Russia: Astel Publishing, 2000, (in Russian).*

not get colds easily. After a regular shower, remain for a few seconds longer and start letting the cold water run over you. After a month of this, you might want to dip for a few seconds into a bathtub filled with cold water and a full container of ice from your refrigerator. All the ice you will save by *not* using ice in your drinks (discussed later in this chapter) will come in handy! The easiest way is to place your feet in a tub of ice cold water for a few seconds only. I am new to this practice, but that is what I do and I love it.

Here is a beauty tip for you: Every morning, immediately after removing your facial masque and before applying a moisturizer, rub an ice cube over your face to close the pores. Apply your moisturizer. The sudden cooling of your skin causes the capillaries to constrict, which is followed in fifteen to thirty seconds by expansion of the capillaries resulting from the warming of the skin.

Skin, the periphery of the body, performs the crucial task of temperature regulation. Skin receptors and blood vessels are part of the body's mechanism for adapting to the outside variables and sustaining a healthy body. To protect internal organs, capillaries respond quickly and efficiently by constricting to prevent heat loss or expanding to cool the body. These actions are swift and dramatic and occur as frequently as needed. Under extreme circumstances, they can occur as many as a hundred times or more, until the the body's internal temperature is stabilized.

There is a dynamic state of stability between the body's internal environment and its external environment. An organism thermoregulates, keeping its core body temperature within certain limits. Even though we breathe cold air, lung temperature will remain the same. Even when temperatures outside the body differ drastically, inside the body the organs remain at a relatively constant temperature, around

37°C (98.6°F). Any variation is an indication of a disease state, unusual activity, or extraordinary environmental conditions. When the temperature of the vital organs is outside this range, body tissues can be damaged.

The body's internal organs are less capable of withstanding temperature changes. Hypothermia occurs when the body's temperature drops below 35°C (95°F). Fortunately the temperature of the body's inside organs does not directly depend on climate. Even when super-cooling occurs, at first a prolonged gradual temperature drop will take place in the skin, and only after some time will the temperature of the inside organs be affected. The body goes to great lengths to protect itself from temperature fluctuations on the inside. This alone can make it obvious that drinking ice water is an assault on human physiology.

Ice water is excellent for tempering your body on the outside. But ice water does not belong inside the body. Take animals, for instance. None of them seem to drink liquids or eat foods that are either very hot or very cold. Nature's message is obvious and one to which we should give careful attention — we should avoid extreme hot and cold temperatures in our food and beverages.

One of the worst digestive offenses is drinking ice water or other freezing cold fluids with meals. "No ice, please!" Say that in a restaurant, and it's enough to mark you as an oddity. Try telling the waiter, "No water, please!" and watch their reaction. They react as though you were speaking Greek (or Russian, in my case!) and cannot understand. I've tried different tricks — turning my glass upside down, moving it to another table altogether — but to no avail. In seconds, a fresh glass of Antarctic ice water appears from nowhere, directly in front of me.

My son, who worked as a waiter through high school, explained to me that they are required to place a glass of ice water in front of every patron, so I shouldn't waste my breath. Until nutritional science says so, our attempts to save the country's water resources will be ignored. The question remains: With all its knowledge of the digestion process, why doesn't nutritional science condemn this restaurant industry standard? It ought to know that we'd greatly improve the health of the nation if we didn't drink Lake Superior with our dinner.

Good digestion is a key to good health. It is a nutritional fact that infusions of iced anything on a stomach full of food will constrict the tiny ducts which secrete gastric juices, impairing digestion and permitting putrefaction and fermentation to take place. By the time the temperature of the stomach contents returns to normal, it's too late for proper digestion.

As we shouldn't disturb the body's *internal* temperature regulation, so we shouldn't disturb — not, at least, as much as we tend to — the systems that regulate the body's *external* temperature. Our wearing extra warm clothes is just contributing to body's loss of its ability for thermoregulation (the ability of an organism to keep its body temperature relatively constant in spite of wide fluctuations of the surrounding temperature).

Tempering the body with cold restarts the mechanism of thermoregulation and you will be comfortable in cold weather. And one day you might even join Victoria in one of her Polar Bear plunges. Oh! How much I wish I could join you both, too!

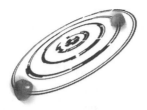

Chapter 22

Essential Truths — and Their Opposites

Do you wish to be stress free? Don't! You might as well be wishing to be dead. Stress can be good and stress can be bad. When we are running around like a chicken with its head cut off, this is bad. However, science is discovering that some stress in our lives is good for us: it boosts our immune system. Some environmental changes produce a "fight or flight" response in our body that stimulates resistance to diseases and aging. Actually, if applied to the latter there is a lot of truth to the saying, "What does not kill us makes us stronger."

"The opposite of a correct statement is a false statement. But the opposite of a profound truth may well be another profound truth." — Niels Bohr, Danish physicist

---

It is true that eating gives us life and the absence of food can kill. But it is also true that while eating increases the degenerative process, fasting elicits an opposite effect — rejuvenation. It is true that food gives energy, and it is also true that food consumption is the main reason we lose energy and functionality. Is it any wonder that the concept of an adequate diet is open to a very broad interpretation? Food intake is always associated with the production of energy, especially for physical labor. Little food intake has been linked to inhibited growth, chronic ill health, and a high mortality rate. Yet numerous experiments with the CR diet prove again and again that calorie restriction with optimal nutrition is the only workable model for achieving the anti-aging effect.

Food is nourishing and aging at the same time. But so is oxygen. It is essential for living, but oxidation produces free radicals that shorten our life. Water is life giving, yet too much water produces water toxicity and becomes life taking. The source of rejuvenation and decay is actually the same thing. So the solution to the aging problem must lie in a *balancing* these two fundamental bodily functions. Of course, this balance point is different for everyone. You have to find your own unique balancing point, if you want to live a life free of diseases and full of youthful vigor.

Characteristically, practitioners of modern western medicine concentrate only on one aspect, one half, of any duality. Medicine sees either the back or the front — never both at once. But quantum physics teaches when we see the front, the back is always there. This view completely corresponds with the Principle of Complementarity.

Recent geriatric research has provided extensive experimental data supporting the anti-aging property of CR. Byung P. Yu and Hae Young Chung[1] propose that "the anti-aging action of CR can be viewed as 'nutritional stress' because the

1. *Byung P. Yu and Hae Young Chung "Stress Resistance by Caloric Restriction for Longevity,"* Annals of the New York Academy of Sciences *928:39-47 (2001) 2001 New York Academy of Sciences*

organism's reduced caloric intake seems to be a stimulatory metabolic response for survivability."

The life-prolonging action of caloric restriction (CR) diets is an excellent example to support the interrelationship between stress and the aging process. CR, as a potent intervention, activates the organism's ability to withstand age-related stress as a survival strategy.

Stress resistance is the body's ability to resist both internally and externally imposed insults. An organism's ability to withstand stress is of utmost importance in promoting anti-aging results. We know that as organisms lose the ability to resist these insults, aging takes place. From that point everything is downhill: Aged organisms suffer even more than younger ones. Thus a prime strategy for anti-aging practices must focus on activating the defense systems that guard against abuse. Take advantage of your body's survival defense system because it is your trump card when dealing with aging. To ensure survival, an organism's defense system must be maximized to its full effect through well-coordinated networks of diverse biologically responsive elements.

If the "nutritional stress" (CR) regimen provides such impressive anti-aging results, could it be that other environmental stresses such as "water stress," "oxygen stress," and "temperature stress," when administered with great care, could be just as beneficial? Not only did I prove so in my own case, but each of these environmental stresses (holding your breath, dry fasting, and tempering your body with ice cold water) have been around for decades. These practices have also produced numerous followers who have shared their techniques with optimal results while developing their own rules and suggestions.

Can the restriction of biological needs prove beneficial? Actually, experiencing deprivation in any form for brief periods is always health inducing. When thoroughly mastered, such deprivation techniques — fasting is perhaps the most familiar example — can be most enjoyable. The notions of deprivation and deriving enjoyment from deprivation are well known in many cultures — even at the level of common humor: "Why are you banging your head against the wall?" "Because it feels so good when I stop."

Under adverse circumstances, these kinds of deprivations are called environmental stress: dehydration, nutrient deprivation, and extreme temperature. Under specially designed conditions we call these dry fasting, calorie restriction, and cold-tempering. These are in fact some of the best rejuvenating and invigorating practices known to man. You end up being more nourished, better hydrated, better oxygenated, and warmed up to a greater extent.

The very idea of voluntary deprivations embodies the notion of yin/yang or counterparts. Indeed, it's only in western cultures that we see these things as dead opposites, as contraries. In fact, they're more like complementaries. Eating robustly (according to the cultural and personal practices we follow) is our norm. So deliberately *not* eating for a while is the complement of our normal practice. We're not *ceasing* to eat — not permanently! We give our digestive system a well-deserved rest. We are creating balance. Eating without fasting is unbalanced!

So much of life comes in pairs: man/woman, left/right, on/off, yes/no, living/dead. In creating and following rational patterns of "opposites" — again, better to say *complements* — we do no worse than to reflect this ever-present duality.

Quantum Eating is about bringing balance to your body and mind and to life in general. Science is catching up to confirm that these so called "deprivation" practices are, in fact, raising your body's stress resistance, which is essential in fore-

stalling aging. They are not just useful health inducing procedures, they are more about recovering and rediscovering our
natural mode of living and seeing things differently.

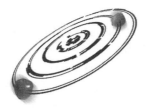

Chapter 23
Living Upright in an Upside-Down World

J ust before the writing of this book, Victoria Boutenko came out with a newly expanded edition of her *12 Steps to Raw Foods: How to End Your Dependency on Cooked Food.* In this engaging, heartwarming, and caring book, Boutenko talks about the survey she conducted, pursuing her interest in what foods people crave in response to stress. She noticed that there was a direct correlation between how people were raised and how they cope with stress. One of her interviewees was "Jonathan," who did not seem to have any attachments to any specific foods. Isn't it a shame we aren't all that lucky? Jonathan recalls from his childhood that his mother never called him to eat if he was playing with other kids. She believed that playing was more important than eating. Food was never used as a reward or punishment. As a result, his life was never centered on food. In fact, he can go for hours without ever thinking about food.

When I read this passage, memories flooded over me. During my early childhood, my paternal grandmother looked after me while my parents worked. She was a tough woman who had lived through two revolutions and two world wars. She never called me to eat, either. There was no such thing as lunch- or dinner-time with her. After surviving several famines, she never worried that I was in any danger of starving if I didn't eat all day long. She knew that when I was hungry I would come and ask — which of course I always did, sooner or later. Her menu was limited: fried potatoes or a large piece of white bread generously covered with butter and sprinkled with sugar. Her attitude toward *my* meals was a subject of constant argument between her and my mother, who in complete contrast thought feeding me was the ultimate purpose of motherhood. Mom was the happiest when I was eating. When she came home from work, she compensated for my grandmother's inattention many times over.

When I became a mother myself, I somehow duplicated not my mother's, but my grandmother's pattern. It just felt right to me, but I was often rebuked for not being a good mother!

True, I did not feed him regularly or often but I prepared nutritious food even though I was hard pressed to compete with America's fast food goodies after we came here. Junk food became an addiction for all of us that took years to overcome.

However, I succeeded in one thing: my son is not a "foodaholic." I do not know of anyone who has transitioned to raw foods so easily. He often tells me he chooses to be a vegan with a small amount of cooked food just to simplify his social life, and not because he has any attachments, cravings, or bondages to cooked foods — or any foods for that matter.

I do not believe in blaming parents, or blaming *any* external conditions, for our shortcomings. Our parents did the best they could with what they knew at the time. What I am trying to say here is this: We acquired this addiction to food and that addiction can be broken. Our stomach and our brain are not short-circuited. The fact that not everyone has these cravings should be a great inspiration to us. It means this is not a part of the body's makeup. It means that if there is a way in, there must be a way out.

We are living in an upside-down world and, in this world, the loving intention to sustain, nourish, and uphold others is misplaced and invested in cooking. This is a bad investment because not only will it not pay out dividends, but, by creating sickness and decrepitude, it exacts a terrible price.

My husband Nick, after being 100 percent raw for several months, lost 60 pounds. Not only did he lose weight, but his whole body underwent a miraculous transformation. All that extra weight was bad for his health and for his self-image. Nick was so excited about the transformation he was going through that he decided to go back to his homeland, Moldova, to visit old classmates and friends whom he had not seen for sixteen years. The man I've known for thirty years, who had never bought a piece of clothing for himself, was shopping for clothes for the whole week before he left. The fact that he was shopping in regular stores, not at Big and Tall, made the whole experience even more exciting for him.

When he got there, all his friends were impressed at how good he looked. They liked the new Nick. Sort of. But what they really wanted was the old, familiar, chubby Nick. Food, they thought — *that's how we'll get him back!* They immediately began force-feeding him as though their life's mission were to put weight back on him. He even took a picture of himself when he was at his heaviest in an attempt to derail their inclinations, showing them that it was really a big victory for him. But to no avail: They tempted him with an enormous variety of delicacies. Let me ask you this: How can you explain why these intelligent, obviously caring people act so irrationally, even insanely? I cannot blame them: they were acting under the influence of cooked food.

Nothing like this will happen with people who are on or transitioning to raw foods. When Nick showed them that his belt size was 10 inches smaller during our raw food presentations, people cheered and applauded.

When my husband returned from visiting our homeland, he brought back many videos. How painful it was for me to see my mom not looking a day younger than her 70 years. I was dismayed but I was also indignant. Why would she not listen? I had been pestering her about raw foods for ten years! The most painful thing a loving parent can do to a child is to age prematurely. Still we have to exercise great caution not to impose our lifestyle on others. In the upside-down world you, yourself, must adjust your attitude to others.

People generally feel guilty when indulging in junk food. At the same time during your dieting phase, you may feel self-righteous when others make the effort to avoid it. Those who master their appetites often behave like fanatic religious converts. Before you know it, you go from a period of guilt to feelings of moral superiority. With the zeal of a new convert, we begin dishing out our never solicited but always pungent opinion. This will promote a false sense of spirituality grounded in being "good," meaning superior.

Realize that none of these reactions is good. Only when it becomes a permanent lifestyle, after achieving great enjoyment in eating less, will you begin to truly respect others' eating habits. It is when you achieve the sanctity of your own eating habits that you will develop a greater acceptance of others. Only when I accepted my Mom's eating habits unconditionally, did she actually began to show some interest in my eating peculiarities. I wish I knew then what I know now.

Just because you've discovered the way does not mean that everyone will be able to follow your path. Others must do their own exploring. I am disturbed by emails that say: I *do not know anything about raw foods, but I want your results. I have lots of health problems and I need someone to prepare food for me, give me support, and to tell me what to do.* These pleas always sound to me like an invitation to carry them on my back, while they dangle, their feet and hands idle.

A health seeker must be *in charge,* not a passive recipient of support, encouragement and information. People must be pro-active to improve their health and well-being. When people come to you and ask for your help, be kind and open, show them the way. But never, never pick them up and carry them piggyback. They will begin experiencing detox symptoms, be discouraged, and feel overwhelmed by disappointments and frustration. These are all feelings they are not ready to deal with. They'll begin blaming external forces — namely you — and rightly so, because you had no business elevating them to your own level. You can never carry them long enough or far enough. The day will come when you will have to put them back where they belong. They might be hurt and they will be angry. These people were not ready, and carrying them on your back did little to implement their growth.

Show them the way to the information and leave them to make their own decision without any pushing and shoving from you. Understand that pain and suffering are an important part of growth. Often crisis is needed for people to change. Your presence was needed as a catalyst, not as a carriage. They must live their own lives and walk their own paths.

Answer all their questions, encourage them by your own experience, but never push them onto your path. Understand, that some are not ready to take the leap. Be supportive and empathize, but don't try to convince them to change — they are not ready just yet. And that is okay for them. Accept them as they are. By never forcing our convictions on others nor withholding encouragement, we not only live who we are, but we also give others permission to be who they are.

Our beliefs weave a canvas for our life like an ancient sampler stitched to tell us the rules. To change the neat pattern of stitches is always distressing. Not everyone is willing.

One of my readers told me that her live-in boyfriend is not raw. "I always tell him if I become too weird, you can always leave me!" First, if she does not want him to oblige, she should never even mention the possibility. Second, she has to shift her perspective to see that her boyfriend is a lucky man. By trying to take care of her body, in particular, and her life in general, she has become a source of positive energy not only for herself, but for him.

If you are in a similar situation, you must realize that just being close to you will cause people to experience emanations of good energy. Positive exchanges of energy take place between individuals. People will sense that you possess a special aura that they don't. Your awareness is more intense than theirs and they will gravitate to that facet of you. Others literally live off the energy you are emanating. As the frequency level of your energy grows, people will be pulled into your orbit. They are privileged to have you in their midst. Even if they do not join in your dietary choices, they know you are special, whether or not they ever admit it. Do not be concerned that your family and friends scorn your lifestyle. By being an example, you are reminding others to eat better, to *be* better. They might resist, but you can be sure they are watching you.

In my first book, *Your Right to Be Beautiful,* I wrote that you will begin counting your life not from birth but from the day you went 100 percent raw. I feel my life took a new direction at that point. I took "the road less traveled," as

Robert Frost called it. I look back at the events, the emotions I experienced before I went raw, and it feels as if I were leading someone else's life, someone with whom I now have no connection. On raw foods we are open to new ideas, bound by no restricting ties to past experiences. Our beliefs are more flexible and easily changeable if they are a hindrance to our growth. Quantum Eating may force you to disengage from socially conditioned patterns of thought and behavior. You will question accepted ideas and theories on lifestyles, nutrition, spirituality, and much more — all with eagerness.

As we adopt the raw food lifestyle, we gradually acquire a new point of view. Life assumes a fresher, deeper, and more satisfying structure. It is impossible to make the uninitiated understand the raw food lifestyle if they have no experience to draw upon, just as it is impossible to describe colors to the blind. Do yourself a favor: Tune out the negative comments of those who have never been 100 percent raw. *Health* is an empty word to them. Do your children and grandchildren a favor: Do not be afraid to flip the conversation around and claim, that playing *is* more important than eating. Remember, by adjusting *your* perspective you are affecting *their* destiny.

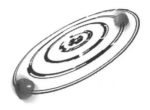

Chapter 24

Stretching Your Benefits: How Yoga and Raw Foods Work in Tandem for Superior Health

I learned to crochet and cross stitch long before I learned to read and write. I remember sitting on the porch at age five with my grandmother, watching the other kids chasing the wind on their bicycles, playing hide and seek, and doing cartwheels. My grandmother and I shared not only our passion for needlework but also a constant awareness of our bodies. She was old and arthritic, and my hips were damaged at birth.

I did not discover yoga until after I had written my first book, *Your Right to be Beautiful*, about my experience with the raw food diet. Had I found yoga earlier, there would now certainly be a chapter about the benefits I've received from this ancient discipline. Yoga, however, did find its way into my second book, *Beautiful On Raw*, and my ebook *100 Days to 100% Raw*.

Bikram yoga, in which original yoga poses (*asanas*) are performed in a particular sequence in a hot room, is my favorite exercise these days. To restrict and then release the blood flow to a specific organ or joint, you stretch one side and compress the opposite one in what is known as the tourniquet effect. Wikipedia gives the following definition: "A *tourniquet* can be defined as a constricting or compressing device used to control venous and arterial circulation to an extremity for a period of time." The term *tourniquet effect* is used to describe any garment that blocks or slows blood circulation or lymph drainage. It sounds scary and like something to avoid at any cost, unless you are injured and it becomes necessary.

Bikram did not invent the poses used in this style of yoga. He did develop a special series of twenty-six poses that he felt would be the most beneficial to bring the body into top condition. What Bikram brilliantly observed was the similarity between a tourniquet and the positions he favored — hence the *tourniquet effect*. In his new book *Bikram Yoga: The Guru Behind Hot Yoga Shows the Way to Radiant Health and Personal Fulfillment,* he explains: when you hold a pose, certain areas are constricted to reduce blood flow, as if bandaged. After holding the pose for ten, twenty, thirty, or sixty seconds, the pressure is released and fresh blood rushes to the affected area. This greatly facilitates healing and reduces recovery time. Organs, joints, and ligaments are cleaned out, flushed with new blood and oxygen. Blood rushes through vessels after they've momentarily been squeezed shut. The tourniquet effect also helps cleanse the lymphatic system.

Tendons and ligaments are composed mostly of collagen fibers — cells that are not generally repairable or replaceable. Structural proteins such as collagen are not subject to renewal. They remain constant during our lifetime without ever being broken down or replaced. They are the most stressed and vulnerable area for aging: Many of the most dramatic deteriorations recognized as part of aging take place in these long-lived, non-renewing tissues. The tourniquet effect is the best way to bring new blood and rejuvenation to these areas.

For example, Bikram describes in his new book what happens when doing one of the poses in his series, called the Standing Separate Leg Head to Knee Pose. During this pose, the pancreas is compressed and blood is drained out of it, as if squeezed from a sponge. At the same time, "the blood driven by the excited heart is approaching the pancreas like a flood. But it can't go in; the flood is blocked because the gates are closed. So outside the pancreas the blood level is rising and rising. It's like the Hoover Dam! Then after 20 seconds in the posture, the blood's volume and pressure have reached maximum capacity, and what do you do? You come out of the pose, open the gates, and blood rushes in and floods the pancreas. Boom! In this way you reenergize, revitalize, and clean it in a brief period of time through this one *asana.*"

This vivid description is my favorite passage in the book because it can be used as analogy for the central concept of this book. This tourniquet effect can be used for all other bodily functions like eating, drinking, breathing, and thinking by temporarily cutting off food, cutting off water, cutting off the constant stream of thinking, and, now, cutting off blood flow! The ultimate effect of the tourniquet maneuver is that you end up being better nourished, better hydrated, more mentally balanced, and having better circulation. The changes in pressure ensure a dynamic exchange of blood that flushes out toxins and debris, increases circulation, and releases stress. Pathological bacteria, infection, germs, and viruses hate this achievement.

However brilliant a man may be, he cannot know every-thing. Bikram admits: "I love to eat at McDonald's and my favorite food is cheesecake with blueberries on top. My stu-dents who know that bring it to me all the time. I love it — so don't worry, yoga is not about eating one 'right way.'" Interesting, coming from a person who insists that his way is the only right way to do yoga. He also writes: "If you're not eating like pigs, then you are eating like goats, munching raw foods or organic foods because you think it will make you healthy. If your engine is broken, what difference does it make what kind of gas you put in your tank?"

Goats? That is us! I never met the man, but I love him dearly because of what Bikram yoga is doing for my legs. But when I read this, I had twitches. Bikram says he likes to fix junked cars and junked human bodies. But that is where the similarity between a human body and a car stops. Raw foods *will* make a big difference. Obviously, his knowledge about raw foods is not just minimal — it is prejudicial.

Bikram also writes in the same book: "So what is the best food in the world? *No food.* Don't be scared. I'm not telling you to go on a starvation diet. Without dieting or deprivation, your body becomes extremely efficient at processing, trans-porting and creating fuel ... Take me: I eat very little, usually very late. I enjoy food, but actually *need* to eat very little."

Needless to say, when I read this, Bikram's eating concept completely rehabilitated in my eyes! (As if he cares!) I was even ready to accept that he craves the "occasional bacon-wrapped hot dog," that will make him sick afterwards. He has been practicing yoga for fifty years, still has a 28-inch waist and can fit into pants he wore forty years ago. However, his face has changed. He looks younger than his sixty years, but the young man in the earlier pictures is unrecognizable. Cheesecake will do that to you. Raw foods would never have the same impact on the face, no matter your age.

Look at aging faces. They look like a toxic wasteland — deposits of fat, accumulations of retained fluids, sick tissues, lumps and bumps cover the landscape. Even with yoga and very little food, cooked food will continue to ravage the face. Check your photos on raw food, and you will see you look better than when you ate cooked food, even though you may have been years younger. You may not appear younger, but you will be more yourself. The real you is uncovered when freed from the waste.

I firmly believe that yoga practice has to be an integral part of the raw food lifestyle and vice versa. For example, if the ligaments or other fibrous connective tissues are shortened as a result of injury or inactivity, raw food will definitely make stretching easier. But your food won't do your stretching for you. On the other hand, there are many people who do yoga regularly yet still struggle to achieve their optimal weight. Because I travel a lot with my raw food presentations, I visit Bikram yoga studios all over the country. Everywhere I go, I see some people who are incredibly flexible but still overweight. Adopting a raw food diet will make a world of difference. Both practices — yoga and the raw food lifestyle — have their limits. As great as the benefits of each practice are, they are finite benefits. For the best possible results, use them in tandem.

Yoga teaches you to find comfort in discomfort, not to run from pain and limitations, but face them head on and move gradually through and beyond them. Raw foods teach us the same thing: You feel bad before you feel good. This develops tenacity and perseverance, everything you need to get to your best health possible. There is no easy way to health! If drugs, supplements, or surgeries could do it, we would be a society of healthy individuals. Unfortunately this is not our reality. But you can achieve your Rawsome health and beauty because you know the way!

Another famous yoga teacher, B.K.S. Iyengar, wrote a very wise book, *Light on Life, The Yoga Journey to Wholeness,* in which he tempers his beliefs about life in general and yoga in particular with social grace, serene dignity, and a grandfather's love. As I read his book, I was greatly impressed by numerous similarities between the practice of yoga and the raw food lifestyle. Both purify and heal the body. Both offer powerful therapeutic effects in dealing with physical and psychological problems. Both promote radiant health.

So many things Iyengar describes about yoga directly relate to raw food experiences. He says: "What we are really doing is infusing dense matter with vibrant energy. That is why good practice brings a feeling of lightness and vitality. Though the mass of our body is heavy, we are meant to tread lightly on this earth." This attitude easily translates to the raw food diet. Another analogy between yoga and raw foods that I learned from this book is that "you are fully within yourself, not outside yourself looking in." As with yoga, the raw food lifestyle initially asks us to exert ourselves more as the resistance is greater, because our flexibility is less. At some point, you reach a state where the effort becomes effortless.

Initially in yoga and in the transition to raw foods, there is discomfort. It is a "good pain." When you begin yoga, the unrecognized pains come to the surface. When you begin the raw food diet hidden problems resurface. When we purify our bodies, the pains disappear, and problem areas heal.

I lived for forty-five years with my right leg shorter than my left. As a result, I was fused like a badly sewn dress. When I began practicing yoga, my legs would not meet. My pelvis was askew so that my left hip stuck out. I have lived like the Leaning Tower of Pisa for so long that when I am straightened, I feel as though I will topple. My yoga session was not about rehabilitation to restore something that was once there, but to create a symmetry that had been shifted at birth.

After years of pain and numerous operations, I guarded my hips as though they were gold nuggets. During my yoga poses, whenever my legs (especially the right one) were expected to respond independently, my whole body rushed to assist. Some muscles in my legs have atrophied from many years of inactivity. As yoga practice was bringing them to life, they were giving me all the pangs of rebirth. The soreness persisted for many hours, even days, afterward, but it was a promising pain. At first I could only go to one class per week. I knew that to really get results, my stubborn muscles needed more. My happiest day was when my hips allowed me to do yoga every day.

But physicality was only part of the whole new experience. Yoga poses pushed me beyond my core being through the darker places and into a comforting light, expanding and healing my emotional self. It seemed that the tight, inflexible muscles were limiting not only my motion but my emotions as well. As everything that was crooked gradually straightened, everything that was weak strengthened, everything that was tight relaxed. I felt as if a wave of new feelings surfaced. My body was a bunker holding me rigid while it held my shattered dreams and unfulfilled expectations captive. As I expanded my mobility, I released my fears, the bitterness trapped inside me, and all of my deep seated insecurities. Suddenly, new possibilities exploded around me.

So if you have a problem, count it as a blessing! B.K.S. Iyengar remembers two students in his class who were trained ballet dancers. They could achieve "every position without exerting any effort, so the journey to the final posture could teach them nothing." He had to become really creative to design routines that would create resistance in their bodies, allowing them to work at the point of balance between the known and unknown.

The same thing is true with raw foods. Detox symptoms are only the birthing pains of the up-coming health: rejuvenation. If the detox symptoms are hard for you, then you are, in fact, fortunate to experience the journey when your body consciousness extends and expands beyond its present state. It is your limitations that allow you to work on the frontier of the known toward the unknown, expanding your body's awareness by learning about your body, about yourself.

Pain is a teacher. It is through struggle that we learn. We learn to see good in pain. Do not avoid the inevitable pain that is part of all growth and change. As raw foods and yoga take you back to health, you will develop greater tolerance of body and mind so that you can bear stress more easily.

Yoga and the raw food diet offer many similarities in the ways they make you feel. Yoga books describe the same euphoric experiences I have found in the raw food diet. Yoga and the raw food diet are alike — liberating, energizing, and exhilarating. Each practice complements the other, bringing many of the same physical and mental benefits.

Yoga and raw foods are both meant for purification of your body as well as for the refinement of your appearance and clarification of your mind. Yoga increases your strength, stamina, and flexibility. Combined with raw food nourishment, yoga releases tension and relieves pain even more effectively. You'll find the results startling: the enhancement of your looks, improvement in your posture, and better skin and muscle tone. You'll feel your vitality brought to a new lofty height by yoga practice.

Raw food will make you less rigid, but it is yoga that will stretch your tissues. Raw food furnishes the body with the best material for optimal health. Yoga helps the body to make the most of it.

Email brings me many questions addressing what seems to be a huge controversy regarding whether yoga should be practiced by Christians, even as a form of physical exercise. I understand these concerns, have shared my own encounters with yoga, and have offered some practical advice. Shortly after I distributed my newsletter, a woman wrote that she was going to unsubscribe from my newsletter, because she considered the matter ridiculous and was outraged that I even responded. She wrote, "I am tired of people who bring God to everything they do. Why can't they just enjoy the benefits of yoga? After all, love, that is all there is!"

"I agree with you completely," I replied "'Love, that *is* all there is!' Therefore, I love people, who 'bring God to everything they do' and I love people who are 'tired of people who bring God to everything they do,' and I love you for unsubscribing."

My attitude toward yoga and Christianity can be summarized by a passage from B.K.S. Iyengar: "Philology is not a language but the science of languages, the study of which will enable the student to learn his own language better. Similarly, Yoga is not a religion by itself. It is the science of religion, the study of which will enable one to better appreciate his own faith." I cannot see how one can explain this any better. I have found Iyengar's book enlightening and illuminating on many levels.

I was disappointed when I read in Bikram's new book, "Next came bizarre props ... Iyengar uses so many props in his method that he's called 'The Furniture Yogi' in India." I have been greatly helped by both yoga systems. These two remarkable men have contributed so much to the health of millions of people in the West. What a great example it would be if they practiced love and compassion towards each other. "After all, love, that is all there is!" Study the different forms of yoga and find the one that feels right for you.

I am absolutely sure yoga, in one form or another, is for everyone. If I can do it, you can do it!

I have had a great deal of physical therapy in my life. For me, yoga is a physical therapy with a new dimension. As a result of my yoga practice I walk better and better without pain or limp, and I have seen my own faith strengthened by my yoga practice. It works for me. Yoga has made me more centered and reflective and better able to pray and meditate.

I want to share with you a great joy I experienced this past Christmas. After doing yoga almost every day for three years, either in a class or a private session, I finally achieved a half-lotus pose! Well, admittedly, I was only able to hold it for two seconds, after forty minutes of warm-up stretching. For those of you who are not fluent in yoga poses, the half-lotus is the most commonly depicted yogis' meditation pose and the one often done by young people who sit cross-legged this way without even knowing it *is* yoga. For me, however, it was a revelation. Nothing I have ever accomplished in my life was harder. When I attempted it for the first time, my buttocks must have been at least one foot off the floor. My hips were damaged during my birth, so trying to stretch the tissues and ligaments in the hip area is like working with wood.

Next to the raw food lifestyle, yoga is the second best thing that has ever happened to me. However, I do not think it would have even been possible to achieve this incredible moment if I had not moved to a 100 percent raw food lifestyle. Some of you might want to visit exotic places or win a marathon. Not me. My biggest New Year's resolution was to be able to sit in the cross-legged position for a pro-longed period of time without tedious preparation.

Those of you who have never done yoga are probably thinking: *What a silly wish! Why would anyone even want to do something so frivolous?* In fact, that was the reaction of my husband. Especially when he learned I was going through what yoga instructors call "good pain," there was way too much of it for him. Nick will never do it and, for the life of him, cannot understand why I would pursue it.

One of the reasons I pursue this discipline — apart, that is, from my sheer stubbornness — is that flexible joints are essential for good health. I not only spend my precious time on doing yoga every day, I also wiped out our 401(k) savings on private sessions to get me through the toughest periods in my healing process. I have no regrets. I feel such a lightness in my body that I would do it again. My husband, on the other hand, is not convinced it was worth it just so I could sit on my butt on the floor. A chair would have been cheaper!

One lady told me that I could not do yoga because I could not even get on the floor without some help. If you *cannot* do it, this is the very reason you *should* do it! Yoga is changing my hips one tenth of a millimeter per day! My favorite saying is by Lafcadio Hearn: "All the best work is done the way the ants do things — by tiny but untiring and regular additions."

Or, in the words of the old Sinatra song *High Hopes*: "Oops, there goes another rubber tree plant!" So, if you are looking for a shoulder to cry on, whining that Rawsome beauty changes are not happening fast enough, look elsewhere. If I can get there on an ant's legs, I am going.

And so should you.

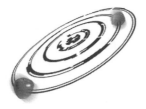

Chapter 25
Rawsome Beauty:
Not a Privilege for the Few,
but a Right for All

Recently I spoke for over two hours to a lively audience
at a ladies' retreat. I spoke on three topics: my spiritual
journey from atheist to Christian, overcoming my physical
adversity, and never giving up on my dreams. The ladies
laughed at funny stories of married life, my Russian heritage,
and the culture shock of coming to America. When I felt I
had their trust — and though they'd just lunched on hotel-
standard chicken Kiev and a sugar-laden dessert — I hit
them hard with my raw foods message. Their response was
great. Later, at dinner, I heard a veritable chorus of "Oh, just a
salad for me, thanks!"

Days later, I received an email from one of the retreat's
organizers. *I've been asked some questions,* said my correspondent, *that I'd like you to answer in more detail.
Personally, I think you look fabulous and certainly
healthier and more fit than most of us* — I'm just quoting,

folks, not boasting! *But someone said they thought you had cosmetic facial surgery. The person was,* my correspondent went on, *concerned about how that would affect the integrity of my testimony regarding what the raw food diet has done for me.* Then came the forthright question — Had I undergone cosmetic surgery? *Please forgive my asking,* she said, *but it's important that I affirm the honesty of your proposed healthy eating plan.*

How was I supposed to feel now — annoyed, or amused? Searching for the words to reply, I decided to proceed gently and factually. *Thank you for asking about cosmetic surgery,* my own email began. *I am flattered. I have never had any cosmetic procedures done. I have* never *been in a cosmetologist's office. I do not even go for facials. I do them at home myself. Externally, I only do what I discuss in chapter 28 of my first book.*

Don't feel bad about asking, readers! I get these questions all the time. My husband even jokes about it. "No, she's never had a face lift," he likes to say. "But if I miss one little job she's told me to do, I definitely get some raised eyebrows."

Women whom I interviewed for my second book, *Beautiful On Raw,* all told me they've been asked the same question again and again — *Have you had something done?* In fact, I consider this question a big compliment, a great testimonial that this lifestyle works. Prove it to yourself. Do what I recommend in my books. You'll soon have people looking at you and asking you the same question.

You cannot fake the glow that arises from the raw food lifestyle. It's internal. It's what happens when a person goes on the raw food diet. She begins to glow. In our own local support group, we see these transformations all the time. That glow of health and vitality is a genuine miracle, one that can happen for everyone — especially you. Raw food will work this magic for you, *without* a surgeon's intervention. Nothing can go wrong with anesthesia and there is zero chance of trauma from surgery when you embark on your raw food adventure.

The word *natural* is extremely overworked in the beauty field. *Natural beauty* has been appropriated by cosmetic companies to promote their artificial enhancements, and have destroyed the very concept in the process. *Rawsome beauty* is a term I coined in my first book, *Your Right to Be Beautiful,* to describe the simple attractiveness that emerges on the raw food lifestyle. This look is free of superfluous elements. Rawsome beauty is an expression of natural laws that, without raw foods, would be hidden from you forever. It is a phenomenon that takes place in people's lives when their personal interaction with food transforms from energy into radiance.

When I titled my first two books *Your Right to Be Beautiful* and *Beautiful on Raw,* I actually proclaimed myself beautiful. If any of the famous beauties of the world had done such a thing, people would hate their guts. Remember the ad campaign, "Don't hate me because I'm beautiful?" We did, didn't we? And yet I was able to get away with it. In fact, in just the first five years of my website's operation, I have received thousands of emails full of kind words about my work and expressions of gratitude for influencing lives in a most profound way.

Why? First, because I did not violate the main principle of encouragement: Do not tell me how much you achieved unless you tell me first how much you had to overcome. And second, because people understood that it is not about me, it is about exciting new possibilities for all of them. It has nothing to do with exhibitionism. (What is there to exhibit?) I *earned* the right to be beautiful, and people were eager to learn from my experience. My claim to beauty is more symbolic of real hope for all of the men and women who are called plain, physically imperfect, or disadvantaged in beauty heritage. My victory is a victory for all of them.

Was it scary for me to call myself beautiful? Very! At first I was quite insecure. I never advertised my author status at my yoga or Pilates classes. My performance was so pitiful, I was afraid people would laugh. *You? Beautiful?* Only when I was able to detach myself from all the baggage that the word *beautiful* entails, was I able to feel relaxed about my position. I finally understood that it was not about my receiving recognition, but about my helping other women to achieve their own beauty. If I, disadvantaged in so many ways, was able to solve the beauty dilemma for myself, how much more could others do? I felt I owed it to other people, especially women, to tell them what I had learned. I marvel at how much my body is reshaping itself on raw foods and daily exercise. I am so grateful for all of these wondrous transformations that I want others to achieve the their own beauty potential.

When you have a serious, maybe even life threatening, illness and are fighting for your life, it sounds completely disingenuous to suggest that now might be the time to bring out your Rawsome beauty. Yet this is exactly the assertion that this book explores. All diseases are a violation of beauty.

In the Gospels of Matthew, Mark and Luke, the Pharisees asked the disciples of Jesus, "Why does your teacher eat with tax collectors and sinners?"

On hearing this, Jesus said, "It is not the healthy who need a doctor, but the sick." Such an obvious fact was this that Jesus used it as a simple device to explain the more complicated conceptual issue of his teachings. It may have been obvious in Biblical times, but it certainly is not as clear now as it was then.

It is considered a norm of our time that health has to be validated by medical professionals. An individual may *say* he is healthy but his claims have no validity unless his doctor concurs. A medical doctor will order multiple tests and check the results against medically established standards. He will analyze the patient's energy level, measure blood pressure, blood sugar, cholesterol level, and then examine his vision just to name a few.

Physicians insists we cannot *see* health, mainly because we cannot see our inside organs. And yet …

"You will also learn through experience and observations along these lines that the general appearance, especially the face of the patient will indicate more or less the internal conditions." — Arnold Ehret.

Still, we play doctor all the time when we say *She looks healthy.* Health is when all body's faculties work at top condition. So when we say *she looks healthy,* what we are saying is that she looks as if all her organs are functioning at their best. We evaluate the limited number of organs that we do see and draw our own conclusion on the condition of the inside organs. What we are really doing is estimating the degree of Rawsome beauty achieved.

If we could see our inside organs, we, like the doctors, would be able to tell the condition of an organ by its shape, color, and consistency. A healthy liver looks dark red. A yellow-brown color is a sure sign of a jaundiced liver. And chemotherapy usually makes it look greenish-brown. Many heart diseases will result in an enlarged, flabby heart. Lung disorders make the lungs look like grayish-blue, filthy, water-soaked sponges puffed up by edema.

Nothing contributes more to being beautiful than having superb health. Rawsome beauty is a public image of your health, an outward reflection of radiating vitality. Glowing health is an ingenious compound of Rawsome beauty. Rawsome beauty is the radiance of the possessor's superior health that strikes the beholder's eye.

In the book *The Power of Now: A Guide to Spiritual Enlightenment,* Eckhart Tolle writes about loathing his own existence. One night he had a deep longing to end his miserable life: "I cannot live with myself any longer" kept running through his mind. Suddenly he was dumbstruck by the peculiarity of this thought: "Am I one or two?" If I cannot live with myself, there must be two of me. "The next question was: If that is so, then which one is real?"

The journey toward Rawsome beauty is not a struggle; it is an adventure. It begins with accepting your body as it is. You may say, *"I do not like myself."* The conclusion is that there must be two of you. Which one is real?

Do not place labels on your appearance. Don't say *I have droopy eyelids ... my pores are too large ... the bags under my eyes look like cargo trunks.* Things are what they are. "A rose is a rose is a rose," as Gertrude Stein used to say. You are going to dwell in this body and nothing you do is going to enable you to change your address.

Acceptance *must* precede action. Self-acceptance is a starting point which makes positive changes possible. It doesn't mean succumbing to our illnesses, bad habits, and premature aging. On the contrary, self-acceptance involves loving ourselves enough to accept sober truths about our health and appearance.

By accepting your body as it is, you are empowering yourself to overcome obstacles. The way you look is the way you look. Accept it. By doing so, you are set free. By accepting, you can be nonjudgmental and start doing what is best for your body. Only from this perspective can you clearly understand what is best for your body, and not confuse it with what is best for your ego, like breast implants and collagen injections, or a face lift.

Accept your body. We all have signature features that are a hallmark of our appearance, like full lips or broad jowls. Signature features are something Quantum Eating will not change and cosmetic surgery should never touch.

On a raw foods regimen, the phrase *I do not like myself* becomes absurd. *You* cannot be hostile to yourself. No splitting the image. There is no guilt about the past, no expectations of the future — only complete acceptance of the present.

After forty, the quest for beauty *is* a quest for health. Beauty after forty is symbolized by clear eyes, a glowing complexion, and shining full hair, and it is all very rare. At the same time, as far as Rawsome beauty is concerned, we live in a democratic, equal opportunity society. This kind of beauty is available to everyone who dares to pursue it. Rawsome beauty has no favorites and renders no privileges. In this book, beauty is regarded as a right, not as a rare commodity. If health is achievable, so is beauty. Strive for health and you will achieve beauty.

When a person strikes us as Rawsomely beautiful, she displays more presence, she stands out, she glows. After we see our first Rawsome transformations, we gain a clear view of how much ugliness we tolerate. By rejecting beauty, you are rejecting goodness and truth.

In the book *Beauty and Revolution in Science,* James W. McAllister states that many scientists believe that aesthetic criteria for recognizing truths do exist. As Heisenberg said, "If nature leads us to mathematical forms of great simplicity and beauty … we cannot help thinking that they are 'true,' that they reveal a genuine feature of nature."

While working on general relativity theory, Roger Penrose became convinced that theories possessing certain aesthetic properties have a better chance of being close to the truth. While referring to the general theory of relativity, Dirac felt that there are aesthetic grounds for believing that it is basically true regardless of confirmation from experimental data. *Beauty and Revolution of Science* quotes him: "One has a great confidence in the theory arising from its great beauty … One has an overpowering belief that its foundations must be correct quite independent of its agreement with observation."

That is how I feel about the raw foods lifestyle. When done correctly, it performs miracles of healing in the human body and brings out the Rawsome beauty in each individual. Quantum Eating, which is simply another level in the raw food lifestyle, is too simple and too pretty not to be true.

Arnold Ehret followed those instructions, eating only fruit and vegetables. He wrote in his *Mucusless Diet*: "For thousands of years humanity has indulged in dreams and wishful thinking about the Fountain of Youth. I have seen people who became so rejuvenated and beautiful after a Mucusless Diet Cure that I almost didn't recognize them … For the ordinary person is will require one to three years."

The body potentially "has" several versions simultaneously without completely realizing any of them, and then one version materializes as a result of your eating choices. When you are adopting the raw food lifestyle, two opposing processes are at work in your body: the old you is leaving, kicking and screaming, and the new you is growing, rejoicing, and getting more confident. Rawsome beauty must be conceived biologically, so to speak, and not intellectually. It has to be deep inside every cell. When you have Rawsome beauty, you realize that nothing you ever do could possibly improve what you already have.

When I was writing this book, I received an email asking me if I would be interested in giving consultations to beauty pageant contestants. I was excited and flattered but at the same time an uneasy feeling came over me. I could not understand my reaction. Sure, I would be delighted to help these young women to learn a healthy way to beauty, so what was bothering me? I was perfectly okay with the means for achieving beauty — it is the final end that was making me uncomfortable. Rawsome beauty is incompatible with competition, because Rawsome beauty encompasses much more than physical transformation, it encompasses spiritual growth as well.

If modeling is all about *looking* beautiful, Rawsome beauty is all about *being* beautiful — deeply. Modeling is about *being seen*. Rawsome beauty is about *being*. Rawsome beauty is nothing more and nothing less than what is seems to be. Rawsome beauty is all about preferring truth to artifice. There is a profound nobility in Rawsome beauty. Its eternal source is health. When we experience Rawsome beauty, there is a sense of homecoming. Rawsome beauty holds up the mirror of compassion and acceptance. Competition is removed; contentment and completion are reached.

Morcover, Rawsome beauty brings a feeling of plenty. No one has to lose in order for you to win. You do not need judges to proclaim that you are beautiful. You do not need fans to give you constant reassurance. And you do not have to worry that it will be taken away by someone younger next year.

Before going 100 percent raw, I was never called beautiful — maybe "pretty," when I used a lot of make-up — but now almost every day someone tells me I am beautiful. At fifty? I do not believe it either! Am I beautiful in the way Catherine Zeta-Jones is or Elizabeth Taylor was? Of course not, but I am beautiful in the sense that I have reached *my* full potential with nothing but raw food and determination. I am about to reveal to you a big secret: You need the courage to say "I am beautiful" for the first time. But once you say it with conviction, no one challenges you and no one realizes that this is the first time you have declared it or that you have no clue where it will direct you. If you *act* beautiful, no one will presume differently.

It has become the sign of our times to mistake glamour for beauty. But glamour is artificial. Rawsome beauty is entirely authentic. My two books started a beauty revolution. For the first time in history, you do not have to be born beautiful to enjoy the designation. I know the day will come when public admiration will shift from lanky six-foot models and glamorous movie stars who are size 0 to Rawsome beauties who achieved their looks by the virtues of moderation, discipline, and diligent attention to their health. I see it coming in the same way new money has overtaken old money. Enterprise and ability have succeeded as the influence of status and titles waned. We might even see it happen in our lifetime. The more you improve your eating patterns along with external care of your body, the more you contribute to bringing that time closer. Every time another person reclaims the right to be beautiful, there is one more on our side.

During the last four years, cosmetic surgeries performed on teenagers has nearly doubled to 244,124 — including about 47,000 nose jobs and 9,000 breast augmentations, according to the American Society of Plastic Surgeons (ASPS). And it has become trendy for nose jobs, breast implants, teeth whitening, skin resurfacing, and liposuction to top a grad's wish list, says Dr. Roxanne Guy, ASPS president. Even in light of these alarming statistics, I see a new trend developing, and it is getting stronger.

The paradigm shift in human consciousness is obvious. After many raw food presentations on my book tours, I am approached by teenage girls wanting to have their pictures taken with me. It makes me very happy to see that these girls value health over the popular fads of artificial boobs, lips, and who knows what else? What they represent is an emerging consciousness that no matter how old you are, health is always beautiful. Nothing is more beautiful to me than seeing sixty- or seventy-year-old women who exude a natural radiance.

More and more people are beginning to see beauty my way. Which is to say: More and more people are seeing beauty *their* way, from *their* own perspectives. Those who e-mail me for the first time, those who hover around the lectern at presentations, often begin by asking questions from the perspective of the world. Worse, they ask from the perspective of a pop culture whose image of beauty is *constructed* — cobbled together from lipstick ads in magazines, rakishly thin Milan runway models, TV stars glued together with cosmetics, botox, and collagen injections. Real beauty, *your* beauty, is not to be found on the television screen, but in the mirror. Look … See … Accept … and Begin.

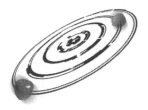

Chapter 26

New Portal to Spirituality, or When Did Beauty Become the Eighth Deadly Sin?

"The greatest truths are wronged if not linked with beauty, and they win their way most surely and deeply into the soul when arrayed in their natural and fit attire."
— William Ellery Channing

When I was ready to publish my first book, *Your Right to Be Beautiful*, I asked for an endorsement from a prominent authority in the raw food lifestyle. As is customary, I provided him with samples to make it easier. The suggestions were tied to his personal field of expertise to give them immediate relevance to both my work and his.

The endorsement came back and everywhere I had used the word "beauty," he changed it to "spiritual beauty." I could not believe my eyes! It made me think: "When did physical beauty become a villain? What is so wrong with physical beauty that he did not even want to be associated with the concept?

Needless to say, to my disappointment, I could not use the endorsement. First, because the change was misleading to my potential readers and second, because I felt he had missed the whole point. I also refused to consider that being beautiful had become so vilified that it was no longer politically correct even to suggest that women could desire it, let alone pursue it.

When I wrote my first book, I determinedly called it *Your Right to Be Beautiful.* I quickly discovered that I had committed an unforgivable sin. I had suggested that women not only *could* be beautiful, but that they had the *right* to pursue being beautiful.

We hear it often now: Beauty is how you feel inside. It is not something physical. It is a kind of spiritual snobbery that makes people think that it is beneath them to strive for physical beauty. Living most of my life with a leg infirmity, I have a very special appreciation for physical beauty. But since I wrote my book I get dozens of emails and letters every day from women sharing their concerns about getting old and feeling unattractive. It happens to be a widespread concern. The reality is that there are a great number of middle-aged women who are scared and insecure, in the face of old age, who are giving in to society's imposed belief that you are no good past a certain age. For many women, not to be beautiful is synonymous with being invisible. Those with homely features should keep home. I was one of them, and these are the people whom I wanted to help most with my books.

I write a regular column, "Raw Beauty," for *Get Fresh! Magazine.* The magazine published an interview with me which is reproduced in my second book, *Beautiful On Raw.*

One reader wrote back:

"Tonya Zavasta's philosophy (*Get Fresh!,* Summer 2005) made uneasy, if not disturbing reading. 'Any woman can fulfill her dream of being beautiful' — ? But what about those with inoperable, incurable birth deformities, or faces disfigured in accidents? How will reading this interview improve their sense of self-worth? Plastic surgery? Many cannot afford it, so beauty, and its dream, hinges on money.

"Am I the only Fresh Network member to detect a thread running through many of the views expressed through the magazine, namely a preoccupation with perfection, and control over it, that goes beyond the desire for health and happiness? ...

"The ultimate perfection is no death, for all natural death is preceded, sooner or later, by a winding down, and a rotting corpse is not beautiful. If you read the poetry of the Japanese Zen masters, you will find there not a restless quest for perfection, but a serenity in the face of what life is: transitory, and made of light and darkness. And a humility in being a leaf on the tree, not the tree itself."

Best wishes,
Steve M.

My answer to Steve M.:

"Dear Steve!

"From the tone of your letter, I can say with great certainty that you are neither deformed from birth, nor disfigured from an accident. Nor do you seem to have enough experience being among afflicted people to know that there is nothing they dislike more than to be given special considerations or a blanket pass to do nothing whatsoever to improve their adverse fate.

"I, on the other hand, speak from personal experience. Being afflicted from birth, I used to feel pain every time I saw a pair of beautiful healthy legs. Women who have had a mastectomy told me they feel the same way about cleavage. Should others be forbidden to wear mini-skirts or décolleté only because they make some of us feel our own limitations more sharply? Where do we draw the line? It is futile to try to be fair to everyone. However, life is fair to those who dare!

"I have great respect for some of the Zen teachings, but does choosing Zen ultimately mean accepting the status quo? If I had made that choice, I would still be a cripple in Russia, unable to walk or to even pray for strength. I chose the path that altered my life. I came to America, had extensive corrective hip surgery, and in my search for health and acceptance, with the true fervor of oppressed spirituality, I found my life's calling by introducing other women to the Rawsome lifestyle I adopted to help me achieve my lifelong goals. There are things about us that can never be changed and must be accepted, but the pursuit of health, happiness, and personal beauty are not among those lost ideals. Is it less humble to want to be a green, healthy leaf than a shrivelled brown one?

"Neither in my books, nor in my articles, have I ever called for perfection. In fact, my books are a celebration of imperfection. My second book is dedicated to plain, imperfect, and physically underprivileged women who dare to be beautiful. I do, however, encourage people to be their best, since we come to this Earth to fill that place which no other soul may fill so well. Under any circumstance, simply do your best, and you will avoid self-judgment, self-abuse, and regret. In this view, happiness means attaining the lasting contentment in the best possible imperfection.

"I am interested in helping people, not in assessing their degree of spirituality. When women ask me how to eliminate excessive wrinkles, acne, bags under the eyes, or varicose veins, should I rebuke them by telling them that they are not spiritual enough or they should not care about such trivial things? Should all hope of beauty be relegated to vanity? Is it nobler to come to the raw food lifestyle fighting cancer rather than hoping to improve your looks? Should we look down on millions of women who do care about their appearance? Or should we remember that the beauty industry would never be so successful if it hadn't resonated with the natural instinct of every woman to be beautiful. It is said that teachers must meet students where they are. And most will not match the spirituality of Zen Buddhist monks.

"According to Toltec wisdom, nothing you or I can say can hurt another person: she has wounds that I can touch by what I have said. By achieving Rawsome beauty, women heal their own wounds by dealing with their body image at every level. Thus, women are no longer vulnerable. Rawsome beauty brings them liberation. That indefinable beauty that comes from superior health, enthusiasm for life, and contentment — a beauty that is nothing more or less than a harmony of imperfections enhanced by the living food lifestyle.

"Nothing lasts forever, nothing will ever be perfect, and nothing will ever be finished. Since wisdom is a science of happiness, it is also the realization that beauty is transitory. Shouldn't we still enjoy the beauty of a flower even though it is short-lived and will wilt and die? A Zen master named Ikkyu Sojun (1481) once professed, 'The appreciation — the savoring — of beauty in all its forms is true Zen.' We should dedicate ourselves to enjoying every minute while it lasts, and certainly should do nothing to speed up its demise.

"The paths are many, but they all lead to the ONE. Let it be a consolation to you that there is actually a way from Rawsome beauty to spirituality ..."

Tonya Zavasta

In the remarkable book, *The Power of Now*, Eckhart Tolle defines spiritual enlightenment as the ability to live in the present moment. There's a story told about the great Zen master Rinzai: In order to take his students' attention away from time and bring them more deeply into the now, Rinzai would often raise his finger and slowly ask: "What, at this moment, is lacking?" My husband Nick, a trucker by trade, says (tongue in cheek) that drivers he encounters on the road often display to one another the Power of Now.

Your progress towards Spiritual Enlightenment very much depends on your not lacking anything at any given moment. This state is more easily achieved with money, possessions, or relationships. But it is much harder to silence the body's problems, such as pain or dissatisfaction with some aspect of your body. When your body is not at its best in health and appearance, your mind wants to escape the now, and dwell either in past (when present problems didn't yet trouble you) or in the future (where they might have disappeared).

Remember that ugly pimple on your nose. (Always on date night!) You hated it and you remembered how good you looked before it appeared. How wonderful your life would be if it disappeared! It was *just* a pimple, yet it had the power to ruin your present. What happens when this pimple becomes extra weight, a double chin, a distended stomach, or real pain that does not let you enjoy the now fully?

You want your body to be different. You do not like what you have. You long for the body you once had, or you hope for the body you might have. Either way, the *now* — the only slice of time you really have — is wasted. As Eckhart Tolle says, "You are losing the present, if you are never present." You are living torn, split. And since there is nothing else but now, your life is not lived to the fullest, if lived at all.

The Power of Now describes several portals into deepening your spirituality. Of course, beauty is not one of them. None of the spiritual teachers have come to discover spiritual enlightenment through achieving Rawsome beauty, but I insist that it is a way! After following the raw food lifestyle for several years, I was amazed to discover that my body is no longer an obstacle to spiritual practices such as meditation, prayer, and self-realization.

> "Spirituality ... is not ethereal and outside nature but accessible and palpable in our very own bodies. Indeed the very idea of a spiritual path is a misnomer. After all, now can you move toward something that, like Divinity, is already by definition everywhere? A better image might be that if we tidy and clean our houses enough, we might one day notice that Divinity had been sitting in them all along. We do the same with the sheaths of the body, polishing them until they become a pure window to the divine." — B.K.S. Iyengar, *Light on Life, The Yoga Journey to Wholeness*

Natural beauty. Ironically, this phrase is often attached to ineffective, overpriced products. Costly and health-disregarding products often masquerade under the name of natural beauty. That contributes to the attitude that there is something degrading about being a seeker of physical beauty, an attitude similar to that of a gardener toward artificial flowers.

For physical beauty to be natural and harmonious, health must be ubiquitous. Quantum Eating is the ultimate way to your best health. Rawsome beauty is a reflection of your superior health, and, therefore, is all about individuality. There is no absolute standard of natural beauty emerging on the raw food diet; which is precisely the reason that its pursuit is so intriguing. It is when imperfections become beauty, as shadows are to light. It is when the autumnal face has even more grace and exquisiteness in its fading than either spring or summer beauty can ever exhibit. When health contributes and sustains beauty, beauty stops being Nature's boast, but becomes a sacrament, almost to the point that neglect of it constitutes some kind of sin. That is why I feel that the pursuit of physical beauty is a sphere of activity which needs redemption in the eyes of naturalists.

Do you wonder whether beauty and taking care of your body have anything remotely to do with God, the meaning of life, or happiness? I discovered that it has everything to do with it! Brought up as an atheist, in a society rooted in materialism, I would never have found my way to spiritual awakening if not for beauty. There is a pass from gaining Rawsome beauty to spirituality. I took this pass. There are many other women out there who have done so, too — and so can you.

Vanity is a positive virtue if it forces us to improve our health as well as our looks. Vanity, which often accompanies beauty, is excusable as a stimulant or motivation to start experimenting with raw foods, but it rarely persists when Rawsome beauty is achieved.

Reasons for our initial involvement may be vain, but they lose importance as we move deeper. And, like many things in life, we can never know in advance the full impact something is going to have on us. Eventually it changes your perspective. You find yourself instinctively embracing a larger, more accurate perception of who you are and how you should look. You start seeing things differently, with less distortion — which results in better health, peace of mind, more enthusiasm for life, and an ever-glowing authentic sense of inner well-being and, yes, physical beauty. Beauty becomes so natural and genuine, so much a part of you, that it carries over into all of your life. Makes you feel absolutely fabulous for no apparent reason.

You will be more present in your body. You will inhabit your body totally. Instead of *having* a body, you will experience *being in* the body. Your stomach is empty and it is pulled into your frame as much as you ever remember. You feel weightless, you love the now so much. There is no other place you would rather be but in your body. You want to savor it. It is rare, it is precious. This creates a euphoric feeling, the ecstasy of enjoying the now.

We feel most alive when we have achieved Rawsome beauty. Even if you have never been a spiritual person, you have no choice but to become one. You will live in a state of blissful existence. You will realize that your body never will be better than it is now. It offers an essential serenity that never goes away. You are dwelling in a state of indescribable bliss and intense joy. Sometimes it is so strong that other people comment on the peace that you project.

When you master not eating, not thinking during meditation comes so much easier. Not that Quantum Eating requires the practice of spirituality, but that it leads to the elevation of one's consciousness to a higher level. Of course, you can achieve this state through spiritual practices. But with Quantum Eating, you will find enlightenment without even searching for it. One day your own body will deliver you to this state.

There is no part of you that will be left untouched by Quantum Eating. It will not only reshape your body, it will also exalt your soul. This act of awe when you are struck by the miracle that your body has performed can become, for many, their first spiritual experience and only then will they redeem their spiritual destitution and discover the meaning of "spiritual beauty." Enlightenment is a state of wholeness, of being "at one" and therefore at peace. In the end, it does not matter which portal you took to get there.

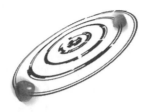

Chapter 27

Creating Your Own Reality — as Easy as Riding a Bike

I was born, as some of you already know, with hip problems. My first seven years were spent in and out of hospitals for surgery after surgery. Many normal childhood activities were taboo for me. More than anything else I ached to ride a bike. My mother, always protective, would never allow me even to try. She felt utterly certain I'd fall and hopelessly aggravate my existing damage. Saddened, but obedient, I stood at the roadside, longingly watching other children as they rode by, smiling, laughing, enjoying the breeze on their faces.

Time passed. I turned forty. *I'm a big girl now,* I decided. *I'm going to learn to ride a bike.* It was now or never! I was afraid, but my husband Nick kept egging me on. *You can do it!* Sure enough, I did. We rode on weekends. The speed gave me that wonderful thrill everyone feels when they first learn to run. It was a delight I'd never experienced before.

One day, after almost a year, the fun ended. I asked Nick to go back to the car and fetch my sunglasses to keep the gnats out of my eyes. Without him there to encourage me, I panicked. I fell off the bike on a stretch of dead-flat pavement, landing on my elbow. Shocked, I saw that the lower part of my hand was screwed almost 180 degrees. Bone protruded through the skin. I knew enough about dislocations to realize I would never have a normal hand again. There would be more surgery, more scars — as if I hadn't enough already.

I lay on my back, no other soul around, only the endless sky embracing me, anguish and grief consuming me. I wept. I raised my good hand — my last intact limb — sending a silent request to Heaven for the fulfillment of one wish: I wanted my normal hand back! In an instant, my life was reprioritized. My limp didn't matter anymore. If only I could rewind my life five minutes. Back to where there was still time to say thanks for the blessings I'd so carelessly overlooked, so that this wouldn't be happening now.

It wasn't God I was angry with. I was furious at myself. For so many years, whenever I looked in the mirror, all I'd seen was my one shorter leg. *Never* had I ever noticed my two flawless, healthy hands.

During the several years of grueling physical therapy needed to unlock my frozen elbow, I couldn't shake the feeling that *I* had *created* the accident myself. I was so afraid of falling that I had pictured the fall in my mind again and again. In my head, I'd heard my mother admonishing me never to get on a bike or I'd fall off and hurt myself. My bike accident, it seemed, had materialized from my thoughts and fears. I expected it. I attracted it. And it came — the perfect self-fulfilling prophecy.

Robert K. Merton explored the concept of the self-fulfilling prophecy in his book *Social Theory and Social Structure*. His inspiration stemmed from the Thomas theorem: *If men define situations as real, they are real in their consequences.*

Merton believed that the more a person concentrates on a merely possible event, the more likely it is to become reality. His fictive example was actually echoed in the American depression of the 1930s: A bank collapses owing to rumors of its failing. The bank is solvent until enough customers believe in the rumor to withdraw their money, causing a bank run that leads to its failure. We call this the Law of Attraction. The Law of Attraction responds to all kinds of "vibrations," just as the law of gravity consistently responds to all of the physical matter making up a planet, or electrical laws consistently respond to all electrical charges.

You know the times when *everything* goes wrong. Trouble seems to come when you're already down. Numerous proverbs, folk tales, and fables perpetuate this familiar idea — they're part of our universal human experience. Even the most scientifically minded among us sometimes think it: Bad news comes in threes. We put the thought out of our mind — *That's silly,* we say to ourselves, whistling in the dark. *It's irrational,* we say. *Snap out of it.* Yet back it creeps: Trouble attracts trouble.

Quantum physics explains this phenomenon. Quantum physics teaches that we are not only the *observers* of reality but also *participants.* We get what we *don't* want because we expend more energy focusing on negative aspects that *might* happen instead of focusing on what we *want* to happen. As the result you bring about what you the most fear.

If you looked at yourself under a powerful electron microscope, you'd find you're made up of chunks of ever-changing energy in the form of electrons, neutrons, photons, and other elemental particles. So are your bedroom slippers, your Uncle Bob, the Ford Focus in your driveway, and everything else in the known universe.

What we experience as the physical world is actually a vast field of flashing, flickering energy. Nothing is literally solid. In a way, it is our *attention* that assembles and holds together this ever-changing energy field, letting us perceive the "objects" we see.

The longer you follow the raw food lifestyle, Quantum Eating in particular, the more you become aware of your own vibrational nature. It's as if the energy you're emanating is of higher frequency and larger amplitude, the longer and more faithfully you follow good eating practices. Your intuition, your ability to visualize and predict outcomes, your capacity to make your dreams materialize, all become more developed than when you ate cooked food. Once you know how the micro-world works, you can use this knowledge to your advantage. You can literally fashion your own reality.

The Law of Attraction says that like is drawn to like. Bear with me as I give you an ultra-simplified version of this phenomenon from a quantum physics prospective. Remember: You must not skip it! Without understanding the basic premise, you will not have a clear mental picture. And without that clear mental picture, you will not be convinced that the Law of Attraction works. And as long as you lack belief, you won't be able to make the Law of Attraction work for you.

Molecules contain atoms. Atoms contain electrons. Think of these electrons as being attached to the atoms by springs. Drop a pencil on the floor, and it vibrates. Pluck a guitar string, it vibrates. Everything in the universe, material and non-material, is energy that vibrates at a particular frequency or a set of frequencies when dropped, struck, plucked, strummed, or otherwise disturbed. These are called *natural frequencies*. An object can have more than one natural frequency. But even a big, complex object can be especially subject to one specific frequency — its resonance frequency. Take the famous example of the Tacoma Narrows Bridge, nicknamed "Galloping Gertie." In 1940, just four months after the first Narrows bridge was built, it was buffeted by especially high winds. These winds "found" the natural resonance frequency of the bridge's main span. The span began to bend in response to the wind, twisting wildly this way and that, finally breaking, and sending cars, steel cables, and massive girders plunging into the waters below.

Resonance occurs when two interconnected material or non-material entities share the same vibrational frequency. Consider two tuning forks of the same natural frequency. A vibration in one will subtly induce vibration in the other, nearby fork. Soon, both will vibrate together in unison. When one of the objects is vibrating, it forces the second object into vibrational motion. This makes the oscillation's amplitude grow larger and larger — exactly what happened in the Tacoma Narrows Bridge case. This is called resonance, or wider vibration. Resonance is what transmits and receives wireless communications, including radio, television, and cell phone traffic.

We all know what it is to *tune in* a radio station. Vibration is a periodic motion, and all periodic motions can resonate with an external force at the correct frequency, as the Tacoma Narrows Bridge resonated with the wind. What makes a radio tune in to a specific frequency? The circuit is designed to have a natural frequency of vibration for its alternating current, which is adjustable. When adjusted to match the frequency of your favorite radio station, resonance occurs and the radio will pick up energy from the radio waves and build up a large oscillation.

Resonance works in radio, television, and cell phones. There's no reason why it shouldn't work in your thinking. Thoughts and feelings, beyond being biochemical impulses, are electromagnetic patterns of energy that will externally resonate with everything having the same frequency. When you vibrate emotions of particular frequency, everything of that same natural frequency will be activated.

Similar entities have the same natural frequency. Everything having the same frequency as your vibrating thought will pick up energy from your thought waves and build up a larger wave. When your thought's frequency matches the natural frequency of an object, that object will begin to resonate. Your desire (vibration) adds energy at just the right moment during the oscillation cycle so that the oscillation is reinforced.

Let me give you a simple analogy to remember whenever you want to apply the Law. Pretend you're in many-tongued Babel.[1] You desperately need something, if only to find the way out of this crazy city. You cry aloud in English (the only frequency you have) hoping *someone* will understand. If you know another language, you might try it, too. In this case, you will be vibrating at two frequencies. Suddenly, you hear your native tongue. In this sea of babbling, you recognize a word or sentence you can understand. You get excited, just as the person who heard you does, and you both begin speaking even louder. The two of you have just made a connection at a frequency very different from the sea of shouting people surrounding you. You attracted the person who speaks your language. In the same way, vibrations of similar frequencies recognize each other and create a resonance. In this way, what you need to fulfill your highly desired dream — whether this be a person, a book, or an idea — will be revealed to you.

The Law of Attraction is impersonal. The Law sees to it that *all* thoughts with matching frequencies find one another and stick together. When you hold the image of your goal in your mind, you are vibrating in harmony — in *resonance* — with every particle of energy necessary for the manifestation of your image on the physical plane. Everything needed to manifest your desire will reveal itself.

---

1. *Readers are reminded of the Tower of Babel in Genesis 11:1-9 — the origin of diverse human languages.*

The connection is established whether or not you're aware of it. We might call it the Law of *Amplification* or Law of *Connection* rather than the Law of Attraction, because the attraction is happening through the *amplification* of all you need to reach your goal and you are *connecting* to it. Concentrating on something "invites" that something into your experience. The subject of your attention will begin moving toward you.

"Thoughts create a new heaven, a new firmament, a new source of energy, from which new arts flow." — Paracelsus, sixteenth century alchemist

---

Look around you at material things. Do you see a chair, a table, your shoes? Every item in your world was someone's idea before it materialized and became your possession. Even in Genesis, before each act of creation, there was first an intention. It was always "And God said" before it was actually done.

You are a cause for everything in your world. You can change course at any time. You can modify your "vibrating" desires and create a "vibrational resonance" with everything that can help you to achieve those desires. Have you experienced a strong excitement about a new project and suddenly all the needed information came your way? This is the Law of Attraction working full force. By being excited, believing in your new endeavor, you become a kind of magnet, drawing toward you events, people, and objects with vibrations similar to your own.

Through your observation, you are actually creating a vibration. Thinking about something is inviting this something into your experience. The subject of your attention will be drawn toward you. Your intense focus on an object or desire becomes a laser ray which activates that vibrational content, turning it into your point of attraction. If you want something, allow it to vibrate within you, without restriction or reservation. Let yourself *burn* with this desire or want. Obsess on it. Without a hint of *no*. Without the negativity of *but what if?* This the only way to make it happen. But if at the same time you have been letting fears or insecurities slip through, you'll create other, conflicting vibrations that negate the positive force of your dream. Our thoughts are energies that determine how we experience the physical world. This explains why positive thinking, prayer, faith, creativity, goal-setting, and visualization all work in our creation of our own worlds.

Constantly focusing on the negative is nothing more than a bad habit. Break it. The essential thing to remember about the Law of Attraction is that is *does not discriminate* between what you do want to happen and what you don't want to happen. The Law responds only to the strength of your wanting. If you expend your energy on intense thoughts and emotions, they'd better be positive, because you are disrupting their energy fields and drawing them to you. Whether you're thinking *I want this* or *I am afraid of that* — it's already on its way! Your life is what you think it is. Your thinking makes it what it becomes. Be safe. Don't think negative thoughts. The best way to start is by avoiding negative words. Steer clear as much as you can of "not" words: *can't … won't … don't.* Replace them with their positive, affirming equivalents: *I can … I will reconsider … I will change.*

"And let the peace of God rule in your hearts, to which also you were called in one body; and be thankful. Let the word of Christ dwell in you richly in all wisdom, teaching and admonishing one another in psalms and hymns and spiritual songs, singing with grace in your hearts to the Lord. And whatever you do in word or deed, do all in the name of the Lord Jesus, giving thanks to God the Father through Him." — Colossians 3:15–17.

We must live in a continuous state of gratitude. To feel unloved and unworthy is to *resist*. Give up feeling like a victim. To allow yourself to feel blessed and worthy of good things is to allow more good things to come. Every time you give thanks to God, you're saying you want more of similar blessings. Be in a state of grace, appreciation, and thanksgiving. I stopped long ago praying for things that I do not have. I only give praise for what I do have. As soon as I adopted this attitude, the frequency of "bad" things happening dropped tenfold.

Gratitude opens your life to overflowing blessings. When you give thanks for everything that comes your way, even the bad things, you acknowledge that good always triumphs. Whenever there is a problem, there is always a solution. Whenever life throws you into a pit, there is always a ladder hidden somewhere for you to climb out. No matter how much may be lost to circumstance, there is still so much left to appreciate. Someone said: *If you can't be thankful for what you receive, be thankful for what you escape.* Think of all the sufferings that have not been inflicted upon you.

Pain brings us back home. We start to appreciate what we do have. That moment of gratitude for what you have is the time to reappraise your values. Sometimes the misfortunes of others can do the same thing for us. When we hear about other people's hardships, don't we feel fortunate to be spared them? Selfishly, perhaps, it is our own pain that makes us sharply aware of just how fragile our blessings are.

Sometimes we need to suffer so that we can appreciate what we do have. Now, after so many operations, I am aware of every step I am taking. I notice that each footstep is totally unique in feel and pressure. I am completely present in walking: aware and grateful. Words are inadequate to express this feeling: oneness with overwhelming love fills every cell of my body. This must be how the divine presence of God felt.

Ever since I have been following a Quantum Eating program that has elevated my consciousness, I have had moments when I've felt a subtle emanation of joy arising from deep within — the joy of being. This joy has no opposite, no "anti-joy." Call this sensation by whatever name your religious leaning leads you to. Call it the presence of Holy Spirit, call it enlightenment — the point remains the same.

Our final goal is the joy of being one with God. God wants us to experience this joy no matter the price. Many of us can learn to surrender, to accept, to forgive, to *let go,* only through traumatic experience. Often it is human drama that teaches us to distinguish between what is real and unreal in our lives. It is often the end of pain that is perceived as pleasure. Failures are stepping-stones to success. Illness, for many, becomes a springboard to health. These are cycles of up and down. They are neither good nor bad. They simply *are.* When you find yourself in this vibrant tapestry of non-resistance these ups and downs become nothing more than ripples in the fabric. You will notice them, but they will not shake your inner peace.

By thinking positive, loving thoughts, you send a message: You have learned your lessons. By being grateful, you are vibrating that you are *already* in the state of grace, that you do not need more suffering to bring you to a blissful state of contentment. Have a thankful heart! It will be your guardian angel. Quantum physics supports the observation that what we are most grateful for *stays* with us, and what we have been taking for granted is most likely to leave us first.

"Better to lose count while naming your blessings than to lose your blessings to counting your troubles." — Maltbie Babcock

Guess what? I'm back riding a bicycle. These days, I do not allow myself a single negative thought. Never mind that now I ride a tandem bike with my husband. Nick says he's not going to take any chances — he's still learning the power of positive thinking! He assures me that he's not letting any thoughts of our making bicycle pirouettes enter his mind. Never mind that we two look like a Russian circus act — a bear and a monkey riding a bright blue, comical bicycle. Watch us, and you'll see we're having the most marvelous time. Life's a circus for all of us. But, Lord, it's lovely if you let it be.

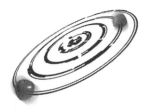

Chapter 28
Think Ageless

My husband's first job in America was working for a real estate investor preparing houses for new welfare tenants. This job included everything from structural repairs to cleaning bathrooms. Nick, fresh from the Russian steppes, was at the time — he's since been domesticated — a very "manly man." No knee-pads or scrubbing brush for this self-styled Cossack, no sir. Thus the cleaning portion of the work fell to me. As I scrubbed bathrooms on my knees and collected roaches by the bucket, did I regret coming to America? No. We knew we were in a country where poverty could be cured by hard work. We believed things would get better. It the meantime, I had my own pretensions to think about. A former university instructor, I was unaccustomed to such intimacy with toilets, bathroom tile grout, and the mélange of aromas which met me there. Seeking psychological escape, I occupied my mind in dreaming about how I would live and look one day.

During this early time in our new country, a couple from church invited us every Saturday for pizza and a movie. During one of our visits, the TV show *Dr. Quinn: Medicine Woman* premiered. Jane Seymour was so gorgeous. I wanted to look just like her. I didn't picture myself *being* her, exactly.

Instead, I appropriated particular features I coveted, like her long, straight hair, her high cheekbones, and her small waist. My fantasy image was as far from the real me as you could get. New to America and the endless, grand luxuries of its supermarkets, we sought to try every fancy boxed and bagged food item available. Frozen this, ready-to-eat that. Seduced by the "suggested serving" pictures on packages, I gained weight. My face became round and fleshy, and I always wore a perm in an effort to hide its chubby rim with curls. Since I did a lot of hard, manual labor, my limp showed more than ever. Only later, and gradually, did I really come to understand that what I was doing to my body, what I was putting into my body, was having effects far deeper and more potent than extra fat alone. Jane Seymour and I, for the time being, were to grow even farther apart. Still, it was the fantasy that triggered a new reality — a new lifestyle which — while it ultimately neither let me be Jane Seymour nor made me wish to be — allowed me to become the prettiest, the most attractive woman that *I* could be, and in my own way.

Let the raw food lifestyle facilitate a body makeover for you. Let yourself dream. Go ahead — dream about just how you want to look. Let your mind run free. Your dreams don't even have to be realistic. What's important is that your dreams present *clear* images of what you want. On one level, my fixation on looking like Jane Seymour was silly. I wasn't ever going to look like her. I'm not ever going to look like her. And — now — I don't want to. But my dream *worked*. It worked because the image was clear. Vivid. Particular.

To lure anything into existence, you must begin with thoughts — clear thoughts — and then create an intense desire for them that will make them come true. The bare-bones version of this notion is already familiar to every reader of this book. Thanks to Dr. Norman Vincent Peale's *The Power of Positive Thinking,* this idea has been part of the warp and weft of western — especially, American — culture for decades. I seek here, however, both to expand your understanding of this notion and to particularize it to the realm of health. There's more here, and I invite you to reflect upon some of the many expansions of the *positive thinking* which I and other, later authors have added to the potent seed which Peale planted among us. It's the very familiarity of Peale's idea which makes it difficult to work with: Simply utter the phrase *positive thinking,* and everyone tends to believe he knows exactly what you're talking about, often shutting down their analytic faculties on the presumption that they've "got it." For this reason, I generally don't use phrase, and preferring the more subject-specific phrase *think ageless.*

A book is a mirror: If an ass peers into it, you can't expect an apostle to look out. — George Christoph Lichtenberg

---

A book — a *good* book — can give you only as much wisdom as you, the reader, are capable of receiving. With life in general, it's pretty much the same. The world is literally your mirror: It enables you to have a physical experience which is a reflection of who you are — your thoughts, your beliefs, your desires — of the vibrations you are sending out, and the energy those vibrations are drawing in. If you want to change your life experience, change the vibrations you are emanating. What dominates your thoughts *becomes* you. What you imagine and believe becomes your life. Beliefs create the most powerful vibrations. Limiting beliefs will instantly place an upper limit on life. Examine your beliefs every once in a while — see whether you aren't fencing yourself in unduly.

Quantum physics tells us that the act of observing an object actually *causes* it to be where and how we observe it. An object does not exist independently of its observer. It is you, your thoughts in particular, that make your spouse loving, your children respectful, and your own body beautiful and healthy. You just have to feel it in your being: *I desire health, I appreciate my healthy body*. Desire is the beginning of all attraction.

People often ask me to discuss solutions for a particular disease they have. I always say that I am not a doctor and cannot discuss treatments. Not only do I not know anything about diseases, but, in a sense, I don't particularly want or need to know much. However, I do know a lot about achieving and maintaining good health.

In Buddhist writings we find an idea both beautiful and useful: When we want to brighten a cave, we bring in a torch. Darkness isn't a *thing*. We do not "remove darkness." Rather, we simply bring light and darkness is chased away. The same concept applies to our body. We do not remove a particular disease. We simply make lifestyle changes and eat healthy foods and the body's cells, tissues, and organs are encouraged to heal themselves. Invite health into your body and sickness will go away. Just as darkness cannot survive in the presence of light, sickness cannot survive in the presence of health. The mistake that conventional medicine makes, conceptually, lies in distinguishing health and disease as if they were opposites within the same category — as if they were different but opposite "things" — when, in reality, sickness is the absence (or partial absence) of health in a body part or body function, just as darkness is an absence of light. Symptoms must be allowed for health to be achieved. If you are feeling, you are healing.

"Disease [is] not an entity, but a fluctuating condition of the patient's body, a battle between the substance of disease and the natural self-healing tendency of the body." — Hippocrates

How many of you have been told that your health challenges were incurable, that you'd simply have to endure them? I was told this about my hips, my sinus problems, my migraines, and my heart problems — all of them diagnosed when I was a young woman. Yet after I "went raw," my body found ways to cure these degenerative conditions. My problems faded, losing their permanent hold on my body and my psyche.

The condition of my hips has qualified me for disability benefits both here and in Russia. At low points in my life I thought about applying for these benefits, and relatives encouraged me to do so. But I could never make myself do it. Consider: to collect payments, not only do you have to convince others that you are disabled, but you have to continue doing so year after year. I saw such a terrible degree of finality in the prospect of making this repeated admission to the world that I refused to accept the possibility, even before I knew anything about the Law of Attraction. I believe that the reason I am doing exceptionally well is that I kept insisting, telling myself and others, I was *not* disabled, no matter what the diagnosis said.

I know several people on disability because of diabetes or heart disease, or both. I tell them that, after going raw, their tests will improve dramatically. So chained are some to the choice of disability, however, that this prospect strikes horror in them, and they stay away from fruits and vegetables so as not to lose their benefits. This is "voluntary disability behavior." I know, and you do too, people whose whole lives become preoccupation with their illness. To convince boards and committees they are sick, they have to convince themselves first. And by doing so, they push themselves deeper and deeper into an invalid mentality to which the body responds by providing all the symptoms they'll ever need. This way, such people build a wedge between themselves and their well-being. It is the saddest thing that our otherwise sound disability benefits system actually *supports* sickness and provides *no incentive* to get well. Even sadder is the mind's ability to deliver whatever the body needs to maintain this status quo.

We know that our cells replace themselves. Our bones, our tissues are all different from the ones we had several years ago. Imagine replacing a different part each day on your car. After a couple of years, not a single one of the original parts would remain. In one way, then, it's a different car than the one we drove off the lot. But we'd still call it "our car," even "the same car." Why are we, our physical selves, the same old, or even older, selves?

We must *change* what goes into the body. Sure, this means food and water — we must consume different, better food, more biologically active water, in different quantities and at different times. But it also means that we must have different *thoughts* if we want to have a different body. Your life is a reflection of the power of your thoughts. If you want things to change, change your thoughts. To think different thoughts, learn new approaches to familiar subjects.

All our fears can be traced to one ultimate source: the fear of death. And what is the most common death in the world? Death from hunger. When you train your body to sustain itself on little food, and that food comes from easily attainable trees and plants, you will let go of this strongest of all fears. On a Quantum Eating regimen, it almost feels as if your cells begin to vibrate at a higher frequency and that you are sustained by sun energy. You feel indestructible.

The next most common death facing humankind is death from sickness. Quantity-controlled, highly nutritious eating can remove this vulnerability as well. Quantum Eating leads to relinquishing the fear of death from illness — a marvelously liberating experience.

The idea of physical immortality comes from Leonard Orr, the author of *Breaking the Death Habit,* and was further developed by Mony Vital in his book *Ageless Living: Freedom from the Culture of Death.* Leonard Orr suggested the concept of physical immortality as the philosophy of the "living." Physical immortality might not be literally achievable, but then, not every useful goal *is* literally achievable. It must be convincing. The more you believe, the longer you will be able to practice it. The idea is to aim high enough and not *plan* to miss the mark. The expected effect is: "Reach for the Moon and you will end up among the stars!"

"In truth, one can never achieve immortality — one can only practice it and live it to the fullest extent of possibility. You cannot purchase, it, keep it, defend it, protect it, or win it. It is an ongoing knowing and state of mind you can choose to practice throughout life." — Mony Vital, *Ageless Living: Freedom from the Culture of Death*

I have not graduated to the physical immortality mentality as of yet, but I have been practicing the "Think Ageless" attitude for quite some time. As with physical immortality, you cannot achieve it, but you *can live* it. Some of you probably would disagree and tell me that for decades you had a refrigerator magnet that says *I like the older woman I'm growing into* and one that says *How dare you think I would rather be young!* These are the best comforting sentiments our culture of death had come up with, and they do seem to ease the aging process. But no matter how cute they sound … let them go! You can do better than that!

Whatever you are thinking is what you will invite into your life. If you think you are aging, the mind accepts this and creates the "hard" evidence to match the descriptions and images you have given to it. If you are terrified of gray hair, flab, getting old, becoming feeble or diseased, losing mobility, you are *inviting* these frailties into your life. If you concentrate on pain, aging, wrinkles, you begin to *see* them.

Robert Anton Wilson in *Quantum Psychology: How Brain Software Programs You & Your World* quotes a study that shows that those who score high on "mental health" generally have a number of illusory beliefs: overly positive views of themselves, convenient "forgetting" of negative facts about themselves, illusory beliefs about having more control than they do have, "unrealistic" optimism about themselves and about the future in general, and an "abnormal" cheerfulness.

Give up your thoughts of aging. The fear of getting sick and not being able to afford doctors is a big percentage of our fears for the future. Since you are the creator of your own reality, aging by default occurs when you are unconsciously giving thought and attention to things like retirement, doctor's check-ups, and hospital insurance.

"Dying is no way to live," says Leonard Orr, author of *Breaking the Death Habit, The Science of Everlasting Life.*

Give up your death-thinking. Planning for your retirement is manifesting that you are insecure and you do not trust that you can make it on your own. It is believing that you will be decrepit and debilitated. Buying a cemetery lot is expecting death in the not so distant future. And your body is listening. It will obey your thoughts and make sure it happens exactly as you plan. Instead, think: There is no physical necessity for retirement in your future, and no death, because you are *not* getting old, sick, or debilitated.

When my editor, Bradley, read the previous paragraph he made a note for me: *you make it sound like you are dis-*

couraging 401(k) plans. And I am, in a way! No matter how much you achieve, no matter how much you earn, no matter how much you learn, and no matter how much you save, if you waste your body — the only home on earth you have — you have nothing. I believe that your knowledge, your money, and your possessions must first be used to ensure health. Fortunately your body needs so little.

"The best retirement plan is to be so healthy that you never need to retire. — Susan Schenck, *The Live Food Factor: A Comprehensive Guide to the Ultimate Diet for Body, Mind, Spirit & Planet*

No child plans for retirement or buys a cemetery lot from his piggy bank. The idea would never cross a child's mind. This is how we should feel. Quantum Eating will provide a high frequency vibration — the sheer joy of living. All you have to do is to go along and not allow your peers to drag you back into the culture of death. Do not think about sickness or death. Do not plan for it, do not provide for it, do not even joke about it. The subconscious has no sense of humor. If you need to make a joke, say you will live forever.

These statements to your subconscious need to be delivered verbally, directly, precisely. Any ambiguity can lead to misinterpretation. English is a difficult language. It is always the "little words" — the articles, prepositions, etc. — that make the language difficult for non-native English speakers like me. Consider that you are dealing with your body from the perspective of a second language. Be very careful about the "little words" when you are talking to it. Be sure it understands. If you are not a member of Mensa, your subconscious probably isn't either.

"The U.S. Constitution says we are innocent until proven guilty. Be immortal until proven otherwise!" — Leonard Orr, *Breaking the Death Habit, The Science of Everlasting Life*

You can create your own reality even if you do not realize that you are doing it. Your new reality can occur intentionally or by default. If you know your thoughts and deliberately focus them toward what you really want from life, then you are the purposeful creator of your own reality. Your desires and thoughts are vibrations. You can use them to create your own health or sickness through your single-mindedness.

During your transitioning to raw foods, watch your thoughts. Since raw foods change the body dramatically, try to be in a state of continuing admiration. Appreciate what is happening in your body, even if this includes some of the temporary negative side-effects of the transition, such as headaches, nausea, dizziness, or other detox symptoms. Be grateful for the experience of cleansing and purification that your body is going through.

When we *expect* to be healthy, health tends to win out. When we *expect* to be beautiful, our features become transformed. Vibrational resonance will be established with the exact match of what you wanted. Predominantly thinking about health and non-aging allows your body to reshape itself and to build internal health. Expect health, expect to stay youthful, expect to live a long life, and you will have it all. Talk about health, about Rawsome beauty, about staying fit and being immune to time. The details work out differently — but the final result is very much what you'll have thought about. Your life may not be appreciably longer, but you will appreciate it longer.

If you continue to experience pain, it is because of your own resistance. Eckhart Tolle, in his book *Power of Now,* points out that all suffering, excepting mental-emotional pain, is due to resistance. For example, my husband suffers from low-back pain. Every day that we are on the road, he drives me to some Bikram yoga studio in the area we are visiting. He waits in the car for ninety minutes and then spends the next ninety minutes complaining about how boring it was for him. The solution for his pain is right there, but he refuses to join me, day after day. There is a reason why you are reading this book, so do not resist the information — act upon it.

"The yogi cannot be afraid to die, because he has brought life to every cell of his body. We are afraid to die, because we are afraid we have not lived. The yogi has lived." — B.K.S. Iyengar, *Light on Life, The Yoga Journey to Wholeness*

Remember Mary Carson from *The Thorn Birds* and her indignation: "Old age is the bitterest vengeance our vengeful God inflicts upon us." We are not guilt free ourselves. Most of it, we do to ourselves. Aging is not something that happens to us as to an innocent victim. Aging is something that we, collectively and individually as part of humanity, bring on ourselves by violating God's given natural laws. And the fact that we cannot stop aging entirely doesn't mean we should not take responsibility for trying to slow it down.

As I turn fifty, my friends, family members, and acquaintances speak about ills and getting old. There are so many books, songs, and movies that talk about old age and the sadness that goes with it. While living Quantum Eating, this part of the culture becomes incomprehensible. Because *your* forties, fifties or nineties do not feel or look like *their* forties, fifties or nineties. You cannot relate to their stories. All you see in them is unnecessary suffering, self-indulgent drama, self-imposed limitations. You see clearly that the source of all these attitudes is sheer ignorance. And wise old age does not look so wise anymore.

My father-in-law almost lost his sight to diabetes. At sixty-nine, he is in poor health and acts as if he is well ready to "shuffle off this mortal coil." He shared with us that he often dreams that he is energetic and running his business. The saddest thing, he says, is to wake up an old man. When I hear it, I inwardly want to scream: it does not have to be this way! In contrast, with the raw foods lifestyle you will experience surges of energy that you have never known before, no matter what your age. You will no longer have to wear old-age glasses, to have old-age pains, or have old-age thoughts.

George Bernard Shaw who was a frugal vegetarian eater, lived to be ninety-four. When asked about his youthfulness at age sixty-eight — "So be a good fellow and tell me how you succeeded in remaining so youthful?" — Shaw replied, "I don't. I look my age. It is the other people who look older than they are."

While writing this book, I was invited to be a keynote speaker at Hallelujah Acres. I was delighted to finally meet the legendary Rev. Malkmus, who at the time was seventy-two. He walked as though suspended an inch above the ground. He was like an electron on the stage — one moment here and another there. He was the embodiment of a swirling energy field. One unmistakable impression Rev. Malkmus projects is that he is one happy man!

Follow the Quantum Eating principles and you will never experience the longing of an old person recalling a long-vanished youth. You'll experience no shudder of regret, no sorrow shaking your whole being, because you'll still be *experiencing* your youth. With the raw foods lifestyle, you feel like an alien observing people from another planet, from the perspective of a civilization far more advanced. The

Quantum Eating lifestyle will make you marvel at the intelligence possessed by the body God gave you. You do not feel nostalgic about your youth, or regret the years' passing. Instead, you enjoy the present to the fullest.

My disability made me a warrior. I came in fighting; I fought all the way, and I am still fighting. After I succeeded in walking without a limp, I knew I could do *anything*. This was the most liberating event in my life. From that point on, everything became possible. I believed I could do *anything*, and amazing things began to happen. The skilled people I needed to fulfill my aspirations entered my life. These were who people who not only helped me, but brought out the best of my talents. Guess what? Even my dream to have long straight hair and a small waist, just like Jane Seymour's (silly me!), came true, thanks to raw foods.

Using the Law of Attraction, you invite into existence (and, more importantly, into your personal realm) whatever you are concentrating on. *Want* that dream. Give it more energy than a passing whim; make it the object of your *intense* focus, pulling it into your circle of being and bending it to your will. Focus your desires on your coming years of health, Rawsome beauty, and youthfulness, and these will become reality. Remember … everything is possible!

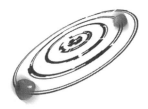

Chapter 29
Simplify Your Life!

"Any so-called material thing that you want is merely a symbol: you want it not for itself, but because it will content your spirit for the moment." — Mark Twain

Several years ago, Paul Nison, author of *Raw Life,* visited Memphis as part of his book tour. I helped to organize a presentation for him to speak to our local raw food support group. It was the second time I'd heard him speak, so I was familiar with parts of his lecture. But this time there was a new topic: he was talking about his overpowering desire to simplify his life. He was talking passionately about how wonderful it is to lead a simple life. How he gave away most of his possessions. How he stopped watching TV entirely. Everything he owns is in his van. I remember finding it all interesting and peculiar, but I did not internalize that part of his message at all. I was sure this was something that was never going to happen to me.

In my internal monologue, I even had an explanation: Living most of my life in constant scarcity of even the basic necessities had produced a natural, psychological response that evolved into the belief that having plenty was a necessity. After all, as an immigrant, I was a part of the most ambitious population, those who strive to achieve and collect material possessions. For us newcomers, success in America was measured by acquired possessions. In our extended family, almost every conversation is about how much it costs and how to get it. God forbid if someone outruns you to the store.

Fancy furniture and accessories were important to me. I wanted to impress, to show off, even to have the neighbors envy me. Little did I know that the raw foods lifestyle was going to change all that. It would, in fact, reduce all my pretensions to zilch.

Seven years into the lifestyle, I got interested in yoga. One of the yoga books I read said this: "The yogi reduces his physical needs to the minimum, believing that if he gathers things he does not really need, he is a thief." When I read this passage, a light went on, and I went on a mission to get rid of everything I was not using.

I believe reading is one of the great joys of life. It doesn't matter whether it's a novel or a biography, a health book or a bestseller — curl up with a good book and it's sheer pleasure for me. I collected books all my life and I brought hundreds of books from Russia to America, only to discover that no one in my household reads them. English books took their place. While in the mood to clear out everything which I don't use, I donated all my Russian books to the local Jewish community, where people from the former Soviet Union can read them. The fact that the books are used gives me more pleasure than when they collected dust in the house.

I used to collect picture frames. Everywhere I went, I bought a nice picture frame. Then I completely lost interest in collecting things. The unadorned present became the most important entity. I gave all my picture frames away as gifts.

My husband watched in horror as furniture, china, skillets, pans, and cooking paraphernalia disappeared from the house. At the time, he resented my throwing away everything he'd worked so hard to obtain. But as I write this book, he has been 100 percent raw for five months. An interesting thing is happening: The man who hoarded junk in the garage has joined me in throwing out things we don't use.

The raw food lifestyle has brought many psychological changes as well. I am detached from my past and, if I visit it in my thoughts, it is more for the lessons I've learned and less for cherished memories. It feels like I am examining someone else's life. Letters, memos, and souvenirs from the past mean less than they once did. Memories mean more than physical objects. I do not collect anything these days. There is no identification with mere "things" — no matter how "precious," materially.

Our own body is the only thing we own in this life. We may not want even to call this *ownership* — it's temporary, more like *renting*. Indeed, Christians and other theists will recognize that God actually owns these bodies we're using. We came with nothing and we will leave with nothing. *Stress-free* is the only way to live that passage in the middle. Simple living is so unassuming. Things don't impinge on or disturb your inner spirit.

The stewardship of material things is far more stressful than you realize. My dear editor, Sharon, has become the guardian of several generations of her family's mementos and now is concerned about who will continue to cherish these things when she is gone. She may never be a complete advocate of the plain life — "I'm not Amish," she insists. But she is gradually separating herself from much of the burden that time has asked her to shoulder.

Just as one should not take things one does not really need,
so one should not hoard or collect things one does not require

immediately. Neither should one take anything without working for it or as a favor from another, for this indicates poverty of spirit. The yogi feels that collecting or hoarding of things implies a lack of faith in God and in himself to provide for his future." — Christina Sell, *Yoga from Inside Out: Making Peace with Your Body through Yoga*

A raw food lifestyle will create a desire to make life simple. You do not feel the loss or lack of anything. You get this reassurance that everything you really need will come to you by itself at the proper time. *God will provide* takes a whole new meaning. You learn absolute surrender to God for what is necessary for your continued survival and serenity. The things we have are for us to appreciate, not to cling to. Only when we use our possessions for our good and that of others will we add to rather than detract from our happiness. You learn how to be satisfied with what you already have. Soon you will see that what you already have is too much, and you'll willingly give it up in the name of sharing.

The correct attitude to our "possessions" is gratitude, not ownership. — B.K.S. Iyengar, *Light on Life: The Yoga Journey to Wholeness*

You will gain the ability to distinguish the real from unreal, the eternal from the temporal, and blissful existence from passing pleasure. The raw food lifestyle brings calmness and tranquility. Quantum Eating will only intensify this feeling.

Therefore I say to you, do not worry about your life, what you will eat; nor about the body, what you will put on. Life is more than food, and the body is more than clothing. Consider the ravens, for they neither sow nor reap, and have neither

storehouse nor barn; and God feeds them. Of how much more value are you than the birds? And which of you by worrying can add one cubit to his stature? If you then are not able to do the least, why are you anxious for the rest? Consider the lilies, how they grow: they neither toil nor spin; and yet I say to you, even Solomon in all his glory was not arrayed like one of these.
— Luke 12:22–27

After I had been on raw foods for some time and was, by then, eating very little, the full meaning of this passage hit me like a brick. Before, it would not have made sense. How could it, with all the cooking and the fear that you will never have enough?

The Jesuit Alphonsus Rodriguez gives a powerful illustration in regard to the virtue of simplicity: "A religious person ought in respect to all the things that he uses to be like a statue which one may drape with clothing but which feels no grief and makes no resistance when one strips it again. It is in this way that you should feel towards your clothes, your books, your cell, and everything else that you make use of ..."

I used to watch *Law and Order* every day. I was addicted. I ate my second meal and watched. I was convinced that this was my relaxation time. However, there always seemed to be distressing interruptions. Because good news is no news, the media rushes to every mishap, tragedy, and disaster. A steady diet of such terrifying events ultimately takes a toll on mental well-being. Your conscious mind knows that you are not going to perish in the teeth of a TV vampire, knows that your couch keeps you safe from train wrecks and cars hurtling off seaside precipices. But your subconscious signals its distress and contributes to your insecurity. Watching the pain of others disasters reminds you that you, too, are vulnerable. The result is a kind of emotional pollution.

As if tornadoes, hurricanes, floods, and criminal behavior were not distressing enough, TV commercials make the raw foods lifestyle very difficult. Constant food commercials bombard you between the small-screen cliffhangers. It's an interesting dialogue between television's entertainment and commercial faces. Your favorite TV detective takes a hit. *My goodness — will he make it?* Suddenly, you're visited by the Keebler® Elves, tempting you to console yourself with chocolate chip cookies.

One day I'd had enough. Who said I have to have a TV in my living room? All of a sudden, I saw the absurdity of these social norms, because you take the artifacts in your living room to be more real than the relations, mental clarity, and serenity of your inner life. Why *does* the TV have to be in the living room? I realized that, when it is there, you watch TV by default. You watch because it is there and everyone does it. Move it out of the high traffic areas and into a room where you have to go looking for it, and you will forget it is even there.

After I took our bed out and started sleeping on the floor, moving the TV to a free bedroom was not much of a stretch. I did not plan to stop watching TV, it just happened. "Out of sight, out of mind" was never more appropriate. Making a special trip to a separate room just to watch TV seemed frivolous and time-consuming. And this is one of the best things that could have happened. Now I eat outside, in total awareness.

For me, breaking the TV addiction was the easiest. Just putting it out of sight in a separate room took care of the problem completely. Now I almost never watch TV unless the program is really good or my husband needs my company. The frustrations, violence, and fear emitted by this box do not attract me anymore. Of course, there are good programs and movies, but nothing that I cannot get from books or by going to a movie theater once in a while. To stay away from the disturbances this box emanates will keep the mind in a state of equilibrium.

As you grow into your new persona, it will be necessary to let go of all your bad and painful memories. You may not be able to forget them, but you should absolutely not dwell on the negative. Try to detach yourself from these old memories.

At one point in my life, I reached a plateau where my legs did not improve, no matter how much I exercised. I kept asking myself: *Why?* The answer came very unexpectedly. During one of my regular phone calls to my mother in Russia, she mentioned with pride that she had kept every scrap of paper, every x-ray from my childhood, documenting all the surgeries, endless doctor visits, and all their reports. She had also kept all of my letters from long hospital stays.

I shuddered.

I pleaded, "Mom! Please! Do me a favor — make a big bonfire in your back yard and burn everything."

It was as if I'd asked her to sacrifice her firstborn child. She felt very sentimental about this whole repugnant collection. She said she looked at this treasure occasionally and cried as she remembered how much I had gone through as a child. It took me a good forty minutes to convince her that it was time to get rid of that stuff. After she did what I asked, my progress in walking and yoga began improving exponentially. This is one of many events in my life that have made me a believer in the ability of our thoughts to create our reality. All these records of my pain and suffering and my Mom's crying over them were creating so much negative energy that it was literally keeping me bonded in my limitations.

You are a spiritual being, first and foremost. You are energy. Center all your thoughts on the necessary or essential. Material possessions in excess of immediate necessities nail you to the ground, lower your vibrations and complicate your life. "Raw and low" eating, if you are not aware of it yet, will introduce a much greater presence within you. Its growth and development will become your biggest concern.

By simplifying your life, you attain a peace which takes you beyond the short-lived pleasure material possessions provide. Success is not measured by what we accomplish or what we purchase. Our success is measured by the moments of joy we experience during our life. Do not fret that you do not have all the material possessions people are expected to accumulate in your life. Ultimately, they are nothing.

Drugs, loveless sex, eating, alcohol, shopping, television — these are just a few of the shortcuts people use to feel good. Our culture feeds the belief that we can rely on shortcuts to happiness, joy, and comfort just by swiping a credit card, picking up the phone, logging on to eBay. On the Quantum Eating program, you realize that a healthy body offers almost unlimited potential for pleasure. The raw food lifestyle will reveal to you that the way to real abundance is only through moderation and contentment.

I am not talking about depriving yourself of material goods that contribute to your pleasure. I love nice clothes. However, we usually wear only 20 percent of our clothes 80 percent of the time. Now my closet is 80 percent less full. It feels great! A friend adopted a practice from a wealthy aunt: Every time she bought a new dress, she donated an old one to charity. The raw food diet makes people generous, compassionate, and indifferent to competition for power and material possessions.

If we are never content with what we have, we will always be poor. Contentment is the key to becoming rich. We become rich by restricting and adjusting our desires, not by letting them loose and chasing after them.

Practicing Quantum Eating, you will realize that you are rich beyond all belief. Your real value is in who you *are*, not in what you *have*. We usually think about acquiring material possessions to secure the future. It means that we do not trust the future to live up to our expectations. I am learning that the less I possess, the more freedom I have to move, to relocate, to go places, to do things unencumbered by my physical surroundings.

When you begin to enjoy *not* eating, you will begin enjoying space and silence as never before. You will come to see material possessions as a major obstacle to growing spiritually. At the same time, do not launch an inquisition against the material acquisition of others. This is a very personal matter and can be resolved only by individuals when they are ready and feel compelled to make changes.

An ancient Taoist adage advises: "Those who strive for longevity should maintain the 'Four Empties.'" The Four Empties are your biggest aid to helping you succeed in Quantum Eating. Here they are, in what I think is the most natural order.

Empty Kitchen. Do not keep enough food in your kitchen to feed your family three times a day through the next ice age. You've seen it — people on TV, given a snowfall warning, hysterically load up their shopping carts ridiculously full. On the raw foods lifestyle, your cupboard is always so bare that the running joke among your friends would be that if they visit you, they had better bring their own groceries. Keeping an "empty kitchen" motivates you to shop more frequently and encourages purchasing fresh, raw foods. This is a variation of the European tradition of shopping at fresh food markets daily, as opposed to the American practice of loading cupboards with processed foods so laden with preservatives that they'll outlast most marriages.

Empty Stomach. While practicing Quantum Eating, your stomach remains empty, yet you do not feel hungry. When faced with the question of to eat or not to eat, you'll have no Hamlet's dilemma. Most of the time, you'll choose not to eat.

Empty Room. Clutter drags your energy down. Clutter and stagnant energy go together, they feed on each other. If you look at a disease as an obstruction of energy, then clutter is to a house as toxins are to the body. Don't you feel good after a good household cleaning? This feeling is real. Because clutter frustrates and irritates like nothing else, you yearn for comfort food. When your space is organized, you eat less. So, clean up your space, if for no other reason than to limit your eating. When you are surrounded by things you use or cherish, the house is a haven that offers you support.

> "I like to say that I provide pain relief to people whose lives are cluttered with too much stuff. Getting your office organized can give you peace, serenity and can really simplify your life."
> — Patty Wolf

Is your house cluttered or treasured? Do the clutter test. Ask yourself two questions: Do I love it? Do I need it? No other reason is good enough to hang on to anything. What if I need it later? Remember — you create your own reality. Whether you cling to it or give it away gracefully will determine the end result. If you let it go thinking someone else will appreciate it more, you won't ever need it again. Try it. You will see — it works!

Does it give you a good feeling when you look at it? If not, it has to go. Keep nothing that you associate with painful memories. By eliminating the things you do not like or use, you invite harmony into your life. On the raw foods lifestyle, you will become a different person and you will not need mementos to remember happy times. Nothing compares to how you feel now. Your belongings must reflect your present state. If your only pleasure is in the past, you need to re-examine your entire mental attitude.

Empty Mind. You need to rest your mind. Even during the sleep, the mind keeps churning out random, often fantastic, thoughts in the form of dreams. It never shuts down. Like a computer, it goes on standby — everything is still running in the background, but the screen is blank. An "empty mind" is the ultimate goal of meditation. Many meditation books tell you that you can begin meditation immediately to relieve stress. However, I agree with B.K.S. Iyengar's observation that true meditation "cannot be done by a person who is under stress or who has a weak body, weak lungs, hard muscles, collapsed spine, fluctuating mind, mental agitation, or timidity."

If you think meditating means just learning to sit quietly, think again. You deal with stress by learning how to relax your brain. Only then will meditation be possible. You need to achieve this state as a foundation for meditation. Physical and mental weaknesses have to be eliminated to prepare you for meditation. Raw foods bring your body to a superb condition and make you ready for the "fourth empty." When you get rid of junk food and junk stuff, you will be free from junk thoughts. Keeping your mind free of mental clutter is the best rest you can give it.

Do not dwell in the past or the future — only the present. Try to keep your mind free of needless worry about the future. This mental pollution will drain your vitality. The future will definitely come, but it can be enjoyed only as present. Face the present and deal directly with present realities. Try to be "here and now" at all times.

If, in your mental dialogue, you are telling me that, like Sharon, there are collections from your grandmother that you simply will never be able to let go, please understand that I am not urging you to do it. All I am saying is that if you stay on the raw food lifestyle, especially as you go "raw and low," as with Quantum Eating, that is what is going to happen. You may not get rid of your grandmother's china, but you might decide to use it and get rid of your own. I promised to tell you what to expect. You will want to simplify your life more than anything.

I might sound to you just as Paul Nison's message sounded to me at the beginning of my raw food journey. *Not me!* you may say. If you don't connect with the feeling and emotions I've described here, that's absolutely okay. But when it does happen, don't tell me I didn't warn you!

Simplify.

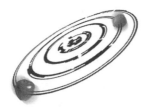

Chapter 30
Sunning and Mooning

My son got his driver's license when he was 15, about eleven years ago. His very first week of driving, the police called to say he had been detained. My husband and I are Russian — we don't take calls from the police lightly! I was frightened. Then embarrassed. You see, the officer had called to tell me my son had been stopped because a policeman in a patrol car had observed somebody's bare butt sticking out of the back window of *my* car. I was now beyond fear and embarrassment. I'd moved straight to mortification.

Fresh from the Old World, I'd never heard of such behavior. In Russia, we didn't let our teenagers drive — no such thing as a "spare" car for us. Driving, in Russia, would have been such an honor that any 21-year-old allowed behind the wheel would have put a professional chauffeur to shame. My imagination ran rampant. I thought about how horrified the drivers in the other cars must have been at this shocking display of flesh.

I tormented myself with questions. Where did I go wrong? Am I a failure as a mother? My one consolation: My sweet son Nick Jr. was the one driving, so it couldn't have been *his* posterior exposed to the blazing Southern sun for all to see.

Things couldn't get worse, I thought. I was mistaken. My darling son, my pride and joy, showed not a hint of remorse! Being the worldly American teenager he now believed he was, he told me quite matter-of-factly that this is what American boys do … for recreation, no less! There was even a name for it, he said. They called it "mooning." Coming to grips with such a revolting rite of passage, I had to admit that I could certainly see how a large circle of shining flesh could be called a "moon" — smooth, glowing, and wrinkle-free!

This regrettable little slice of American Pop Culture 101 comes to mind whenever I see a midlife baby boomer zooming about in a convertible with the top down. Here is another cultural peculiarity I can never understand. I find it unnerving that this sight always triggers this association, but at the same time, I do like the term "mooning" — I can see the connection.

From the beauty perspective, exposing your face in an open car with the sun glaring down and gas fumes smothering your pores is an even more absurd practice. Your face is another body part you want to keep from the open car window and sun unless you want it to look like a desiccated prune.

Do you ever feel a twinge of envy for these men and women in their open Ferraris? Don't! I can't help feeling sorry for such folk. They are trying to recapture their youthful image — an entirely human and understandable thing to hope for. But the fact is that every prolonged exposure to direct sun inevitably results in wrinkles and spots that totally destroy the very illusion they're trying to maintain. We don't want our faces to get wrinkles. But think about this: Our butts never do!

The reality is that excess sunbathing turns your skin into "beef jerky." Under sunlight, plants develop precious substances through the chemical reactions of photosynthesis. The gentle peach and the broad, robust banana leaf, the delicate fern of the Amazon and the dark, hidden violet of the Congo jungle floor, the windblown grasses of the African veldt and the Great Plains of the North American continent, given consciousness, would all acknowledge their debt to the sun. All of these plants depend on the sun, and all "know" how to live with the sun, unharmed by its rays, indeed thriving because of those rays from the star which gives us life. Sun doesn't hurt the gentle leaves of trees or the delicate petals of flowers. So what's gone wrong with us humans? Why does it seem the sun has turned against us?

Medical and health professionals have begun, in recent years, to demonize sunbathing. Sunshine bears the blame for all kinds of evils, putting it on par with booze and cigarettes as the enemy of long life and good health. *Damage ... danger ... protection* — thcsc are the kinds of words that "pop medicine" applies to the sun, as if it were inherently like some kind of enemy marching toward us, intending to mount a siege. We blame freckles, liver spots, red blotches, wrinkles, and dryness on the sun. And the older we get, the more ammunition we use against the sun.

I abhor the phrase "sun damage." The sun *per se* does not create these problems. Toxins present in the body are what does the damage. The sun did not *create* skin damage, but simply made it visible. That's what light does — it makes us *see!*

"Unless one has a proper diet, sunlight has an ill effect on the skin. This must be emphasized: sunbathing is dangerous for those who are on the standard high-fat American diet or do not get an abundance of vegetables, whole grains, and fresh fruits. Those on the standard high-fat diet should stay out of the sun and protect themselves from it, but at the same time they will suffer the consequences of both the high-fat diet and the deficiency of sunlight." — Dr. Zane Kim, American nutritionist and sunlight therapist

Light gives luminosity and warmth. But there is so much more to sunlight. Light is life itself. The discoverer of Vitamin C, Nobel Prize winner Albert Szent-Gyorgy, said, "[A]ll the energy which we take into our bodies is derived from the sun." His studies furthered the belief that humans are actually living photocells which gain energy and nutrients from sunlight. Plants find their most powerful supplies of "negative entropy" in sunlight. Plants store energy through photosynthesis. Humans and other animals absorb and assimilate this energy when they eat plants.

Solar energy makes us whole, as do the plant foods we eat. When we consume and digest any plant, it is metabolized on an elementary level into carbon dioxide (CO_2) and water. However, the sun energy that is present in photosynthesis will be utilized by our body. It is possible that when we eat plant foods, we take up the photons of light and store them. We extract the CO_2 and eliminate water, but light, an electromagnetic wave, becomes the source of energy for all the molecules in the body.

And God said, "Let there be light" — Genesis 1:3a

Matter is not converted energy — it *is* energy. Einstein's equation, $E=mc^2$, means that any piece of mass or matter is energy that can be calculated by multiplying that mass by the speed of light (300,000,000 meters per second) squared. We are literally made up of light. How come? Sunlight is non-material, right?

The first sign something was wrong in Newtonian paradise was the discovery that something was missing in our mechanistic picture of light. How did the sun's light and heat reach the earth? We talk about light as being dually particle and wave. Often, the grade school or first-year college science teacher introduces the wave concept of light by analogy with waves in the ocean. The trouble with this analogy is that an ocean wave travels through water. The ocean wave *is* water. The wave of sunlight travels 93 million miles to reach the outer limits of earth's atmosphere, but it doesn't travel *through* anything. It's fairly clear, when we think about sunlight, that there's no observable trail of particles tracing a path between the sun and earth. The space between the sun and the earth is empty (compared, at least, with the ocean), but somehow heat and light from the sun can travel, as waves, without there being any appreciable substance to make waves *in*.

But waves must move through *something*. They don't travel in a vacuum. This was obvious to the scientists of the nineteenth century. They had found that when they placed a ticking clock inside a glass container and gradually evacuated the air, sound waves vanished as soon as a vacuum formed in the enclosure. Sound waves travel in air. Not light waves! Quantum physics confirms that sunlight — electromagnetic radiation — is special. In fact, in the subatomic reality, many paradoxical situations originate from the dual particle/wave nature of light. Light can take the form of electromagnetic waves or of particles.

Newtonian classical mechanics describes matter in motion as a continuous chain of changing positions. An object moves gradually from one position to another. Quantum mechanics shows that things move by "jumping" from one place to another — without necessarily ever appearing anywhere between the two places. It's counterintuitive, at first. It seems so uncertain. But it's true. There is so much we don't know about sunlight.

Now may be the time to return to an older way of thinking. The Greek sun god, Apollo, was also the god of medicine. His temple at Delphi carries two valuable inscriptions for a healthy life and a healthy attitude toward the sun: *All things in moderation* and *Know thyself*. The Greeks worshiped a god of medicine because, since earliest Greek Classical times, they practiced some form of healing and preventative medicine.

So with the Romans. Fresh air and sunshine were the Roman sources of good health. But with the fall of the Roman Empire and the subsequent rise of Christianity, Europe abandoned sunlight therapy — not because it didn't work, but because the sun had served as gods to the Greeks and Romans (as to the Egyptians before them). The sun thus became, in the southern European Christian mind, a pagan evil. Still, European society remained largely rural for a long time. Lacking strong interior lighting, most people got a fair share of the sun simply by working outdoors, without deliberately sunbathing. Mere circumstance thus forced a certain level of sun exposure.

Things continued more or less in this way until the nineteenth century, which saw the Industrial Revolution and the advent of electric power. The sweeping effects of Edison's technology and subsequent change in lifestyle gradually brought people indoors, spending more time away from exposure to full-spectrum sunlight. Even so, until antibiotics arrived in the early twentieth century, medical people and popular writers alike advocated sunlight and fresh air for improving general health and as cures for such diseases as tuberculosis. Post-WWII prosperity allowed Americans to afford health care, and it became commonplace simply to take a pill for whatever ailed you.

The sunbathing panic started with malignant melanoma and the great scare that equated sun with the occurrences of this life-threatening skin cancer. Further studies, however, have shown that sun exposure doesn't necessarily increase the risk exponentially.

Current studies quoted in the books *Light Medicine* and *The Healing Sun* are also starting to show that sunlight — in moderation — is both healthy and necessary to human well-being. Benefits once again, we're told, outweigh hazards. And while melanoma is a real threat, the death toll from non-melanoma cancer is much lower than that of the death rate of, say, breast cancer (which is now believed to be partially prevented by a sun-nourished body). It may just be that more people die from the lack of proper sun exposure than are felled by too much sun.

Dark-skinned people experience less risk of melanoma from sun exposure. But they, too, suffer from melanomas. So other risk factors must be involved. Current research even suggests that countries with more reliance on sunscreen have a higher instance of melanoma.

It may be that even the current predilection for UV 400 (ultraviolet-blocking) sunglasses is doing us more harm than good. The inability of the cornea and retina to receive the necessary light energy to stimulate brain function and release hormones within the cell structure may be causing blindness and eye disease rather than protecting against it.

Even beyond this, more researchers are discovering that our eyes have not only a perceptual function, but an absorptive one: Not only do they see, but our eyes also absorb light and energy from our surroundings.

"The lamp of the body is the eye. If therefore your eye is good, your whole body will be full of light." — Matthew 6:22

The endless poets and philosophers who have considered the eyes to be the "windows of the soul" and a bridge between the physical and the spiritual worlds would be heartened by today's findings concerning the importance of light.

The eyes not only send images to the brain but also stimulate the hypothalamus gland, which is responsible for secreting serotonin — the mood and sleep regulator for the body. This is why bright artificial light has come to be used as treatment for SAD (Seasonal Affective Disorder, a form of depression caused by lack of sunlight during winter) and is recommended for everyone during long, dark winters. Even small adjustments in light level can profoundly affect health and well-being. It is becoming more and more obvious that we are truly creatures of the light.

Sunlight carries nearly the full spectrum of light, but its energy peak is highest at the blue-green end. Common electric light, by contrast, is weakest in the blue-green range. Ultraviolet light is a nutrient the body needs. Nonetheless, UV rays are currently demonized by modern science. Scientists have said UV has caused cataracts and skin cancer in lab animals. Such studies may involve too much attention to extremities, however. Scientists' proclivity for giving lab rats cancer with everything in the known universe is rarely offset by explaining that the quantities required to create such effects in humans would be massive.

Healthy humans also need vitamin D, which the body manufactures using sunlight. The label *Vitamin D* is something of a misnomer. D is not technically a vitamin, but actually a hormone capable of being produced by the body. It is this ability to produce its own D that allows the body to fight, and in some cases prevent, degenerative and infectious diseases. The body is better able to use the D that it produces itself rather than the D it ingests (in, for example, popular vitamin pills). The sun's ultraviolet rays activate the body's production of this hormone, which in turn is necessary for growing healthy teeth and bones, and for a healthy immune system. In the final analysis, we are much more likely to get sick from too *little* sun than too much. (Science hasn't studied, incidentally, the effects of exposure to moonlight. Depending upon what you mean by "exposure" in this case, however, I urge you to consult again the cautionary tale at this chapter's beginning, and in particular the possibility of police involvement.)

The mainstream medical and cosmetic advice for your face is: "Protecting it from the sun is of utmost importance. So, avoid the sun and apply a good sunscreen — the most important product to use." I agree with the first point. I quite disagree with the latter.

Though manufacturers promote using sunscreens as a public health measure for preventing skin cancer, there are good grounds for avoiding sun blocks. The introduction of sunscreen in the '60s allowed people to stay out longer without burning, but offered no protection from what really causes skin damage and early wrinkling. The idea behind sunscreen is that the SPF (sun protection factor) permits a person to stay in direct sunlight in direct proportion to the SPF indicated. Suppose in a given setting you'd sunburn in, say, an hour. A 15 SPF allows you to stay out 15 hours before burning. But there is evidence that prolonged exposure of this kind may actually increase the risk of both melanoma and non-melanoma skin cancer.

Use common sense as your sunscreen. Do not overexpose. Be aware that the majority of suntan lotions use PABA,[1] which the FDA has warned can be carcinogenic in the sun. PABA, while it is used to block UV rays, can also

---

1. *PABA stands for para-amino-benzoic acid and works by absorbing UV rays in much the same way as oxybenzone.*

cause genetic damage to the DNA, which in turn can stimulate the growth of cancer cells.

Instead, build up your exposure *gradually*. Your skin will darken naturally. By giving your skin a chance to adapt slowly, it will release the proper amount of melatonin to adapt to healthy exposure without burning.

Eating plenty of fresh fruits and vegetables helps your skin to adjust to sun exposure, making sunburn less probable. Careful! You can't switch to raw foods for a month and bake beside a Las Vegas pool all day with utter immunity. Humans may be simpatico with plants, but none of us is a saguaro cactus! We thrive on *partial* sun. No matter how well we eat — which in this book means how raw, how lightly, we eat — we still must and do eat. *Whatever* we consume, we will still carry *some* toxins in the body. Too much exposure to UVB radiation will bring these toxins into play. We release a lot of toxins through the skin. Sunlight greatly accelerates this process. Toxins are drawn to the surface, and if there are too many of them, they will be fried. That is what "cancer caused by the sun" actually is. If not cancer, then the result will still be what we call "premature aging."

I'm sorry to bring up the subject again so near to the end of this chapter, but consider: Buttocks do not get wrinkles! I do not think many of you use sunblock on your own posteriors. Faces are different. Since you want the same smoothness for your face that your bikini-bottom region already possesses, keep your face covered! Exposing the rest of your body to the sun is actually a very healthy thing — and an absolute necessity once you embrace a raw food lifestyle.

Many young raw food promoters passionately advocate nude sunbathing. Some even perform nude scenes in nature on national TV and, by association, scare "proper" folk away from the raw food lifestyle forever. Ten years later, I'm still not sufficiently "liberated" to embrace nudism. I may never be, and dearly hope that widespread "mooning" will never become *de rigueur* as a sunbathing technique. If you're an "old fashioned girl" (or guy) like me when it comes to nudity, let me assure you that *partial* sunbathing will give you all the benefits of sunlight you'll ever need.

I make sure I get at least fifteen to thirty minutes of direct sun exposure every day. Usually I get just a dash of partial sunbathing early in the morning when I have my morning vegetable juice outside in the yard. As for our faces, however, a return of ladies' hats would be the best thing that could happen on the fashion scene! When you wear a hat, your eyes will still get enough indirect sun.

Get your exposure in the early morning or late evening, when it is not so bright that you need to wear sunglasses. If you wear tinted sunglasses, get gray ones. They offer a better light balance. Avoid pinks, blues, and reds. Tinted contacts hold the same dangers of unevenly balanced light. If you can find your way around the block safely, do not wear your contacts or prescription lenses. "Let the sun shine in." Treat sunlight as the most important non-food factor in your raw food lifestyle.

Some spiritual leaders encourage us to develop a conscious relationship with the sun and the moon. One of the spiritual practices is watching the sunrise. The claim is that it gives you vitality and strength that lasts all day. Another spiritual practice is staring at the moon. There are spiritual leaders who believe that staring at the moon can heal all the diseases of the mind and body. Would one call such a practice "mooning"? Too bad the name is taken.

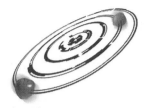

Chapter 31

Go Raw and Meet Your Destiny

Most yoga practitioners have a mantra which is, at most, a few syllables long. Not me. Mine goes like this: *If you have not achieved your optimum health and appearance, you have not met your destiny.* Like mine, your destiny may be elusive. I strove to be a teacher. For many years I studied mathematics. I was good at both learning and teaching. However, the more education and degrees I attained, the fewer students I had in my classroom, and the more unhappy I became. Only after going 100 percent raw did I finally discover that what I really wanted to do is motivate people to be the best that they can be. I like public speaking, especially making people laugh. I wanted to be in front of people. My subconscious sent me signals, but I misinterpreted them. After my surgeries corrected my limp, and after I greatly improved my appearance as the result of raw foods, I became more confident and was able to realize my heart's desire.

Life's goal is to fulfill one's intended destiny, a destiny that will make the world a better and safer place. The yardstick of success in life is not money or possessions. The real yardstick of success is how many exhilarating moments make up your everyday existence. You have to be your own person. It is only by reclaiming our dignity that we find our destiny.

The challenge of finding that person when you eat cooked food is that you are affected by artificial stimulation. There is the difference between being drunk and sober. A drunk is not a true representation of the person when sober, though elements of that original person remain. Cooked food affects the psyche in a similar but subtler way. You do not have drunken blackouts but you will raid the refrigerator when you have no business doing so. Your mind is impaired. You are not yourself.

Once you have control of your body and its aging process, you will realize that Quantum Eating is not just about eating, not just about staying youthful, but goes much deeper. Quantum Eating can be the beginning of a whole new experience. It can raise your spiritual consciousness to perfect harmony with your Creator. You begin to *feel* that God's love is the underlying fabric of the whole universe.

Quantum Eating snaps you out of the dull, debilitating habit of waiting for your life to begin. Practicing Quantum Eating will create a sense of peace in your heart, a feeling of security about the future. You'll feel no foreboding about the future, no pain from the past. You anticipate the excitement of every new day. You gain a sense of direction in life. You will know the right steps to take to achieve fulfillment and joy in your life.

My husband once listened to *How to Make Money in Real Estate* and promptly declared that he'd always dreamed of being a landlord. I am big on fulfilling dreams — if not mine, then someone else's. I got involved in real estate to fulfill *his* dream. To my dismay, he misread his feeling! He hated being a landlord, and I was stuck with handling the rental properties and dealing with tenants. How many of you out there have found yourself trying to fulfill someone else's dream, a dream dumped on you because the other person did not know what they really wanted to begin with? Learn from my mistake: Try to help people realize their dreams through encouragement, but be careful not to become a horse in their stable.

I would place an ad to rent a place, but when the phone rang I would think: *Oh, no, not another prospective tenant!* I was writing my first book then and wanted most of all to be left alone. The thought that I had to leave my creative work on my book to show the property was so disruptive. While everyone else got rich in real estate, I only succeeded in becoming a complete flop. Prospective tenants probably picked up the negative vibes I was sending, and I had a very hard time renting our properties. I drove them off through sheer ill-feeling. However, all the hardship I had to endure dealing with tenants is a topic for another book, *Stay Out of Other People's Dreams* (which I am never going to write).

I was gloriously happy to see those properties out of my life, even though we sold at a loss. I have never been sorry for the money we lost, but I sincerely regret the eight years of my life I spent doing something I had no business attempting in the first place. The raw foods lifestyle will help you to avoid such situations. You will clearly see why you are here and what you should be doing.

We have a tendency to put limitations on ourselves. Our accomplishments, our physical body, our creativity — every aspect of life has an upper limit that we feel we do not have the knowledge, confidence, or ability to achieve. Now, on raw foods, all barriers are down because it is not solely your doing. There is a greater power, a greater force, a greater love supporting you.

By embracing your right to be healthy and beautiful, by discovering the powerful self-confidence that comes from knowing yourself, this lifestyle will make it clear to you who you are, what you're here to do, and why it's important. Not only your body, but your values, your perspectives, and your aspirations will change. While you are on cooked food they are like a broken compass, always pointing the wrong direction. On raw food, you will become inner-directed, following your own heart. Fulfilling your destiny becomes the *raison d'être* behind each step you take.

I know why I am here — to encourage people. Inspiring people to achieve their better selves is the only gift I have in abundance. God made sure I learned firsthand from a variety of hard experiences preparing me for my life's mission. When you are mapping the path of your destiny, you operate as a living entity without limitations.

You owe it to yourself to find out who you really are. When you eat cooked food you are standing outside the boundary of understanding your essence. Raw foods will help you to cleanse yourself and ultimately realize who you really are. Quantum Eating is bringing the body to a place of awareness, to a place of knowing the truth. You will act and think and speak from that designated place.

My convictions were focused and reinforced when I read, *Personality Types: Using the Enneagram for Self Discovery* by Don Richard Riso with Russ Hudson. This book was recommended to me by one of my readers. I was especially interested in how the Enneagram (a nine-pointed geometric figure) was used to describe nine personality types. It was Pythagoras who first believed that the geometric figures, the Enneagram in particular, could be used to describe any natural phenomenon, any piece of knowledge. Geometric figures provide a workable topology which offers elegant representations of living structures. Modern research confirms that in all of science only mathematics is a match for quantum reality.

At the same time, I was never able to find a clear fit in any of the studies about character types, temperament types, body types, blood types, etc. Having failed miserably to fit into *Eat Right 4 Your Type,* I approached this book with suspicion. But there I *found* myself! I am a Motivator.

I recognized myself immediately — it was an epiphany. Still, I was not ready to accept the book as entirely right. The results, I thought, could be mere coincidence. I applied the book to everyone I knew well enough to serve as a subject — especially my dear husband, because after thirty years I had to know him better than complete strangers in a book. To my surprise, the book described him better than I ever could. Our lives would have been much simpler and serene if I had known all of these things about him from the start, instead of lurching through life by trial and error.

In this book, the descriptions of the personality types range from the highest levels of health and integration to the lowest depths of neurosis. The Enneagram allows fluidity to show how one personality can integrate with other types and move between the subtypes. There are three subtypes: healthy, average, and unhealthy. The most interesting observation I made after I checked it on everyone I knew was this: On the raw foods lifestyle, people's personality characteristics would shift into the healthy subtype, even if they initially showed traits from average and unhealthy subtypes. Not only does your health improve, not only does your emotional state improve, but you actually become a better person. The raw food lifestyle is bound to effect a change in the moral structure of one's personality. After going raw, read this book and you will be pleased to recognize yourself in a healthy subtype.

What you are meant to do in life doesn't have to be heroic. In fact it can be humble, but it is still an important piece in life's puzzle. As Helen Keller said: "God has given each of us a task which we can perform better than anyone else. We must find out what that task is and how to do it in the best way possible." Whatever limitation we have, it comes to full fruition in some extraordinary ability within us. In other words, whatever your weakness is, remember that you are blessed in equal measure by some other quality which you have in more quantity than anyone else. And, rather than being distressed by your liabilities, search for what is special in you, what only you possess, what you were compensated with, because for everything we have been deprived of, we have been given something else.

Successful people know how to put their strengths to use. Happy people know how to put their weaknesses to use. Your strengths predispose you toward a certain vocation in life, but it is your weaknesses which make you indispensable in your chosen work. You are a special human being, and the greatest thing you have to offer the world is *you*.

To earn your living without compromising your ideals of good, love, and compassion is a blessing you will strive to attain. Your vocation is right if it does not require you to take a vacation from your conscience while performing your obligations. If you do not know what you should be doing in life, it is because you do not have enough information. Read, learn … and everything will reveal itself.

The most important thing for us to remember is that we are nothing but energy. Learn as much as you can, but then trust your intuition. When one follows the natural order, acting spontaneously and trusting the future is the best reward. God's will is done though physical laws and psychological interactions with other people. You will almost feel with your sixth sense what situations to avoid and which person is there for you to learn from.

Ask yourself a question: Does your chosen work come easy, does it bring joy and satisfaction, or does it feel like you are carrying a heavy burden? When work is an extension of your lifestyle, work becomes joyful to perform. Your vocation is rewarding and fulfilling. There should be no struggle, no sacrifices. You may be very busy, but you enjoy every minute of it. It becomes an avocation because you do not want it to end. You are less concerned with the final result of your actions and more with your accomplishments in the present moment. What tempted you into that pursuit is the exhilaration you experience when you're doing what you were entrusted to do.

When you honor your physical body as a living temple and you do not engage in behavior which sacrifices its integrity, your public image and inner presence will converge. Getting ahead, seeking recognition, distinguishing yourself in any way becomes of no importance. Using your talents and position to make a contribution to a better world assumes primary importance. You will gravitate to the job that is directed toward helping or serving other human beings, helping others to change and move in a direction that will transform their lives for the better.

"He who, forgetting self, makes the object of his life service, helpfulness and kindness to others, finds his whole nature growing and expanding, himself becoming large-hearted, magnanimous, kind, sympathetic, joyous, and happy; his life becoming rich and beautiful." — Ralph Waldo Trine

Spirit is the breath of life. Spiritual moments occur when you feel God's presence in a way you've never experienced it before. This is when you feel more alive, more real, more authentic, more your true self. We are also totally aware, not only of where and who we are, but also why we are.

Archimedes said, "Give me a place to stand on, and I can move the earth." There is actually a place for you — a place where you can change the world and make a profound difference in people's lives. There is for you some unfound field where all of your talents will be sown in fertile ground, producing a marvelous crop. *Here* is the place where you perform the utmost service to humankind and fulfill your purpose. You will actually receive occasional confirmation, through the feelings of excitement or elation, that you are in the right place, doing the right thing.

We receive guidance from a higher level. We have spiritual input to help us make difficult decisions, to guide us through tough times, to give us inner peace. Do not resist going in the direction life is pulling you and you'll achieve the energy level that synchronizes with your destiny. When you find your place in the world, you are likely to feel a sense of ease, contentment, and satisfaction.

Here is where your energy will peak. Here is the realm of maximum excitement, where you will be launched like a rocket. Seek out the direction that raises your vibrations, that gives you more energy. *That's* where you need to be. *That's* where you need to go. That's the place where your power to "move heaven and earth" resides.

If you ever get the feeling you're in the wrong place in life and you should be doing something different, then you *are* — and you should! The raw food lifestyle will make things crystal clear.

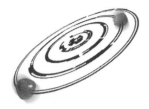

Chapter 32

Supplements or Stimulants?

Many people want me to sell their supplements on my website. Some can be very forceful, assuring me that theirs is the most natural enhancement and will give me the most energy. I am safe from these temptations — this very promise turns me off like nothing else.

To promote such elixirs of youth, the ads will say: "Declining energy is at the root of numerous problems associated with aging and reduced quality of life." They have it backwards: It is the numerous problems associated with aging that lead to declining energy.

Let us look at two real things that promote health and longevity that have been around for many centuries — fasting and yoga. What does fasting do to you in the beginning? It actually makes you miserable because you must endure detox symptoms. The same thing happens with raw foods. What happens when you drink a big glass of vegetable juice? You feel a buzz, accompanied by some dizziness. Sometimes you will feel like lying down for a few minutes. Boundless energy, lightness, and good moods all come later. The same thing applies to practicing yoga.

Bikram's words are repeated day after day all over the country in his famous Bikram Yoga Studios: "Welcome to the

Bikram Torture Chamber! Kill yourself for 90 minutes, so you will have a healthy body for 90 years!" and the other "What would you rather do: suffer for 90 minutes or suffer for 90 years?" And oh! how good you feel 20 minutes after you leave the Chamber!

Consider the following scenario: Your body has no energy. You are sick and tired. Your system is full of toxins and is fighting degenerative conditions. Now you take a supplement and all of a sudden you feel great and have a lot of energy. What exactly has happened? The toxins are still there, the degenerative problems are still there, but now, for some reason, you feel great. It is because you whipped your body to work. You pushed it to perform. You forced it into submission. You made it "behave" with the ingredients present in supplements. If they were as natural for your body as raw foods, you would have to be sick and tired before the rush because the toxins have to be eliminated first.

Long term health must be earned. There are no shortcuts. No magic pills. Everything that promises quick and easy ways to energy is an *artificial* stimulant. Stimulants are like bank loans — the body always pays interest.

When something wholesome and natural is artificially concentrated, it automatically becomes a stimulant. Any natural product can be turned into a stimulant. Just remove some water and you get a stimulant. Some, of course, are milder than others and do not contain toxic substances. But they still give the body unwarranted energy. Why do you think a whole fruit or vegetable has a particular water concentration? It is because that is what our body requires. Nothing concentrated grows for our immediate consumption. Wholeness is present only within the defined boundaries of apples, carrots, celery, and the like.

The consistency and shape of the vessels in which nutrients appear are essential. Nutrients are fleeting. Air, heat, and light destroy nutrients. The moment an apple looks like anything but an apple, at least some of its nutritional value has been lost. The best way to maintain nutrition is by biting into it. Even when we cut it, some nutrients are lost. You cannot encapsulate whole foods. The moment concentration is changed it is no longer whole food.

Supplements you take for a long time will always throw your body out of balance. When you take supplements, there is so much to remember. You need a degree in nutritional science to use supplements safely. Some vitamins and minerals interact with one another, or with other medications, decreasing their effectiveness. Calcium and iron, for example, if taken in separate pills, should be taken at separate meals. If you take thyroid medication, you should not take calcium or iron at the same time. When it comes to micronutrients, more is not necessarily better, because too much boosts your risk of potentially dangerous side effects. Too much zinc, for example, can lower high-density lipoproteins, "good" cholesterol. Too much vitamin B_6 may cause numbness in the legs and other neurological symptoms. Taking potassium supplements without medical supervision may be dangerous. When you eat raw foods you do not have to worry about any of these problems. Trust your body — it knows best.

We trumpet the benefits of supplements in uniform tablets, capsules, and potions, and we praise science for its ability to squeeze numerous nutrients into them. But the initial fruits and vegetables they used are left without glory. They are spectacularly simple miracles. Take nutrients on their terms, not yours, and you will discover their incorruptible goodness.

Nutrients in a piece of fruit are living and fluctuating. And just as a living entity is characterized by self-organization, nutrients also act as a unit. At the same time, nutrients are open-ended. A continuous stream of information is going not only within them, but also between them and the external environment. Nutrients in raw food interact not only with the cells of your body, but with the air you breathe, the water you drink, and the emotions you experience.

Everything living in nature has a will to multiply, to reproduce — in short, to continue. Fruits that we eat would have continued to ripen if left on the table. Vegetables, if you cut a piece and place it in the ground, will sprout. The seeds and nuts we eat, placed in soil, will reproduce. When you eat something that grows essentially without human interference, the innate intelligence of your body is able to connect with the driving force in the living food and assist your health to prevail. Life persecutes death with all its mighty power. Wouldn't you want to have life on *your* side?

Wikipedia defines life thus: "Life is a condition that distinguishes organisms from inorganic objects and dead organisms, being manifested by growth through metabolism, reproduction, and the power of adaptation to environment through changes originating internally."

Ask yourself the following questions: Will any supplement do any of those things? Will it sprout like a carrot top placed in the ground? Will it reproduce like a raw nut or seed planted in the soil? Will it adapt to its environment? Will it stop ripening when refrigerated, but swell with juice when left in a warm place? The answer to all these questions is obviously "no." That supplement you're about to take is ... dead.

Supplements are conceptual solutions to your well-being. It is a reflection of someone else's brainchild — no matter how vast the intellect, that knowledge is always finite. When the complexity of living is reduced to powder in a pill, it is only an approximation, never *real* life.

There has never been a single supplement that has survived the test of time. What supplement has been around for a millennium, a century? How many even for a decade? None of these highly praised manufactured concoctions are still touted. When was the last time you took *Lydia Pinkham's?* Some company changes a name, shuffles supplement contents, and everything is branded as a new miracle.

Throughout the centuries there have always been people who have lived long healthy lives. But there have always been variables which made it difficult to draw linear conclusions. One century-old individual may have had a shot of whisky and a cigar every day while another never touched either. How can you formulate concise rules, given such inconsistency? The usual claim is that a certain supplement is "the one." Yet there are still people who live long lives without ever taking such an aid. Where's the proof?

It is both naïve and arrogant to dismiss the wisdom of previous generations as superstition while believing that modern scientists with their technological advances are wiser and better equipped to find an anti-aging remedy. Yes, science sent a man to the moon. It had never been done and seemed impossible. But the feat had concrete problems that submitted to technological solutions. Aging is not a problem with concrete solutions.

There are probably a thousand other natural stimulants, whether so labeled or not. Whether caffeine or energy enhancers, they are still stimulants. Though no adverse reactions have been determined for a given stimulant, it may be only a matter of time. If it walks like a duck, quacks like a duck ... well, you get the point!

Say a person is sick and tired and feels like an old horse. She takes a supplement and now she is full of energy. Did she get younger and healthier overnight? Certainly not. She is still an old mare, whipped by a stimulant into perform-ance. Such practices are outlawed in the racing world. So why would someone voluntarily succumb to a practice that the law refuses to allow for an animal? Only because you cannot see the actual whip!

"Our own physical body possesses a wisdom which we who inhabit the body lack. We give it orders which make no sense."
— Henry Miller

Adenosine promotes sleep. Normally, adenosine attaches to special receiving areas on cells, or receptors, and sets off distinct reactions. Stimulants block adenosine, and as a result induce alertness. Animal studies show that adenosine acts on specific receptors that line the surface of cells to induce slumber. Therefore, compounds that block the receptors increase alertness.

Do you *really* have more energy, or do stimulants only make you *feel* as if you have more energy. Stimulants, whether caffeine, guarana (common in energy drinks) or yerba mate tea, all work by blocking the effects of adeno-sine, a brain chemical involved in sleep. When these stimu-lants block adenosine, this causes neurons in the brain to fire. Thinking the body is in danger, the pituitary gland initi-ates the body's emergency mode response by releasing adrenaline. This hormone makes the heart beat faster and the eyes dilate. Most cardiologists will tell you that a burst of adrenaline was beneficial in the days when a person had to outrun a saber-toothed tiger but can actually damage the heart of our more passive, sedentary society. Stimulants also cause the liver to release extra glucose into the bloodstream for energy and affect the levels of dopamine, a chemical in the brain's pleasure center.

All of these physical responses make you *feel* as though you have more energy. However, the increased stamina and "boost" performance that vendors promise is more like a physical "swan song" with the body forced to use its reserves. When the body expels toxins, either through the raw food diet or fasting, the body will experience withdrawal symptoms from internal stimulants and you will feel bad.

Stimulants fall into the category of substances that temporarily increase bodily functions to simulate energy. The quality of this temporary energy burst is artificial, temporary — like the false, brief energy boost you feel in the wake of a highway accident narrowly averted. And about as healthy.

I receive a lot of questions about noni juice, goji berry juice, Mona Vie, and other nutritional supplements that promise unique and exceptional anti-aging results on the body. I have never used these products, so I have nothing to say for or against them. From what I have read about these products, I am sure they can be beneficial for people who eat cooked food. If you absolutely cannot be persuaded to eat only raw foods, you might consider using them.

But the elixir of youth cannot originate from extracts, tinctures, or tonics. Such concoctions are usually made by removing water, producing strong extracts which become stimulants because they are so condensed. The stimulation tells the body to heal here and now in this particular area, or to target particular receptors. Thus, a concentrated potion can be beneficial as a crisis measure, but never as a continuing anti-aging remedy. Such potions encourage the body to work faster than it otherwise would. All supplements increase the metabolic rate — and we already know that this is not the way to achieve longevity.

A supplement or stimulant can help with memory, potency, and energy levels, just as the label promises, but only at the expense of something else. Supplements have their place in restoring your health, but they will not provide long term anti-aging results. They can help to speed recovery in a particular area, but always at the expense of other bodily functions.

Usually, these products contain some rare ingredient: an exotic plant such as a mushroom discovered on the Tibetan plateau, or Brazilian guarana berry, or even Sea Buckthorn berries from Siberia, to bait the hook. I do not believe a loving God is so selective that He has placed the solution for rejuvenation in far away places, inaccessible to most of us. Not that there is anything wrong with exotic plants. In fact, they do have some medicinal properties — my own cream contains Sea Buckthorn oil — but miracles are in *all* living raw foods, not some rare, inaccessible Shangri-la. I freed myself from medical dependence — why would I put myself at the mercy of the merchants of supplements?

"We will never extend our lives significantly, to 150 or 200, by loading ourselves with even the most potent antioxidant supplements. On the contrary, antioxidant supplements might actually make us more vulnerable to some diseases." — Dr. Nick Lane, honorary senior research fellow at University by College London, *Oxygen: The Molecule that Made the World*

Dr. Nick Lane postulates that extra antioxidants may be responsible for cleansing out free radicals that could hurt proteins and DNA, which in turn would weaken the individual cells, affecting the overall strength of the body. It may be also that minuscule doses of toxins present in fruits and vegetables can put the body on emergency alert and cause the production of stress fighting proteins.

Nick Lane, in *Oxygen: The Molecule that Made the World*, writes, "Clearly, fruits and vegetables are filled with goodness; yet, perhaps surprisingly, this is about as much as we know for sure. The depth of our ignorance is conveyed pungently in an article by John Gutteridge and Barry Halliwell: 'Twenty years of nutrition research have told us that, for "advanced" countries, the way to a healthy lifestyle is to eat more plants, a concept familiar to Hippocrates. What it has not told us is exactly why.'"

Natural toxins are found in parsnips, carrots, celery, and other vegetables and greens, toxins such as psoralen, xantho-toxin, and bergapten — three chemicals toxic to humans. The doses are so small that they do not present a toxicological risk to humans. These toxins are designed to prevent fruit from being eaten before it is properly ripe, or even from being eaten at all. The fruit is, after all, designed to reproduce, not to offer nourishment. Perhaps it is the balance of antioxidants and mild toxins that confers the benefits of fruit.

The benefits of fruits and vegetables cannot be reproduced simply by taking antioxidant supplements. In plants, even toxins might be beneficial in the whole realm of things. Plant toxins, if palatable, are likely to have beneficial effects on our immune system. The effect of supplements does not even come close to the benefits of the real thing.

All of our advances in biology and medicine will, in the end, I believe, do nothing more than explain the wisdom of nature. While I was working on this book, a study was published in the *Journal of the American Medical Association* (vol. 97, pp. 842–847) about how antioxidants may be linked to a higher risk of death in the general public and people with certain conditions. A group of Danish researchers analyzing the available evidence on antioxidant supplements found that several of them may be responsible for premature death. They conducted about seventy trials with about 230,000 participants. Originally, the research targeted the question: Can these supplements reduce the risk of cancers in the gastrointestinal tract? What they found, to their great surprise, was a trend toward increased premature mortality. Dr Christian Gluud, head of the Copenhagen Trial Unit at Copenhagen University, says that you "either do not obtain any benefits from antioxidant supplements or that you may bring on hazards by taking them."

When these researchers looked at all the antioxidant supplements together, they found no significant harm, but neither was there a significant benefit. When they subdivided the trials and studied different supplements separately, they saw an increased mortality of about 7 percent from beta carotene, 16 percent from vitamin A, and about 4 percent from vitamin E. They saw an acceleration of atherosclerotic vascular diseases and an acceleration of cancer. The analogy they use is that you're sitting in your car, heading for your final destination, and antioxidants put the pedal to the metal.

Does that surprise you? It shouldn't. Everything that speeds our metabolism will eventually reduce longevity. However, the way the experiment is done is very unfair toward the manufacturers of these supplements. All prescription drugs speed up the metabolic rate. When you take any drug, you are dropping a heavy brick on your gas pedal. If the research were done against control subjects who take medicine, the result would be an increased longevity.

This type of research will allow traditional medicine's dream to come true, providing a reason to set very restrictive standards on the use and consumption of nutritional supplements, resulting in your not being able to buy or consume many supplements without a doctor's prescription. Your right to buy supplements is in danger of being taken away from you. So you may have no choice but to go raw, because even concentrated vegetable juices might fall into this category. How long can it be before medical science decides that there is a dangerous level of beta-carotene in a carrot and it should only be available by prescription? Is this an exaggeration? I can only hope so.

By applying drug-type risk assessment models to nutritional supplements, what the researchers are saying is that the more concentrated a natural product is, the more potent it is, the more it acts like a drug. I wish they would follow this logic all the way to the end and say that since cooking removes water and concentrates natural products, it too acts like a drug. But that is only a wish. They will never carry their logic that far: Eliminating cooked food would reduce the need for medicine for most degenerative conditions. Subsequently, doctors would become educators instead of prescription writers. Medicine and supplements have their place in *some* situations, to be sure. But they *always* work against longevity and negate anti-aging benefits.

I recently read promotional copy advertising for yet another miracle anti-aging supplement. The ad copy said: "It has been known for years that we need at least ninety nutrients to maintain our health. These nutrients include a minimum of seventy minerals, eighteen amino acids, and three essential fatty acids. To obtain these nutrients we would have to eat at least fifty-seven different sources of food each week."

This is not exactly the case, as shown by C.L. Kervran in his remarkable book *Biological Transmutations*. After presenting numerous relevant experiments and analyses, the author discusses the special property that living organisms have — the ability to transform not only molecules, as chemistry shows, but atoms themselves.

Life cannot be entirely explained in terms of the laws of chemistry and physics. In chemistry, it is assumed that during chemical reactions nothing is lost, nothing is created. Transmutations are rendered impossible! In accordance with the Second Law of Thermodynamics, energy always breaks down, there is only positive entropy. Life defies these laws.

C.L. Kervran talks about a famous experiment conducted in 1600 by Flemish chemist Jan Baptista Helmont. He planted a willow sapling in a clay pot containing 200 pounds of oven-dried soil. Over some five years, he watered the tree with nothing but rain or distilled water. By the end of the experiment, Helmont removed the tree and weighed it. It had gained 164 pounds, while the weight of the soil remained approximately the same. The plant obviously turned water into wood, bark, and roots.

He goes on to quote another observation which is irregular from the chemical viewpoint. French chemist Vauquelin documented the fact that chickens which receive only grain for feed produce more calcium than they ingest. The eggshell they produce is composed of more calcium than is contained in their feed. Chemically, this is impossible, unless the chicken is able to produce calcium within its own system whether or not it consumes it.

There is no limit to what living organisms can do. There *is* a transmutation of matter: One element changes into another. The human body is a skilled alchemist. It cannot turn dross to gold. But it can turn almost anything it is given into a life force.

One experiment that C.L. Kervran quotes is particularly relevant to me. He writes: "Dr. Plisnier cities in particular a case of a person over sixty years old who had a fracture in the femur neck. The classical methods of treatment had failed to heal it, in spite of two operations and a diet rich in calcium. A specially formulated diet, poor in calcium, brought about a recovery." This is what happened to me after my hip replacement operations. Green juices and salads made my bones heal very quickly, *without* my consuming any traditionally calcium-rich foods.

"Hundreds of experiments in reputable laboratories undoubtedly demonstrate that transmutations of atomic nuclei occur in living matter. It may be impossible, but it seems to happen. Sodium changes to potassium, calcium to potassium, and vice versa. In certain cases, silicon plus carbon gives calcium." — Jerome Cardan

---

The miracle of the transmutation of elements is closely tied to the miracle of life. Possibly, it is more apparent when the body is cleansed from all the toxins.

Scientists seeking magic nutritious potions are searching in the wrong places, the wrong ways. Great anti-aging benefits lie not in getting *more* nutrients, but in being able to clean your body to sustain itself on less. Whatever we do eat has to be the most wholesome and nutritious food, because we can get away with eating less of it.

Health is a state of mind that guarantees that the thought of "popping" a supplement will never cross your mind. Health is energy with no ointments, potions, or poultices. No supplementation is needed for the healthy body to feel great. If you are not energetic, you are not healthy — taking a pill is not going to change anything permanently.

The only way to get pure energy is to remove toxins. Cleansing the body of toxins can be quite unpleasant. Therefore, raw foods and fasting have a redemptive quality attached to them. After an initial low, they deliver a blissful high, but not before! First, you actually *pay* for all the abuse you put your body though. Everything that gives energy without cleansing to make the body healthier is a stimulant.

There are cases of deficiency when supplements can be very beneficial. Some supplements, such as those in the "Super Foods" category, have been praised highly for their health benefits. I will not tell you not to use them — just do not tell me they are better than the real thing.

Women often ask me about natural hormones. So-called bioidentical hormones were promoted by Suzanne Somers' book *The Sexy Years.* At fifty, I do not have any menopause symptoms. My near vision is perfect; I sleep like a baby, and I have never had hot flashes! I do not understand what all this fuss is about. When women go raw, hot flashes, irritability, breast tenderness, water retention, and sleeping disorders all disappear or never start. However, programming is hard to overcome. I know women on raw foods who have none of these symptoms but still think that they might *need* to take *natural bioidentical hormones.*

I cannot say whether bioidentical hormones are helpful or not. I do not know; I have never taken them. I will only tell you why I never considered using them. Let us get it straight: Suzanne made a decision to take natural hormones because she had every menopause symptom in the book. And the "healthy cooking" she promoted before her fascination with bioidentical hormones apparently did not help.

These hormones are supposed to be much better than the synthetic estrogen from horses' urine. Bioidentical HRT is synthesized in a lab, made from plant extracts. (They definitely have more cachet than Premarin®, which is made from mare's urine!) The claim is that bioidenticals replicate exactly what our own bodies produce. So? Just because the body produces it, should we conclude more is better? How presumptuous to think we know how much the body really needs and are qualified to increase natural quantities.

Hormones, natural or synthetic, were never meant to be introduced into the body in the form of a cream, pill, or anything else science might think of to make a buck. Such intrusive methods create an imbalance in the natural order.

Premarin®, for example, introduces a foreign substance into your body. Premarin® is for horses — and you aren't one of those! The body reacts as it often does, by increasing its reaction through inflammation. After extensive studies, medical science concluded that long term usage in women could contribute to heart disease and Alzheimer's.

In Somers' book, she indicates that, at one point in her life, she was extremely stressed. Her hormone levels needed to be kept elevated, so her doctor kept changing her doses, yet her hormone levels stayed the same. Her body was absorbing it. When her stress stopped abruptly, the hormones level was too high for her. All of a sudden, the results were a high estrogen effect and excessive bleeding. Suzanne called the doctor who decreased the doses and got things back in balance again.

Her doctor explains how the hormones work: "If you wake up in the morning and your thinking is a little foggy or uninspired, and you don't feel motivated, then you would take a little more of the estrogen cream. If, however, you wake up in the morning and you are a little uptight, and your breasts are tender, take minimally less." Suzanne enthusiastically concludes: "We are doing this in concert together, and it helps me to feel that I am in control of my health and my body."

In control? Not the way I see it — this sounds to me more like being on a leash. She drives three hours to see her doctor to see if she's foggy or uptight. Did she consider that there might be other factors at work besides her hormones? Maybe the big premiere the night before accounts for some foggy-mindedness, or a quiet night in is responsible for being alert. Who wants to let your doctor and your hormone level conspire to dictate every mood swing? How about the occasional chorus of "So you had a bad day"? When you are truly in control, you do not need anyone, least of all a doctor, to make you feel great.

Her doctor says: "The beauty of bioidentical hormones is that they talk to you: if you give too much, you have side effects; the same goes for testosterone, DHEA, HGH, thyroid, and the adrenal hormones." No wonder she's confused — all those initials-only hormones shouting from the peanut gallery!

Let me remind you what Jesus said, "It is not the healthy who need a doctor, but the sick." I do not want to visit a doctor, or call a doctor, or even think about doctoring as a profession on a regular basis. I certainly don't want to depend on them for a drug prescription or for adjusting my hormone levels by administering "natural" hormones that need endless monitoring. In fact, I do not want to depend on *anyone* else to stay healthy. Can you blame me?

It is economical to be healthy. When you are healthy, you do not spend money on medicine, doctors' visits, therapy, or supplements. It is a great feeling to have the final say in the health, well-being, and destiny of your body.

Formerly, women were treated with Premarin® alone. Then medical science discovered that many developed breast cancer because the hormone created a dangerous imbalance. Thousands of women died. Now, they claim, they have it right: In the physiology of the body, estrogen always goes with progesterone. Let me suggest a possibility: in the physiology of the body, estrogen always goes not only with progesterone, but also with numerous other interconnected things that they will be discovering for years to come without ever discovering everything.

"No amount of moral fiber, scientific creativity or natural intelligence could have elaborated, from first principles, antibiotics, or steroids, or azathioprine, or indeed virtually any of the cornucopia of discoveries of medicinal chemistry. They were rather 'gifts from nature,' profounder and more complex than human knowledge at the time, and even now, can comprehend." — James Le Fanu, M.D., *The Rise and Fall of Modern Medicine*

Do not let the word *natural* confuse you. When anything natural is isolated and concentrated, it becomes foreign to the body. Cortisone is secreted by the adrenal gland. Mind-altering chemicals such as cocaine and morphine are from 'natural' sources. Aspirin is made from the bark of the willow tree. Drugs like actinomycin and vincristine, and many others, including antibiotics, are all 'gifts of nature.' These are all drugs with serious side effects.

At least eight of the body's major hormones produce less with age, such as human growth hormone (HGH), the sexual hormones (testosterone and estrogen/progesterone), thyroid, insulin, DHEA, melatonin, erythropoietin (EPO), and pregnenolone. The theory is that replacing all or some of these hormones to their original levels will slow or reverse the symptoms of aging. If only it were that simple!

Artificial replacements restore youth the same way that a "trophy wife" restores an old man's libido. In either case, the restoration is temporary, often requiring progressive upgrades to higher dosages or even younger wives until the doses are harmful and the wives are barely legal. But, in the long run, these 'youth' remedies will bring him down. Artificial levels of hormones can damage the body the same way a young wife can damage. In the end, the side effects must be given as much consideration as the benefits.

Suzanne titled the book *Sexy Years,* putting the emphasis on women regaining their sexuality. As estrogen levels go down, testosterone levels go up, and during menopause a woman goes from being loving and sexual to being moody and bitchy. Or so the common thinking goes. Some menopausal symptoms are definitely caused by changes in the woman's body, but much of it may be part of a self-fulfilling prophecy. How much sexuality and sensuality is lost may have more to do with the partner than the woman.

After being together for thirty years, Nick and I are experiencing the best time in our marriage. (The fact that he has been 100 percent raw for several months now has helped. In fact, gentlemen, it will *always* help when you come around to your beloved's point of view.) During the last ten years I have been raw, he paid me many compliments and was impressed by my transformation. Now his transformation is so remarkable that I keep exclaiming: "How good you look!" All of a sudden I am experiencing renewed deep, loving feelings towards him. (Especially, when he withstood incessant temptations while visiting his friends and was able to get them interested in raw foods, not the other way around!) Of course, my getting my own way *always* makes me warm and fuzzy. Our attraction is mutual and without artificial aids. (I only hope that when you are reading this book, Nick is still raw and I will not have to eat my words. There's too much starch in book paper. Besides, it's cooked!) Nothing will revive a relationship better than going raw together!

All these hormones are intended to simulate a calorie-restricted diet. You can get all the benefits by going straight to the real thing — "raw and low" instead of pills and shots! Calorie-restricted monkeys do not show the steep declines in hormone production. The lure of these calorie-restriction mimetics (CRM) to gullible people amazes me. They will do anything, pay any price except to eat less. The simplest, most effective, and, finally, the cheapest solution of all.

One scientist I saw on TV takes 120 pills because he believes that anti-aging research is on the brink of a breakthrough within fifteen years. As dedicated as I am to youth, I would never swallow 120 pills loaded with who knows what unknown toxins daily, especially for perhaps a decade and a half! Convert to raw foods. Let your body decide in its own time and its own way what to rejuvenate and in what order.

Menopause should give pause for thought. And one of the most useful thoughts we might have could be this: In seeking control of our health, what counts is: when we go raw we must trust our body. We must never let our inflated egos substitute our limited knowledge for the innate wisdom of the body. Our fragmented, vestigial knowledge concentrating itself on a pill or cream will be disastrous for this partnership sooner or later. It always is. At first, it might seem that we are smart enough to figure out what hormones or nutrients the body needs, but in the long run, we will create an imbalance and all the problems associated with that imbalance. I believe it is the body that has the ultimate knowledge and it is not our job to put in our two cents worth.

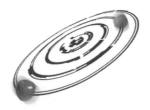

Chapter 33

Crossroads in Searching for Superior Health

I started a raw food support group in Memphis several years ago. One day a gentleman who had read about our meetings in a health food calendar joined us. He said he was fifty-four. He looked super fit. His black with a touch of silver hair was braided in long, thick strands and the whites of his eyes were dazzling. His dark olive complexion was glowing. With such radiance, I was sure the guy could read books at night with no lamp. I obviously went on a fishing expedition to find out what was responsible for such a picture of health. To my surprise, he told us he has been a fruitarian for thirty-five years. He even gave me his theory of why only two types of nuts — pine nuts and black walnuts — qualify for the fruitarian lifestyle.

Members of our support group who had learned from most raw food books and particularly from me that eating greens was absolutely essential on the raw food lifestyle started to rebuke him that all his teeth were going to fall out if he did not start eating greens. He gave us his dazzling smile, revealing all thirty-two teeth intact, and he never came back. He certainly left many questions in his wake and I wish I'd had the chance to learn more from him. He evidently didn't feel that we had anything to offer him.

Do you think he was going to change? I don't think so either. I never felt more ridiculous. Just remembering this episode brings embarrassment. A few facts we did learn about him summed up to the following: He lives in a remote Tennessee village. He had never been sick in his whole life. He never read a book about raw foods. In fact, he used to think he was the only one in the whole world who ate that way. In short, nobody told him it couldn't be done. Now he had the power of his own experience to back him up. I still believe most people cannot make it on the raw food lifestyle eating fruits only. However, this incident taught me never to be rigid in my statements: Sometimes, the reality of someone's experience will teach us that we can be just plain wrong.

Many people complain that the information in different raw food books is conflicting and contradictory. They complain of confusion when they are looking for simple absolutes. I do not believe anyone who writes a book about raw foods is intentionally misleading. They share their experience. Contradictions are an inherent part of life in general and health in particular.

There are people who can live on fruit alone and be healthy. There are others who eat almost no fruits, eat mostly greens, avocados, nuts and seeds, and also experience exceptional health.

Dr. Doug Graham has helped many people on high-fruit, low-fat diets. Gabriel Cousens, M.D., is leading people to health on green salads, green juices, flax seeds, and very little fruit. Brian Clement, at his Hippocrates Institute, helps people to cure themselves of cancer and other serious degenerative conditions on green juices, wheatgrass juice, and absolutely no fruit. There are also private clinics where people are curing themselves of the same conditions on fruits alone, such as watermelon or grapes.

Contradictions? Not really. Only quantum physics at work. Also, I think there is one common thread: It shows that all living raw foods have the power to cure.

Jay Kordich promotes juicing; Victoria Boutenko loves green smoothies. Jay will give every reason why *removing* fiber helps you to get more nutrients. Victoria, on the other hand, gives valid objections on why *preserving* fiber is necessary. Do they confuse me? No, because I do not expect them to give me the absolute formula for *my* best health.

By emphasizing one particular side of reality, they create their own "truth," and it will remain "their" truth as long as it works for them. Every book, especially non-fiction, no matter how objective an author attempts to be, is propaganda — or, at least, subject to criticism. This book is no exception. It is okay as long as you do not place impossible demands upon it to provide you with absolute truth, and as long as you, the reader, are doing your job — to sort things out. Make it right for yourself.

Another example. Meditation is good for your mental health. Stopping your feverish, compulsive thinking for even a little while is very beneficial. Short periods of time when the mind is undisturbed by thought or emotional upheaval are highly beneficial during our hectic lives. How can it possibly hurt? Well, it can! Alan Wallace in *The Attention Revolution* gives an account of a man who decided the ultimate goal of meditation was to stop thinking entirely. Taking the practice to such an extreme, eventually he "didn't think" himself into a vegetative state and had to be hospitalized.

In Russia, we say a fool can whack his forehead even while praying. Some intellectual effort is necessary to reflect and interpret the advice you receive, and especially the results you are achieving. Each person has to reach optimal health through his own individual efforts and creativity.

People often ask me to give them a detailed program of my daily schedule, so they can duplicate it. I am glad to share my experience, but you'll find it a hundred times better to get your own. What is good for me might be too extreme for you. Alternately, your body may soar to heights beyond my results, and my guidelines, if held to rigidly, may limit your growth. There is no one absolute truth that will fit us all. You have to find your truth anywhere between two extremes that work. If this is confusing, sorry — that's the beauty of the world we live in.

I find that some individuals promoting raw foods object to juicing as not being natural. I keep Rawsome beauty as my lighthouse. I make all of my raw food decisions by how healthy they make me look. Appearance is my judge and the mirror that will let me know if there are any excesses or deficiencies in my diet. Yes, I am against cooking, but I would never criticize any raw foods. I never say that I am unconditionally opposed to fresh juicing, greens, fruits, seaweed, or even dry fruits. It all depends where you are on your health journey.

My approach to the optimal raw food diet is based on health conditions shown by appearance. Traveling around the country on my lecture tours, I meet many people who practice raw foods to some extent or another. Several years ago I began a personal experiment on the effects of juicing. I wanted to see if I could identify people who were juicing regularly based solely on their appearance. I am almost always right, because juicers have a certain glow. In short, people who juice look better than people who criticize juicing. I have been juicing for ten years, and it has served me well.

I believe that juicing closely mimics the natural process of juice and pulp separation that begins in your mouth. When we eat fruits or vegetables, we first bite into it, then we masticate. Chewing separates the juice from the pulp. Juice will pass your throat first. If you chew properly, fiber will pass the throat a few minutes later. The nutrients in freshly-squeezed juice will enter the blood almost instantaneously. Fiber, which is indigestible waste, ends up in our feces. We need fiber, no question about that. But chewing hard vegetables and greens all day long will wear out your teeth and place unnecessary stress on your digestive system.

Because I juice, I do perfectly well on two small meals per day with some fruit in between. I do not need to eat a lot of fruits and vegetables to meet my nutritional needs. Having a green smoothie as my second meal provides me with the best source of minerals, vitamins, protein, and fiber. And eating fresh fruit gives me abundant energy.

To come up with one recommendation about raw foods for everyone is a noble object, but any attempt to do so is bound to fail miserably. It ignores the reality of the world we live in, a reality governed by the law of opposites. Whether you choose to implement the information in whole, or to research further, or to test the plan partially, whatever you do will eventually become your reality. By making choices, we create the present we live in.

I cannot take responsibility for your health and well-being. Nobody can, but you. I can only tell my story, detail the books I've read, and convey the feelings, thoughts, and sensations I've had. From that point, take it or leave it. In either case, the results are entirely yours. Let your Rawsome beauty be the guide if you are moving in the right direction. The journey to health is self-exploratory, but the ride is exhilarating nevertheless.

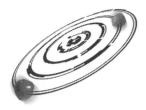

Chapter 34
Recipes:
Energy Meals that Buzz with Power

Just two months before going to publication with *Quantum Eating,* I asked the subscribers to my newsletter to share their favorite recipes with me to use in this book. Because this book addresses an advanced raw food lifestyle and the *highest* possible level of health, I asked that the recipes include no soy products, oils, mushrooms, or any items that must be marinated or dehydrated. The response was great, as you will see from the recipes submitted on the following pages.

These recipes share a theme: *simplicity*. Every recipe included is extra nutritious and easily digested. But there is still room for "quantum leaps" in development. When you decide to take your raw food lifestyle to the "Quantum" level, you should omit certain ingredients. That is why in some recipes, you will see the notation "for Quantum Eating, omit or substitute...." The purpose of this is to help you modify the recipe so that you can take your raw food diet to the advanced level. On the Quantum Eating level, sea salt, spices, olive oil, and even water are omitted or substituted.

Do not ever feel guilt about not reaching the Quantum level at the first attempt. The recipes in this book are very good for your body. So I recommend you use them in their original version first and proceed with Quantum options only when you are ready. Have fun with these recipes and enjoy every step of your journey.

Quantum Eating is very advanced and very simple at the same time. With a little mindfulness and creativity, you can create simple, delicious recipes that will bring your health and anti-aging results to their highest level possible. With all of these variations, your choices are endless. At the same time, remember that the use of fewer ingredients gets us closer to a mono meal (eating one type of fruit or vegetable at a time) which is the ultimate ideal. Less *is* more.

Thank you to everyone who took the time to submit their recipes and share their thoughts with the world. You are an inspiration to me and others as we follow you into the tasty realm of raw foods.

Note about water: *In some of the recipes, water is an ingredient. For Quantum Eating, you will want to substitute it with either fruit or juice. Appropriate substitutes include fresh watermelon, tangerines, pineapple, or coconut water. You can always substitute fresh vegetable juice, as well.*

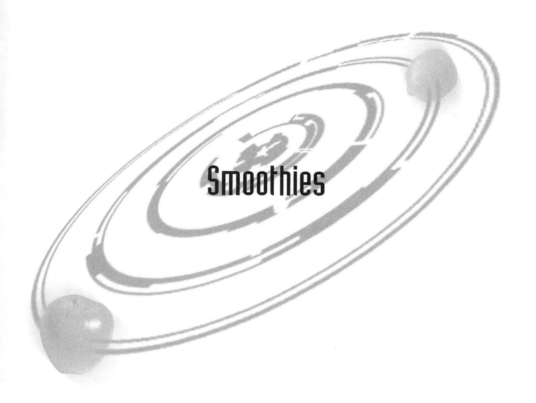

Smoothies

Iced Chocolate

Susan and Les O'Neill of Australia
Prep time: 5 minutes
Servings: 2

1 large or 2 small frozen black sapotes
(chocolate pudding fruit, also called
marmalade plum)
coconut water from 1 coconut
1 large or 2 small cos (romaine) lettuce
1 large or 2 small bananas, cut in chunks
(optional)

Place all ingredients in a mixer and blend.

Pineapple Crush

Susan and Les O'Neill of Australia
Prep time: 5 minutes
Servings: 2

2 cups of frozen pineapple, cut in chunks
1 cup of frozen watermelon, cut in chunks
juice of 1 lemon
coconut water from 1 coconut
1 large cos (romaine) lettuce

Place all ingredients in a mixer and blend.

" I have found that if you add 2 small passion fruit to the pineapple crush and have the drink daily for a few days, your lips will start to plump up. This was definitely not an allergic reaction because my husband's lips also started to fill out a bit more. My friend noticed the change in my lips over a week and asked what I had done. She grows her own passion fruit and decided to try the same drink. The next time I saw her she had a fuller lip line and far smoother lips. My lips have kept their new shape and have not gone down since. We found this quite interesting." ~Susan

Cleopatra's Secret

Susan and Les O'Neill of Australia
Prep time: 5 minutes
Servings: 2

1 punnet frozen blueberries
(approximately 1 pint)
1 large or 2 small bananas
1 cup coconut water
2 cups of baby spinach leaves or 1 small
cos (romaine) lettuce

Place all ingredients in a mixer and blend.

" Green smoothies frozen in popsicle or icy-pole moulds are great for young children. It gets plenty of greens into the kids and teaches them healthy eating from a very young age." ~Susan and Les

Liquid Pizza

Susan and Les O'Neill of Australia
Prep time: 5 minutes
Serving: 2

juice of 1 lemon
1 small avocado, pitted
4 Roma tomatoes, chopped
1 generous handful of fresh basil
6 leaves of silverbeet or bok choy, chopped
1 small chili or pinch of cayenne pepper
    (for Quantum Eating, omit cayenne
    pepper)
1 large clove of garlic, chopped
coconut water from 2 coconuts

Place in a mixer and blend. This recipe is great on a cold winter's night. You experience lovely warm hands and feet about an hour after drinking it. It takes away cravings for cooked pizza.

Liquid Salad

Susan and Les O'Neill of Australia
Prep time: 5 minutes
Serving: 2

juice of 1 lemon
4 sticks of celery, chopped
4 tomatoes, chopped
1 large cup of parsley
1 small handful of mint leaves
coconut water from 1 coconut

Place in a mixer and blend.

Jewel of the Nile

Susan and Les O'Neill of Australia.
Prep time: 5 minutes
Serving: 2
1 generous bunch of cilantro
1 mango, diced
2 small apples, core removed
1 large or 2 small bananas, chopped
2 cups of baby spinach leaves, chopped
coconut water from 1 coconut

Place in a mixer and blend.

This is a very palatable way of getting cilantro into the system to help with removal of heavy metals.

Green Orange Smoothie

Janna Hallman
Prep time: 10 minutes
Servings: 1-7, total yield is 1 quart

2 cups of fresh squeezed orange juice
2 ripe bananas, chopped
1 mango, diced
2 large handfuls of spinach, chopped

Blend together and enjoy!

" My children especially enjoy this green smoothie for breakfast. My family and I are enjoying experimenting with green smoothies. So far, this is one of our favorites. We are raw for the most part, but that cooked food addiction is tough. I believe that we will eventually get there." ~Janna

Green "Power" Smoothie

Charlotte Thuemmel
Prep time: 10 minutes
Servings: 1, yields 1 quart

2 apples, cored and quartered
2 cups cold water (for Quantum Eating,
   use a substitute, see p. 370)
2 teaspoons sesame seeds
4 fresh kale leaves, washed and removed
   from stems
2 tablespoons flax seeds, ground

Lightly blend together the apple, 2 cups of water (or juice), and sesame seeds. Add kale and ground flax seeds to blender and mix on high speed until creamy. You may adjust amounts of ingredients to your taste.

" I love this drink and have the whole quart for either breakfast or lunch every day. All of the ingredients are very nutritious. I like the fact that the sesame seeds and kale are both high in calcium. The inspiration for this recipe came from Victoria Boutenko." ~Charlotte

Two-Step Chai Smoothie Meal

Kelli Haines
Prep time: 10 minutes
Servings: 2

> *1½ cups soaked almonds*
> *3 cups coconut water*
> *2 fresh or frozen bananas*
> *2 medjool dates, pitted*
> *1 tablespoon raw cacao nibs (optional)*
> *1 teaspoon each: cinnamon, cardamom,*
> *   ginger, vanilla*
> *(for Quantum Eating, omit these*
> *   ingredients)*
> *3 romaine lettuce leaves*

Blend the soaked almonds and coconut water well in blender and then strain, reserving the pulp for use in other recipes. Pour fresh almond milk back into the blender and add the bananas, dates, cacao nibs, cinnamon, cardamom, ginger, vanilla, and romaine lettuce. Blend well and enjoy in a tall frosty mug.

" I love chai flavors and try to slip them into anything. This smoothie is a complete meal for one and has it all: fruit, nuts, greens." ~Kelli

Mieke's Ultimate Green Smoothie

Mieke Hays
Prep time: 10 minutes
Servings: yields 6–8 cups

1 very ripe banana
2-3 organic apples, cut up with core and
*   skin (no stem)*
3 medjool dates, pitted
1 bunch of organic parsley
a shot of liquid chlorophyll (for Quantum
*   Eating, substitute fresh wheatgrass*
*   juice)*
dash of lemon juice (optional)
water to fill half of blender (for Quantum
*   Eating, use a substitute, see p. 370)*

Blend well in a VitaMix.

Banana, apples, and dates are my generic staple ingredients, but I rotate the greens, which are parsley, kale, collard greens, spinach, turnip greens, and green chard. Parsley, my absolute favorite green, is said to be very rich in calcium and as nutritious as wheatgrass. This smoothie is delicious!

" This is my favorite green smoothie. It's just delicious and always turns out good with the apples, bananas, and dates, and parsley, my favorite green. Victoria Boutenko inspired me with her *Green for Life* book. I drink smoothies every day. It's VERY healthy and my husband likes it too! I'm so thrilled I get to share my green smoothie. I hope you put it in your book for the whole world to have!" ~Mieke

SMER
A Delicious Green Drink

Mark Hazelwood
Prep time: 5 minutes
Servings: 1-2

6-8 ounces grapes
1 slice avocado, perfectly ripe
2-4 frozen strawberries
agave (light colored) (for Quantum
Eating, substitute raw honey)

Put grapes, strawberries, and avocado in a blender. Blend together. If the grapes are sweet enough and you don't mind grape skins, then it is ready to drink. I like to strain it into a bowl (with a metal strainer), taste it to see how much agave to add (usually a spoon or two) and then mix it quickly one more time.

Notice that the consistency is that of pudding or a milkshake because of the avocado. The taste buds are coated instead of splashed quickly with thin liquid because of the avocado. The avocado doesn't add taste but makes the drink thicker. The frozen strawberries ensure that the drink is always cool even though it has just run through a blender. You can replace the strawberries with any frozen fruit. If there are papayas, mangoes, or fresh figs in season at the time, toss them in as well. Grapes and avocado are always mandatory.

" For me it is the drink of the gods, completely raw, sweet, delicious, and alkaline. If I had to choose only one recipe to live on, this would be it. I can't say I ever drank a green drink that I liked the taste of. I raised my son on this smoothie and everyone who's ever tried it loves it. He's no raw foodist but knows that making a smoothie, staying on fruit and liquid, will get him well quickly without medication. When he got sick as a child, I would fill the fridge with raw food and tell him that was all he could have until he was better. He'd be well in three days. This smoothie is affectionately known between my son and me as a **SMER** (think of it as your **SM**oothie **E**mergency **R**oom).

Most know how good grapes are for you, but grapes can sometimes be sour or bland and who's going to consume them regularly with that in mind? This recipe is very simple and turns grapes into an exotic desert.

Sharing this wonderful smoothie recipe and a few of the details is what may help people stay on raw. Many people need a drink that mimics a thick sweet shake or pudding to replace that craving and thus get over it while never having to give up those taste sensations."

~Mark

Pina Colada Green Smoothie

Doreen Moore
Prep time: 10 minutes
Servings: 2

1 young coconut, milk and meat
½ pineapple, peeled, cored and cut into
  cubes
1 banana, fresh or frozen, cut into 2 inch
  slices
2 cups spinach, 3 kale leaves, or 3 collard
  leaves

Place all ingredients in blender and blend until smooth. Enjoy!

For a nice variation, replace milk and meat of 1 young coconut with the juice of 2 pink grapefruits.

" I like this smoothie because it is sweet and delicious, yet gives me nutritious greens in addition to the nutrition of the fruit. Also, people who are not fond of greens don't mind them in this smoothie because you can hardly taste them. I hope you enjoy this recipe." ~Doreen

Morning Energizer (Grapefruit-Banana Smoothie)

Claudia Ravel
Prep time: 10 minutes
Servings: 2

½ grapefruit, peeled and diced
1 very ripe banana (fresh or frozen)
1 tablespoon ground flaxseed
1 teaspoon ground sesame seeds
2 cups distilled water (for Quantum
*   Eating, use a substitute, see p. 370)*

Peel off only the outer yellow skin of the grapefruit with a knife, removing as little as possible of the white pith, since this is the part with the most nutrients. Blend grapefruit pieces, banana, flaxseed, sesame seeds, and water in VitaMix and blend. Make sure the bananas are very ripe; the riper they are, the sweeter they become and offset the bitterness of the grapefruit. The bananas can be either fresh (which I prefer in the winter, because the drink won't be ice cold) or frozen (which I prefer on a hot summer day).

" I love to make this smoothie before I go to work in the morning because it only takes a few minutes to prepare. I peel the grapefruit the night before and put it in a Tupperware® bowl. This way I just have to throw it in the blender in the morning. It is a great energizer and very healthy. It provides a lot of vitamins and nutrients (vitamin C, Omega 3s, potassium, and calcium) and is very tasty." ~Claudia

Green Smoothie with Pears

Claudia Ravel
Prep time: 10 minutes
Servings: 2

1 big leaf collard greens
3 leaves turnip greens
1 handful of spinach leaves
2 tablespoons ground flax seed
1 tablespoon hemp seed (optional)
½ cup walnuts or pecans
1 very ripe banana
2 ripe pears, quartered and stem removed
1 carrot
1½ cups distilled water (for Quantum
   Eating, use a substitute, see p. 370)

Put all the ingredients in a VitaMix and blend. You can add more or less water, depending on how thick you want the smoothie.

" I really like Victoria Boutenko's green mango smoothie, but I wanted to find a nutritious smoothie that I can make in a few minutes (mango or pineapple tastes very good mixed with greens, but it takes more time to peel and cut the fruit). I don't peel the pears; I just cut them in half or in quarters and throw them in the blender. This smoothie tastes delicious, is very nutritious and it is very quick to prepare.

Not one day goes by that I don't make at least one of these two recipes. I am a working mom and, as you know, preparing raw food can be a little time consuming. These recipes are very quick to prepare, and this is very important for busy people. I love the recipes so much and I am sure other readers will too. I have shared my recipes with a lot of my friends and co-workers and would love to share them with a lot more people." ~Claudia

Apple-Bok Choy Smoothie

Courtney Peterson
Prep time: 5 minutes
Servings: 1-2

½ pound of bok choy
½ pound of Gala, Braeburn, or Fuji apples
   (about one 1 large apple)
20-30 g of flat-leaf Parsley
½-⅔ cups of water to blend (for Quantum
   Eating, use a substitute, see p. 370)

Use both the bok choy leaves and the entire "stalk" when measuring out a half-pound of bok choy. Put all the ingredients in a VitaMix and blend on high for about one minute. Since none of the ingredients are juiced, you want the smoothie to be extremely well-blended. The (mild) bitterness of bok choy can vary quite a bit, so if you have particularly bitter bok choy, increase the relative amounts of apple and parsley. Be sure to use fresh Gala, Braeburn, or Fuji apples;

the recipe doesn't taste as good with other varieties of apples, or with apples that aren't fresh and are old.

Modifications/Variations: For the intermediate version, either juice all the ingredients and omit the water, or blend all the ingredients but only use a quarter-pound of bok choy. For the beginner version, juice all the ingredients and use a quarter-pound of bok choy.

" In addition to the large amount of greens, which are vital for minerals, I love this recipe because of how hydrating the apple and bok choy are together. It's light and refreshing, and the parsley gives it a nice twist. Bok choy is particularly high in calcium, magnesium, and folate. To get my daily serving of greens, I actually double this recipe. I drink it about twice a week on average."

~Courtney

Apple-Dandelion Smoothie

Courtney Peterson
Prep time: 5 minutes
Servings: 1-2

⅓ pound of dandelion
½ pound of Gala, Braeburn, or Fuji apples
  (about 1 large apple)
⅔ cups of water (for Quantum Eating, use
  a substitute, see p. 370)

If your dandelion leaves have particularly long and thick stems, trim off the last 1-3 inches of stem, then measure out ⅓ pound of dandelion. Put all the ingredients in a VitaMix and blend on high for about 1 minute. Since none of the ingredients are juiced, you want the smoothie to be extremely well-blended. The bitterness of dandelion can vary quite a bit, so if you have particularly bitter dandelion, increase the relative amount of apple. Be sure to use fresh Gala, Braeburn, or Fuji apples; the recipe doesn't taste as good with other varieties of apples, or with apples that aren't fresh and are old.

Modifications/Variations: For the intermediate version, either juice all the ingredients and omit the water, or blend all the ingredients but only use ⅙ lb of dandelion. For the beginner version, juice all the ingredients, but use ⅙ lb of dandelion.

" With the dandelion, this recipe is super-charged with nutrition. Dandelion is high in iron, calcium, magnesium, vitamin C, vitamin A, and vitamin E. The apple does a surprisingly good job of masking the bitterness of the dandelion, and as a result, brings to life the best flavors of the dandelion — nice flavors that you never knew dandelion had! The result is surprisingly satisfying, and I sometimes find it addicting. If the dandelion is still too strong, simply add less. To get my daily serving of greens, I double this recipe. I drink it about 1-2 times a week on average.

These are both "advanced" green smoothie recipes, with modifications for the intermediate and beginner levels, and they are super-nutritious!" ~Courtney

Sunflowers with Strawberries in Orange Sauce

Becki Campbell, www.rawfoodfirst.com
Prep time: 5 minutes
Servings: 1-2

½ cup sunflower seeds for soaked 4 hours,
  or overnight, or even sprouted a day
1 cup strawberries, sliced
2 oranges or 3-4 tangerines, peeled and
  quartered

Put soaked sunflower seeds and sliced strawberries in a bowl. Peel oranges and blend in a high speed blender such as the K-TEC or VitaMix. (In a high speed blender, orange seeds are undetectable when blended, but in a regular blender they are only chopped up. If you are using a regular blender, remove the orange seeds before blending.) Pour blended oranges or tangerines over sunflower seeds and strawberries and enjoy!

Variation: Rather than blending the oranges or tangerines, you can juice them. You may need a few more oranges or tangerines if juicing.

" I have been making this recipe for over 20 years juicing the oranges! Now I choose to blend the oranges. Either way, it is delicious. My daughters loved this as a snack any time of day!" ~Becki

Better Than Chocolate Mousse

Tonya Zavasta
Prep time: 5 minutes
Serving: 1

coconut water from 1 coconut
2 ripe bananas, peeled and cut in chunks
2 teaspoons of raw carob
1 teaspoon of white or black raw tahini

Blend in a Vita-Mix

❝ Those of you with a sweet tooth will love it! For a long time this drink was my second meal. I liked it so much."
~Tonya

Tonya's Favorite Green Smoothie

Tonya Zavasta
Prep time: 5 minutes
Servings: 2

2 cups of watermelon chunks
2 banana, peeled and cut in chunks
4 leaves of Kale Lacinato, stems removed
(use stems in your juice) cut in pieces

Place watermelon chunks first, then banana chunks, and finally the kale in a Vita-Mix.

❝ I often use this recipe as my second meal at 2 P.M. It keeps me satisfied until the next morning." ~Tonya

Green Pudding

Tonya Zavasta
Prep time: 5 minutes
Servings: 2

2 ripe mangoes, peeled and cut in chunks
2 leaves of Swiss chard, stems removed
(use the stems in your juice)

Place greens first, and then chunks of mango on the top and process in a VitaMix.

" Nick demonstrates this recipe during my presentations. This pudding is popular all over the country." ~Tonya

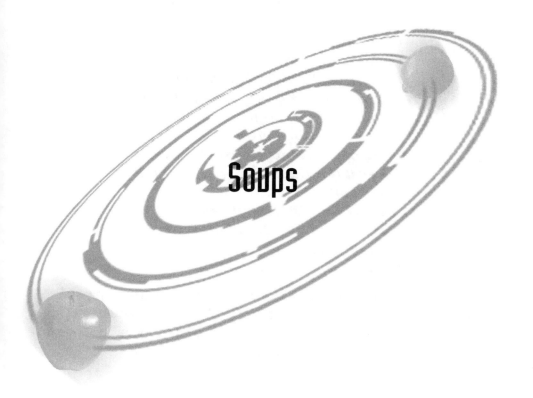

Soups

Sweet Pea Soup

Ken Rohla, President of Fresh and Alive,
www.freshandalive.com
Prep time: 10 minutes
Servings: 2-3

*2 cups fresh or sprouted green peas, or one
10 oz. bag of organic frozen green
(sweet) peas, thawed & warmed in
warm water*

*1 bunch parsley, flat or curly, rinsed in
warm water and finely chopped*

*1 cup warm water (for Quantum Eating,
use a substitute, see p. 370)*

¼ cup lemon or lime juice

*3 tablespoon organic first cold-pressed
olive oil (for Quantum Eating, omit this
ingredient)*

*2 tablespoon Bragg's Liquid Aminos or
Nama Shoyu (for Quantum Eating,
omit this ingredient)*

2 green onions, finely chopped

To serve warm, soak peas in warm water and rinse parsley
and green onion in warm water. Blend all ingredients except
onion briefly, just enough to make a creamy soup with flakes
of parsley visible. Stir in chopped onion and serve.

" I like this recipe because it's tasty and easy to make.
People at raw potlucks often ask for the recipe." ~Ken

Fast Food Hot Soup

Judy Spindler
Prep time: 5 minutes (if fresh vegetable juice is pre-made)
Servings: 1

> 8 ounces freshly made juice
>   (see list below)
> 1 young coconut, meat only
> 1 avocado, pitted and diced
> 1 red or yellow hot pepper,
>   seeds removed, chopped
> 2 cups of any greens

Juice vegetable(s) of choice to make eight ounces of fresh juice: Kale, collards, Swiss chard, parsley, spinach, bok choy, broccoli stems, asparagus, blended with carrot juice. (This is my most important source of energy.)

Blend one 8 oz. juice of your choice, meat of a young coconut, avocado, red/yellow hot pepper, and greens of your choice. (Spinach and parsley are my favorites).

66 I really like this soup in the winter — it warms me right up!" ~Judy

Raw Gazpacho

Tonya Zavasta
Prep time: 20 minutes
Servings: 2

Step 1

1½ cups of tomato juice
1 cup of carrot juice
½ cup of cucumber juice
½ cup celery juice
½ cup of lemon juice

Collect all the juice in a bowl. This will make four cups of freshly squeezed vegetable juice.

Step 2

1 teaspoon of raw honey
1 cup red bell pepper, minced
1 medium cucumber, chopped
3 scallions, minced
2 cups tomatoes, freshly diced
¼ cup fresh parsley, chopped
¼ cup fresh basil, chopped
1 cup fresh corn kernels
dash of ground cumin (for Quantum
*   Eating, omit this ingredient)*
2 tablespoons olive oil (optional) (for
*   Quantum Eating, omit this ingredient)*
Celtic salt and Cayenne pepper to taste
*   (for Quantum Eating, omit these*
*   ingredients)*

Dissolve honey in 1 cup of vegetable juice. In a bowl, combine this mixture with all other ingredients and remaining vegetable juice.

" Gazpacho is a delicious soup that originated in Spain. Unlike most soups, it is served cold and so it is perfect for conversion to the raw food lifestyle. This gazpacho recipe is incredibly easy to make and very healthy. This particular recipe is very popular at the Memphis raw food support group potlucks. We had this soup for our Thanksgiving dinner!" ~Tonya

Russian Borsch

Tonya Zavasta
Prep time: 20 minutes
Servings: 2

Step 1
1½ cups of tomato juice
1 cup of carrot juice
½ cup of cucumber juice
½ cup celery juice
½ cup of lemon juice

Collect all the juice in a bowl. This will make 4 cups of freshly squeezed vegetable juice.

Step 2
1 teaspoon of raw honey
1 cup of beet root, shredded
1 cup red bell pepper, minced
1 medium cucumber, chopped
3 scallions, minced
1 large avocado, chopped
2 cups tomatoes, freshly diced
¼ cup fresh parsley, chopped
dash of ground cumin (for Quantum
    Eating, omit this ingredient)
Celtic salt and Cayenne pepper to taste
    (for Quantum Eating, omit these
    ingredients)

Dissolve honey in 1 cup of vegetable juice. In a bowl, combine this mixture with all other ingredients and remaining vegetable juice.

" Soup has traditionally been served for hundreds of years in Russia as the first course. It is believed that soups promote good digestion. In Russia, there are many types of soups, both hot and cold, and Borsch is one of the most popular. My husband used to miss Russian borsch so badly. Not after he tried this one! My recipe offers a new, raw twist to this ancient tradition. ~Tonya

Lorenzo's Tomato Avocado Soup[1]

Susan Schenck
Prep time: 20 minutes
Serves 2-4.

2 cups water (for Quantum Eating, use a substitute, see p. 370)
1 large tomato
1 ripe avocado
2 cloves garlic
juice from a small lime
¼ onion
½-¾ cup broccoli
1 big red kale leaf
4 small chilies or 1 jalapeño
(optional — omit for hygienic purity)
4-5 stalks bok choy
1 inch fresh turmeric
1 red bell pepper
¼ cup flaxseeds
1 teaspoon powdered sea vegetables
2 tablespoon raw apple cider vinegar
(or substitute lemon juice)

Blend ingredients in Vita-Mix until very creamy.

" A friend of mine serves this soup every time we go to his house, and my husband and I can't get enough! He says he has experimented with it a lot and found that the only crucial ingredients that cannot be omitted or substituted are the avocado and tomato, which is why I gave it this name." ~Susan Schenck

---

1. *This recipe is from Susan Schenck's book,* The Live Food Factor, A Comprehensive Guide to the Ultimate Diet for Body, Mind, Spirit & Planet.

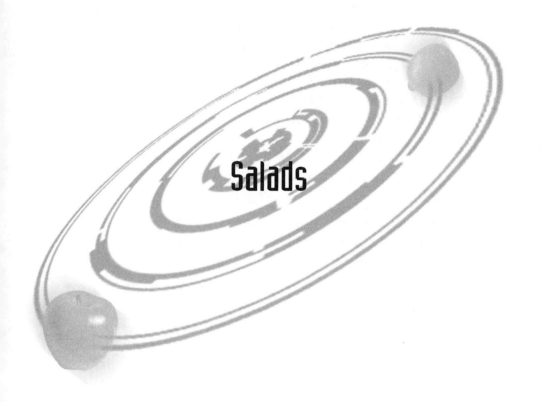

Salads

Sunshine Roll-Ups

Marisol Hanaway
Prep time: 20 minutes
Servings: 7 rolls

7 large Kale leafs, cleaned
1 red bell pepper, julienned
1 yellow bell pepper, sliced
1 avocado, pitted and diced
1 small cucumber, diced
¼ cup red onions, thinly sliced
¼ cup cilantro, chopped
1 tomato, diced
1 cup sunflower greens
1 lemon juice
pinch of Celtic salt (for Quantum Eating,
    omit this ingredient)

Prepare kale leaves by taking out the hard white vein in the center of the leaf. In a separate bowl, mix the bell peppers, cucumbers, tomatoes, avocado, cilantro, sunflower greens, lemon juice, and Celtic salt.

Fill the kale leaf with the mix, roll it up, and enjoy. You can also use beet tops.

" It is really a delicious roll. I am inspired by this recipe because of its simplicity and the wonderfully nutritious ingredients." ~Marisol

Tomato-Basil Salad

Jennifer Turke
Prep time: 10 minutes
Servings: 3-4

2 large tomatoes, diced
1-2 large cucumbers, diced
4 cups dark leafy greens of choice,
*   chopped*
2 tablespoons hemp or sesame seeds
2 tablespoons fresh basil, chopped
1 teaspoon fresh oregano, thyme or both
*   (optional) (for Quantum Eating, omit*
*   this ingredient)*
sea veggie sprinkles (optional)
dash of sea salt (optional) (for Quantum
*   Eating, omit this ingredient)*
juice of 1 lemon
1-2 tablespoons agave or honey (for
*   Quantum Eating, use raw honey)*

Toss all ingredients in a large salad bowl and enjoy!

" The fresh basil really makes this salad. I love using fresh herbs in my raw recipes!" ~Jennifer

Eat Your Greens Salad

Jennifer Turke
Prep time: 10 minutes
Servings: 2

1 large head Kale, chopped small
1 yellow or red bell pepper, chopped
2 tablespoon hemp seeds
2 fresh garlic cloves, pressed
2 tablespoon fresh herb of choice, chopped
*   (basil, cilantro, parsley, etc.)*
juice of 1 lemon or lime
1–2 tablespoons agave or honey (optional)
*   (for Quantum Eating, use raw honey)*
sea salt (for Quantum Eating, omit this
*   ingredient)*

Massage chopped kale with sea salt in a large bowl until slightly wilted. Add all other ingredients and mix gently. Yum!

Note: If you do not consume sea salt you can still enjoy this salad, just massage the kale a little longer.

" There is now so much information available on the benefits of regular garlic consumption. Everyone, including raw foodists could benefit from more dark leafy greens like kale. This salad is a fun and an easy way to get more of both!" ~Jennifer

Lime~Mint Dressing

Jennifer Turke
Prep time: 10 minutes
Servings: dressing for 1 large salad

Juice of 1 large orange
Juice of 1 lime
3-4 inch chunk of aloe leaf, without skin
2 tablespoon fresh mint leaves, chopped
1-2 tablespoon agave or honey (optional)
(for Quantum Eating, use raw honey)
dash of sea salt (optional) (for Quantum Eating, omit this ingredient)

Blend all ingredients and toss over your salad of choice.

" This dressing is very light and cooling. It is amazing over a cucumber salad, and aloe vera is great for the skin!"
~Jennifer

Carrot Salad

Judy Spindler
Prep time: 5 minutes
Servings: 1

2 cups carrot pulp
¼ cup red onion, diced
½ red pepper, diced
1 teaspoon lemon juice
2 cups greens of your choice

Mix carrot pulp, lemon juice, red pepper, and red onion. Serve over 2 cups of any greens.

" Besides juicing, I really put time into "alive food" which I add to my salads. I like counter-sprouting peas, red lentils, clover, sunflower seeds, radish seeds. I like indoor growing — especially in the winter: buckwheat and sunflower sprouts. I like growing unusual greens like Chinese edible mums, sorrel, arugula, chickory, chervil, and purslane. Praise the Lord for His variety that helps us be well.

My motto is 'depend upon God and eat as closely as possible to how God made our food.' I am fifty years young, married twenty-seven years, have four children (ages 24, 20, 18, 16), home-educate the youngest half a day, work at home as a Hallelujah Acres Health Minister, run the church nursery, teach pre-school Sunday School, act as Awana Club Secretary, exercise two to three hours a day, and teach karate three nights a week. I learned from Tonya to eat earlier in the day, which helps with the karate schedule. Most important for me is to make time to have two to three freshly made juices per day." ~Judy

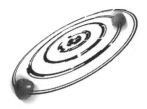

Chapter 35

Show Your Glow: Striving for Perfection in Complexion

Traveling as I make my raw food presentations, I meet many health-oriented people who either already primarily eat raw or are transitioning to the raw food lifestyle. You know immediately there's something special about them. They exude high energy. Their clear eyes emit a light that seems to go straight to your soul. You can feel how they bubble with positive attitude. The catch — you have to be pretty healthy yourself to pick up on those vibes! They're all, it seems, from Missouri — the "Show Me" state. *Okay — just show me this glow!* That's the attitude you'll see in the average person who's checking you out, deciding whether it's worth it to go raw. The fact that you never have a cold or flu, you have so much energy, you can live on four hours' sleep, you never have a hot flash … All good benefits to report, but hard for people to verify. Curious folk want to *see* your health. And where will they be looking? At your largest organ: your skin.

For women, in particular, a word to the wise: The raw food lifestyle doesn't mean an instant transformation from

Plain Jane to Fabulous Babe. Many expect that once you eat raw you should thereafter always exhibit a glowing complexion. This is not always the case. Here, I believe, is one reason why: Many in the raw food community look down on external beautifying procedures. Many believe that a quick splash with water is all that your facial skin needs. But unless you're very young, you probably won't be that lucky.

I'm not that lucky. (And I'm not that young!) I hope to convince you that a little attention to your complexion will take you a long way toward achieving your Rawsome beauty potential.

Your skin's condition reflects your internal health. Skin problems like acne, blemishes, and dryness are signs of an overtaxed system. Just as deficiency and toxicity are the main two causes for illness, they tend to be the same two causes for most beauty problems as well. Poor elimination and poor circulation are two major causes of negative skin conditions. A raw food regimen definitely takes care of poor elimination. But correcting your poor circulation can use some external help.

When your system gets overloaded, your body can't eliminate of all its waste through regular channels. Skin eruptions are excretions of waste materials from the pores. Dry, oily, or sensitive skin, acne, and facial blemishes all result from gut problems, so they do have to be addressed internally. At the same time, you shouldn't ignore external measures that can help you.

Here's a fact that's sure to surprise you. More than half of the dust that accumulates in your house is from your skin. We literally shed our skin and grow the equivalent of a whole new skin every twenty-five to thirty days. This shocked my husband Nick, who reports that he's just tossed out a vacuum cleaner bag full of his discarded self. The funeral, he says, was quite touching, though attendance was thin.

Most people do a dry body scrub, but not many do a dry facial brushing. Though body brushing is not a new concept, it is a commonly held belief by many in the beauty industry that brushing one's face is not necessary, perhaps is not even beneficial. I believe that face brushing is just as important as body brushing. Dead skin cells accumulate on the face, just as they do on the body. Some will slough off naturally, but these flaky, dehydrated cells need some help to "get lost." Body brushing *and* face brushing are essential components of a health and beauty regimen, and should be done daily.

The body is so intelligent that it will take care of our inside organs first. Sometimes, there's not enough vitality to reach the skin. Brushing stimulates *surface* blood flow and tells the body where it needs to heal first. Exfoliation energizes your face and improves circulation. All of these steps result in a better looking complexion.

Exfoliation is *necessary* to get younger looking skin. Mature skin needs exfoliation even more. But the more mature your skin, the more gradual the approach you need. When we look at mature skin, what we see is mostly dead skin cells. These dead cells accumulate on the surface, densely packed, making natural exfoliation difficult. This creates lines and wrinkles, making your skin more prone to problems, like the accumulation of melanin, or of brown and black spots, and small raised beige lumps. Your body's self-healing process can't catch up with years of dietary and environmental abuse. Here's where raw foods and facial brushing can help.

When the outer layer of skin becomes thickened, discolored, rough, and uneven, the best way to help the skin shed built-up layers of dead, unhealthy skin is to use a good brush. Gentle manual facial brushing will speed cell turnover, maximize oxygen intake, strengthen the skin's inner structure, and reverse the effects of aging. Such exfoliation will not only even out skin tone, but will also improve the texture of your skin.

Tiny bacteria live on our skin. If exposed to oxygen, these bacteria would be killed instantly. The easiest protection for some microbes against oxygen toxicity is to hide. Anaerobic microorganisms tolerate oxygen in their surroundings by physically screening themselves from their worst enemy. Their shield? Layers of dead cells.

Exfoliation is the most important element in all skin care. It helps with everything from aging to acne to dry skin. Brushing also helps reduce surface skin oils and can help remove blackheads and other skin impurities, as well as smoothing out fine wrinkle lines. Collagen can only be manufactured in the presence of molecular oxygen by improving circulation — thus brushing might stimulate collagen production as well.

When I am on the lecture circuit, I show people how I brush and "polish" my face. It was a challenge to find just the right brush to optimize my facial routine. All the facial brushes I tried were too soft. This softness actually makes sense when you consider that most people who eat cooked food generally have more sensitive skin. We raw food aficionados need something a little stiffer. I finally found a brush that was effective and appealing. This may amaze you, but … I use a shoe brush with natural horse hair bristles. Though designed for polishing shoes, it is not too harsh for the face.

Two hot tips:
1. Buy a brand new brush. I'm not sure even raw foods can offer much of a remedy for a face waxed and polished to the brilliance of a soldier's drill boots.
2. Don't tell the guy in the shoe store what you're using the brush for. We raw food folk have enough trouble making ourselves credible to the uninitiated.

Many beauty books say you shouldn't exfoliate more than twice per week. But by eating raw foods you will become *different*, so the advice of traditional beauty professionals won't work for you. On raw foods, your skin will become more supple. Less sensitive, too — you'll find your skin heals much faster. At first you must be gentle while brushing, but gradually you can brush more vigorously. Your face *will* begin to glow!

Brushing helps "unglue" dead, dry skin cells from your skin's surface. By brushing, the epidermis is exfoliated, leaving a silky texture. Now that you're regularly ridding your skin of dead cells, the beauty products you use — moisturizers, especially, can be absorbed more effectively. The trick is to use a good nurturing and healing cream to accelerate skin recovery time, allowing you to use your brush daily.

This brings us to the topic of what facial cream to use. Some people, after going raw, decide *not* to use any cosmetics on the face and body. I understand where they're coming from. Many cosmetic products contain toxins. While they're cleansing their bodies on the *inside*, it might seem logical to avoid adding chemicals on the *outside*. In fact, when you eat raw, your body does become even more intolerant of the wrong cosmetics.

Several years ago, I was wandering through the cosmetics section of a local department store. A major cosmetics company was introducing a new anti-aging cream, offering free samples. (Now, me — if it's free, I'll try it. Make no mistake — I may be Russian by origin, but sometimes I'm a red-blooded American consumer.) Because I had used this company's products before, I thought nothing of using the cream that night. When I awakened, my skin was as red as a radish and covered with a rash! I was shocked. Why would my skin suddenly show such a strong reaction? I'd never had allergies to any cosmetic products before. I began to analyze, in hopes of finding an answer.

My conclusion: Changing your lifestyle as completely as you do when you go raw, you become more sensitive to certain outside influences that previously had no effect. Some ingredients, never a problem for a person on a cooked food diet, become poisonous to a raw food person. The same thing can happen with skin care products.

I'm asked constantly what cosmetics company's products to use. Everyone on raw foods seems to want *raw* cream. Many health conscious women are "hesitant about using the laboratory-produced preservative," as one put it in an email to me. And they believe that a cosmetic company should use only vitamins to preserve. All they have to do, they think, is to find that one perfect manufacturer.

No one, I can assure you, abhors processing and preservatives as much as I do. I do not eat *anything* from a box, container, or bottle, and I'll be the first to advise that you should always prepare your own food. I'm a stickler when it comes to women who tell me they want to look good but won't take time to juice or to make a green smoothie every day. You have to *earn* your health, I say. Still, we all have to draw the line *somewhere*. I draw mine at making my own cosmetics. I used to do this regularly. But since writing and appearances take so much of my time, I find that a good commercially made cream works well in conjunction with my stringent eating regimen.

There are some good companies in the "natural organic" cosmetic industry that I recommend in my books and on my website. However, if you imagine that they obtain vitamin C by squeezing lemon juice or get beta carotene straight from an organic carrot, think again. Consider this: A plant food in its pure form isn't stable. Just think how short a time your freshly squeezed juice lasts in your fridge. And how quickly it would go bad if you left it sitting on the counter in your bathroom! All companies, in fact, use a "laboratory-produced preservative."

Extracting the active, beneficial component from a plant almost always requires a process that is synthetically derived (such as obtaining genistein from soy). Further, these food extracts are far more stable than the whole food. In cosmetic production, raw materials must be cleaned or purified by mechanical means such as bleaching, clay, filtration, natural solvents, or heat. Often they are chemically altered by oxidation or hydrolysis.

The reality is that natural or plant-based preservatives have rather poor anti-microbial or anti-fungal properties. To test the stability of a cream sample, the company usually places a jar of the product in an oven at 40°C (104°F) (the optimum temperature for microbial life to proliferate) for several weeks and tests for signs of mold. With no preservative, the mold begins to grow in a short time. Only after I saw it with my own eyes did I finally capitulate to the idea of using a preservative in my own cream. Please consider: If a cosmetic product is contaminated, skin complications could be a serious concern.

I wish we could have a cream without laboratory produced preservatives. One method is the centuries-old base for homemade cosmetics — cocoa butter — instead of water. It is mixed at a temperature below 40°C (104° F). The ingredients (cold-pressed cocoa butter and essential oils) are individually stable with a long shelf-life that extends that of the final product.

Oils are not living products, even when they are cold-pressed. Oils are liquid fat. I do not consume any oils, and I use them very sparingly on the outside. When you mix fats together the resulting mixture is also fat. Your skin does need *some* oil, but it needs water much more. In cosmetics, "moisturizer" is a cream that hydrates the skin. The most obvious way to hydrate the skin is with water. Oils, because of their ability to penetrate the skin, provide a similar effect. However, oils don't really moisturize your skin. Oil repels water. Oils work best after a hot bath or after applying a towel soaked in hot water to your face. Your pores are then open and contain water. The oil keeps the water inside your pores and in your skin by acting as a barrier. A traditional moisturizer contains about eighty percent water. And if you have water, you *must* have a preservative.

A good moisturizer restores normal levels of hydration to the skin, while building a barrier against loss of water through the epidermis, repairing scaly, damaged, or dry skin that results from external environmental aggressions or internal changes. Naturally moist, smooth, and supple skin results from sufficient amounts of water, and some oil. After facial brushing you will have to use either a moisturizer or some oil. It is your call!

If you want to make your own moisturizing cream, I admire you. I'll even provide you with recipes in my newsletter. But be prepared ... you will have to pull out your pots and pans and use your stove. This is another reason I don't make my own creams at home any longer — I just don't like the fuss. The tradeoff is that you will have a preservative in your cream.

I have been 100 percent raw for ten years. Now, even a morsel of processed food (with preservatives or home cooked) will make me sick. However, carefully chosen cosmetics don't. This is the main reason I do not mix "raw" ingredients in my kitchen when I need a moisturizer.

Some preservatives are better than others. Some are used in such minute amounts that their toxicity is actually lower than that of fresh vegetables and greens. (Yes, there *are* toxins in raw foods as well. You cannot avoid toxins entirely.) I believe a good facial cream, after a dry brushing, can do so much good for your complexion that it will compensate many times over for your aversion to the preservative's presence in it. At least, it does for me.

Try different products. See what works for you. Your body, cleansed by your raw food practices, will be a good indicator of what product to use. Trust it!

Let me answer two common questions I'm asked …

Question: *Please let me know whether the appearance of my skin will get worse before it gets better. I've been about 80 percent raw up until ten days ago, after which I have been 100 percent raw. I'm not sure if I am particularly over sensitive about my looks, but in the last few days, my skin feels very dry all over my body. Any advice?*

Answer: Some people, especially those who are thin, notice, when going 100 percent raw, that their skin becomes very dry during the first few weeks. They panic, thinking their faces and hands appear to be aging rapidly. As with other health issues, going 100 percent raw might cause surface indicators to get worse before they get better. When you go 100 percent raw overnight, the introduction of toxins into your body is drastically reduced, and your body will begin releasing retained water. The first several weeks are when the greatest weight loss will occur. You are losing water, primarily. The main reason is that cooked food contains a great deal of hidden salt. Your skin is losing water also, so dryness is the most apparent there. Dry, flaky skin is one of the detox symptoms. You simply have to live through this temporary condition.

Your skin is the largest organ in your body. One of the skin's functions is to regulate salt and water levels in your body. Your body is releasing water it does not need any longer. Dryness of the skin is a detox symptom that will be alleviated when most of the toxins, including salt, leave the body.

Your skin is divided into three main layers. The top layer is the epidermis. Under this is the dermis, and below that is the subcutaneous layer. The epidermis is what we see, but it is the condition of the dermis and subcutaneous layers that determines whether or not we *like* what we see. You'll need to give raw foods some time to work their miracle from inside.

You might need to drink more water during this period. But I believe daily fresh-squeezed vegetable juices and green smoothies will work better. I would recommend during this time continuing to dry-brush your whole body. Do not forget your face.

Question: *Alpha hydroxy acids are seen as the fountain of youth among beauty professionals. This anti-aging treatment offers intense exfoliation. They claim that mature skin will look smoother and fine lines will soften. What is your opinion?*

Answer: Almost every skin care product boasts that it contains AHAs. Alpha hydroxy acid (AHA) is an umbrella term for a variety of fruit acids including glycolic, citric, lactic, malic, and tartaric acids, which are derived from fruit and milk sugars and served up in creams and lotions. These acids work much better from the *inside* when we eat fresh organic produce.

AHA *will* exfoliate your skin. But do not forget that these are *acids* we're talking about — too much can cause a burn. Using these acids as a daily product or a chemical peel results in noticeable redness, dryness, and flaking. Many women tolerate these signs as a price for beauty. The price is too high, in my view, and the attained beauty very short-lived.

Their complaints include severe redness, swelling (especially in the area of the eyes), burning, blistering, bleeding, rash, itching, and skin discoloration. An industry-sponsored study found that people who use AHA products have greater sensitivity to the sun, raising the specter of a greater risk of photo-aging and skin cancer. The "positive" results people perceive when using chemical peels are from the swelling and edema they cause. These will diminish wrinkles and make the skin smooth, but the long-term condition of the skin is hurt dramatically because of this deep irritation.

AHAs are capable of penetrating the skin barrier. AHA products work in a manner similar to that of chemical peels, increasing cell turnover rate and decreasing the thickness of the outer skin. The degree of this effect depends on the product's pH level (a measure of acidity), the AHA concentration, and the AHA vehicle cream, as well as how the product is used (frequency of use and where it is applied on the skin). Apart from your manner of use, you have no way to control the process. *I* like to be in control.

One study looked at the effects of glycolic acid on the production of sunburn cells (markers for UV-induced skin damage). The study followed one group who were treated with non-AHA products while another group used the product with AHA. The study found that the people who received an AHA product and applied it to the skin while in the presence of UV radiation experienced *twice* the cell damage of those who were treated with the non-AHA product during UV radiation.

A fruit masque is one ideal way to benefit from AHA with no side effects. Facial brushing is an easier, more natural way to remove dead layers of skin and achieve the exfoliating effect AHA produces. A brush is also the most cost-effective way to rejuvenate your skin. With dry brush exfoliation you are in total control of the process, which allows you to be gentle with and attuned to your skin's response. New cells grow continually, so if you eat raw foods while using a skin-care regimen including dry brushing, your new skin should begin to show results in about three to four weeks.

Newcomers to the raw foods lifestyle often assume that related beauty and skin care regimens will prove a hassle, involving exotic ingredients and fussy procedures. Not always! As I've shown here, sometimes you can simply brush off your troubles!

For more information about facial brushing, visit my website: *www.BeautifulOnRaw.com.*

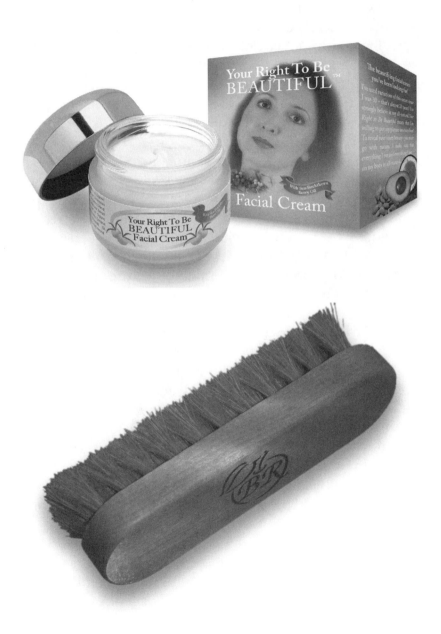

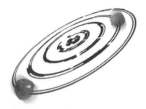

Chapter 36

The Beautifying Facial Cream You've Been Waiting For

I've been using variations of this cream since I was thirty — that's almost twenty years. Because I am committed to sharing my secrets of health and beauty, I now offer this cream to the public. I believe so strongly in my all-natural *Your Right to Be Beautiful™ Facial Cream* that I'm willing to put my picture on every box!

Let me be clear. There is no "magic potion" that miraculously fixes everything. The cream will not flatten your stomach, perk up your breasts, or enhance your sex life. You will have to go raw to achieve these results! However, combined with a raw lifestyle, this cream will nourish and help to heal your skin. It will support you in your goal to look and feel beautiful inside and out.

It is an all natural healing cream containing wild crafted and organic essential oils and certified organic herbs that promote healing and new cell growth. My cream is as close to food as it can get! Its vanilla scent and whipped frosting-like texture smells and looks so delicious that you may be tempted to taste it! And indeed, though it's not intended for eating, it practically *is* a food product; it is that safe! The all-natural ingredients include oils of almond, coconut, mango seed, sesame seed and avocado.

The consistency of this cream is really light and fluffy. These are the main characteristics of the "mousse" style, the latest trend in the cosmetic industry for skin care products.

Your Right to Be Beautiful™ *Facial Cream* is soothing and anti-inflammatory and can be used on any type of skin, including sensitive skin. It can be used as a daily moisturizer because it nourishes and restores dry, dehydrated skin, leaving it feeling firmer and softer. It can be used under makeup foundation or as a soothing after shave cream. It can also be used as an enriching and healing night cream. The cream does not leave film residue, since the ingredients are quickly absorbed by the skin.

What makes *Your Right to Be Beautiful*™ *Facial Cream* so special? There is a "secret" ingredient in *Your Right to Be Beautiful*™ *Facial Cream:* Sea Buckthorn oil. Sea Buckthorn plant (*Hippophae rhamnoides* — no, you won't find this one in your neighborhood nursery) is native to the mountainous regions of Siberia.

When I began making my homemade cream, I still lived in Russia. I would always add Sea Buckthorn oil. It was discovered that the oil aided in the healing of skin damage (from radiation or the sun), acne, skin ulcers, burns, irritated or dry itchy skin, eczema, psoriasis, dermatitis, and wounds. Its nourishing, revitalizing, and restorative action seemed to have no limits.

In fact, the extract of Sea Buckthorn berries has been used for centuries in Asia, Russia, and Scandinavia, where it has been prized for its restorative properties. The value of the annual production of Sea Buckthorn products in China exceeds $20 million, yet the Sea Buckthorn is virtually unknown in the West.

After my move to the U.S., my mother would visit from Russia and wanted to bring something that would remind me of home. I always asked her to bring a bottle of the Sea Buckthorn oil.

The red and yellow berries of the Sea Buckthorn offer several essential vitamins that are usually only found individually. The berries contain a high percentage of vitamins C and E, and beta-carotene (pro-vitamin A). The vitamin C content is among the highest for any plant. Combined, these powerful antioxidants function as part of the body's natural defense system, combating wrinkles, dryness, and other symptoms of aging or neglected skin.

The production of enough of my cream to sell to others meant that I had to consider the perishable nature and short "shelf life" of all-natural products. Oils can become rancid, and natural extracts can get moldy or develop pathological bacteria as they travel between states or sit on a shelf. I needed to find a way to avoid having my cream go bad without using toxic substances.

Even if a truly "all-raw" product could be formulated, it would have the same fate as the fruits or vegetables that sit in your refrigerator for more than a week. The product would have to be refrigerated, and even then, after a few days, mold would begin to grow and it would not be safe to use. My dilemma was to formulate a good cream that would last. I certainly did not want to run to the kitchen to create a batch every time I needed moisturizer!

The goal was to find a preservative that would not harm your skin, would not introduce toxins into your body, and hopefully would be beneficial while preventing the risk of microbial contamination.

Caproyl glycine is the new preservative from Europe that I have chosen for my cream. Caproyl glycine is a lipoamino acid obtained by the grafting of a glycine onto an octanoic fatty chain. Glycine is an amino acid found in vegetables. The octanoic chain is commonly found in nature, primarily in coconut oil, but also in other oils such as palm seed oil. Caproyl glycine also has skin protecting properties.

Creating this cream has been a labor of love. I have carefully selected each ingredient and I am committed to keeping it the best possible quality. After two years of research into thirty companies, I finally have a product that I am willing to stand behind 100 percent!

I have such confidence in the cream's purity and power, that I offer this **absolutely unconditional guarantee**. Try *Your Right to Be Beautiful™ Facial Cream*. Use it regularly, as indicated. It will revitalize your skin, restoring it from the ravages of dryness, redness, and minor inflammation. You will notice how well it moisturizes and freshens your face, accentuating your natural beauty. However, if for any reason you are less than completely satisfied, simply return the unused portion for a full refund (less shipping & handling).

Ingredients: *Organic Infusion of Purified Water, Extract of Organic White Tea* (Camellia sinensis) *Leaf, Extract of Organic Echinacea* (Echinacea angustifolia) *Root, Extract of Organic Nettle* (Urtica dioica) *Leaf, Extract of Organic Rosemary* (Rosemarinus officinalis) *Leaf, Extract of Organic Elder* (Sambucus nigra) *Flower, Extract of Organic Lemongrass* (Cymbopogon citratus) *Herb, Emulsisifying Wax, Coconut* (Coconut nucifera) *Oil, Safflower* (Carthamus tinctorius) *Oil, Sweet Almond* (Prunus amygdalus dulcis) *Oil, Sesame* (Sesamum indicum) *Oil, Caproyl Glycine, Vegetable Glycerin, Mango* (Mangifera indica) *Seed Butter, Grape* (Vitis vinifera) *Seed*

Oil, Avocado (Persea gratissima) *Oil, Natural Vanilla Flavor, Sea Buckthorn* (Hippophae rhamnoides) *Oil.*

Hi Tonya! My very dear friend gave me your facial brush and moisturizer. I am an aesthetician and felt that daily facial brushing is too rough on the skin. I'm not yet convinced this isn't true; but I must say, the bags under my eyes have lessened. And the moisturizer literally smells good enough to eat. My dry skin drinks it right up and was surprised that my husband (who has very oily skin) enjoyed it after a facial as well. It does soak into the skin beautifully. — Alex Rosado

---

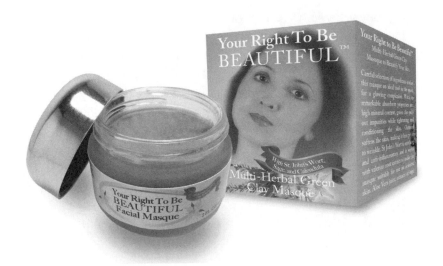

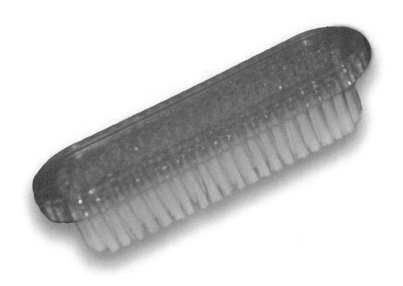

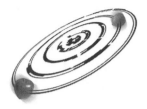

Chapter 37

Multi-Herb Green Clay Masque: "Your Right to Be Beautiful"

When in my first book, *Your Right to Be Beautiful,* in Chapter 28 I wrote about applying a daily masque, I didn't realize I was setting myself up for a barrage of questions. The most common question I'm asked is the most obvious: *What kind of masque do you use?* When I answered, "Any clay masque will do" people got upset; they were unsatisfied. They wanted specifics, an exact brand. That is when I began to feel at first uneasy, and then, inspired.

I've experimented with a hundred different masques over the years. Some I liked more, some less. It's one thing to use a masque on my own face — totally different to recommend it to thousands of my readers.

Dermatologists teach us to make our masque match our skin type: oily, dry, sensitive. If you have oily skin, they advise a clay or mud masque to absorb excess oil buildup. Dry skin? Try a creamy, hydrating masque. If you have sensitive skin, use a light, gel masque.

I've noticed that people who have oily skin have it all their lives. If they have dry skin they are stuck with it forever, and the same is true of people with sensitive skin. There seems to be a finality in having a particular skin type. Once your skin type is determined, it is assumed that it is yours to keep. I see a similarity to the constancy of some medical treatments such as insulin for diabetes, Norvasc for high blood pressure, Prozac for depression and so on. But let's get one thing straight: It is not normal to have oily, dry, or sensitive skin — You should have healthy, glowing skin.

When your system gets overloaded, your body can't eliminate all of its waste through normal channels. Dry, oily, or sensitive skin, acne, and facial blemishes all result from gut problems, so they must be addressed internally. My masque, therefore, does not deal with the symptoms, it is only meant to assist with what you are doing with your raw foods regimen. It cleanses, hydrates, and soothes the outer layer of your skin. The main change must happen on the inside; however, this *does not* mean we should ignore the outside.

Be realistic. If you're hoping I'll promise you that cellulite will be banished, your wrinkles removed, and that last patch of acne will be gone, all from using this masque … forget it! I can tell you, however, that I have seen all of these things happen with my own eyes on my own face, and on my family members' and numerous clients' faces — all by changing the diet to a raw food regimen!

Instead of dealing with symptoms, I insist you eat plenty of raw foods. Instead of trying to develop a masque for each type of skin, I chose a balanced approach to the masque formulation and let the body figure it out. I believe everybody's skin needs to have built up impurities removed, needs hydration, and needs to be treated gently. So I've developed a masque you can use for *any* skin type. For oily skin, this masque contains a clay which is ideal for absorbing excess oil buildup. For dry skin, this masque offers hydrating components. If you have sensitive skin, it is packed with soothing ingredients.

My masque offers the benefit of detoxifying properties and at the same time it is soothing and relaxing. It will tighten, clean, and refresh the skin. Your skin will be hydrated, nourished, oxygenated. The final result is a renewed, rested, and youthful appearance.

The body's first priority is survival. Your skin is the periphery of your body and will be addressed last. Here's where a masque can help. By introducing oxygen and improving circulation, we affect our body's priorities. Let me emphasize here one more time: only when you provide the *best* possible nourishment for the inside organs can you hope for the dramatic results on the outside. Only when your blood is clean do you want to stir it up and bring it close to the surface.

Masques are a wonderful way to make your skin glow, even out its tone, and help it to be supple and youthful. A good masque increases blood circulation and removes toxins. Think of facial masques as the ultimate nutrient delivery system. In general, the ingredients are more concentrated than those in lotions or cleansers, so they produce bigger benefits in less time. A masque is much thicker than a mois-turizer or topical treatment and, because of its extended application time and the inner warmth opening the pores, the passage of nutrients into your skin occurs far more quickly and efficiently. Masques can also remove excess oil, environ-mental debris and pollutants much more gently than astrin-gents, toners, or scrubs, and eliminate them completely.

One of the main ingredients in *Your Right to Be Beautiful™ Facial Masque* is French green clay. Also known as Illite clay, French green clay is a natural, bio-organic mate-rial. Green clay owes its coloration to two factors: iron oxides, and decomposed plant matter — mostly kelp, seaweed, and other algae! (No wonder I chose this particular clay for my masque!) French green clay gets its powers from the very cycle of life that nature uses to regenerate itself.

French green clay is extracted manually from a quarry in Southern France. After being mined, it is brought into the sun to remove excess water. This prolonged exposure to life-giving sunlight endows the clay with its healing powers. Then it is ground with huge hydraulic crushers and pulverized into a fine powder. The highly micronized state of French green clay gives it remarkable absorbent properties. It literally drinks oils, toxic substances, and impurities from the skin. French green clay contains numerous valuable elements, including silica, magnesium, calcium, iron, phosphorus, sodium, potassium, copper, zinc, selenium, cobalt, manganese, phosphorous, silicon, micro-algae, kelp, and phytonutrients, all of which are beneficial for your skin.

High in minerals, French green clay will pull out impurities and tighten and conditions the skin. Oatmeal softens the skin, making it less prone to wrinkles. St. John's Wort flowering herb is soothing and anti-inflammatory. Together with Valerian root extract, it makes the masque suitable for use on sensitive skin. Aloe, sage, rosemary, nettle, and chamomile extracts add calming and conditioning properties. Green tea, calendula, and cornflower extracts stimulate skin rejuvenation. The diverse combination of wild-crafted and organic herbs that promotes healing and new cell growth makes the masque beneficial for all skin types. Avocado oil extract moisturizes the skin and makes the masque suitable for everyday use.

One common opinion is that facial masques shouldn't be used more than once a week. I think of masques like exercise: you won't get the benefits if you only do it once in while. While developing this masque, one of my objectives was a delayed drying time. Plus, by leaving the masque on your face for three to five minutes you get all the cleansing benefits without the drying effect that most clay masques produce. It can be used as often as skin permits, ideally every day. It will leave the skin instantly brighter and clearer-looking.

Directions for use:
1. With clean, dry fingers apply the masque on your dry face and décolletage area and massage for about one minute.
2. Do not wear your masque longer than five minutes. I actually keep mine on for two to four minutes.
3. Rinse it off with warm water and a toothbrush the way I describe in chapter 28 of *Your Right to Be Beautiful*. Ideally, use a specially designed masque removing brush, which comes free with several special orders from *www.beautifulonraw.com*.
4. Follow with a cold rinse. Dry skin with a towel.
5. Finish by moisturizing with *Your Right to Be Beautiful™ Facial Cream*, made with Sea Buckthorn Oil.

Our specially designed "Masque Removing Brush" (*www.BeautifulOnRaw.com*) is made with soft nylon bristles that are just right to gently brush your skin with no pulling or stretching. It not only makes the removal of the masque much easier, it also provides additional exfoliation. It reaches into the pores to lift and remove blemish-causing contaminants. It will leave skin looking and feeling its healthiest.

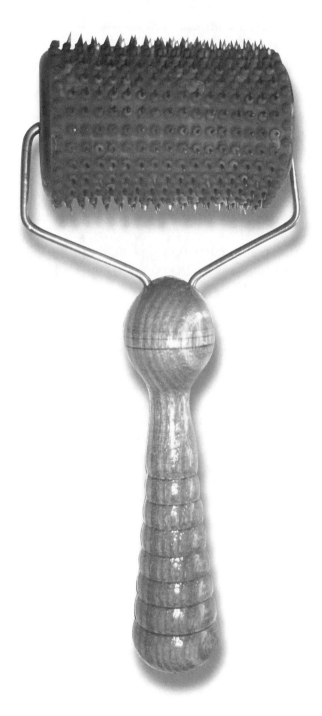

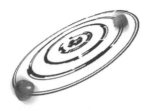

Chapter 38

Skin Rejuvenator: "The Rolling Bed of Pins"

Imagine ... you must look your very best today, and you have just minutes to spare. Maybe it's a date with someone special. Or a job interview when you want your Rawsome vivacity to shine through. Remember what Scarlett O'Hara did on her way to see Ashley? Rouge was a no-no for a nice Southern girl in her time. So she pinched her cheeks for color. Intuitively she was striving for the *blush of youth*. She knew that by increasing blood flow to her cheeks she'd look more beautiful.

You needn't feel the pinch the way Scarlett did. I'm offering you a much more effective solution. I *should* have kept this secret for myself. Sometimes I need a little edge. As I travel on my raw food lecture tours, I know I'm being looked at closely. I have to live up to expectations. People come up to me, look me right in the face, scrutinizing, to see whether (as some have put it) I'm "real." But a promise is a promise. I've pledged to share with you every beauty secret I know or discover. So ... here it is!

You've watched children play. You've seen the healthy blush and silken skin of youth. A child's glow seems to come from inside. Indeed it literally does — blood comes close to the skin bringing its warmth from underneath — like looking at a fire through silk.

Blood is essential for rejuvenation. Blood delivers nutrients to the cells and carries away toxins. Keeping your skin rejuvenated takes good circulation. Stimulation affects blood circulation, allows for the creation and repair of capillaries. Our own blood heals and rejuvenates us.

Because we are eating raw, our blood is clean and healthy — free of nasty abnormal proteins, clusters of platelets, and the parasites that contaminate the blood of those who still consume cooked food. As one doctor said: "If we were to maintain our blood in normal condition and circulation, sickness would be almost impossible." If we can only get our blood into hard-to-reach places, we'd have the elixir of youth at our fingertips.

You've heard about yogis sleeping on nails. And I can hear you thinking, *"Not only do you want me to eat all raw food, and not eat after two in the afternoon. Now you've got me sleeping on a bed of nails? Tonya — you're nuts!"* (And I am, of course. Raw, naturally.)

Well, not exactly a bed of nails, so relax. I'm grateful you have stayed with me so far and I'm not about to press my luck.

Lying on a bed of nails, walking barefoot on broken glass — these practices are very old. Yogis lie on beds of nails as part of their religious tradition. They also sleep on thorns and shards of glass. Physically, the benefits of walking and lying on glass or nails include relaxation and stimulation. Some magicians use the demonstration as part of their shows — just for the fun of it!

How can you lie on a bed of nails and not be injured? The secret to this phenomenon has a scientific explanation. Consider … If you step on a single nail, Ouch! It will pierce your skin. Your whole body weight is concentrated on one nail-point — thus there is extreme pressure, a puncture wound, and pain.

But on a "bed" of nails, your body's weight is distributed over dozens or hundreds of nails. The force you put on each individual nail is drastically reduced. Hence … no injury. In fact, lying on a bed of nails produces a very invigorating effect. It's not magic, it's physics!

Acupuncture works — we know this scientifically now — for much the same reason. But you must have a certified practitioner. Even if you can find one, it's costly. What if we had something for use at home which had a similar effect? The "Rolling Bed of Pins" does just that. This device is unique, and simple — based on the ancient healing traditions of India and China.

The "Rolling Bed of Pins" stimulates surface blood flow using a series of small pins in a rolling action. You roll it against your facial skin in any direction that seems comfortable. Do the same for your scalp. (I used it for a week and noticed increased hair growth.) Actually you can use this device for any area of your body to reduce pain and increase the healing effect of good blood circulation. The deeper the needles penetrate, the more stimulation you receive.

The "Rolling Bed" uses two types of needles — copper and iron. Some of the iron needles are plated with nickel or zinc. Some copper needles are plated in silver. As a result, five different metals come into contact with your skin.

Using the "Rolling Bed of Pins" causes electrophoresis of metals to take place, and the body assimilates the missing microelements. The term *electrophoresis* describes the migration of charged particles in an electric field. *Electro* refers to the energy of electricity. *Phoresis,* from the Greek *phoros*, means "to carry across." Thus *electrophoresis* is the process by which molecules are forced across skin, moved by an electrical current. The needle tips act as electrodes.

The galvanic current produced between the needles of different metals in contact with the skin produces a healing effect. The difference of potentials between the underlying metal of the needle and the metal used for plating creates a galvanic current at the tip of each needle. Galvanic current is also produced between different pins. The intensity of this galvanic current is regulated entirely by the body's electrical characteristics, which directly correlate to your skin's health. During contact with the needle tips, this galvanic current passes through to the deeper skin layers, where biochemical reactions take place.

Your skin is your body's largest organ. And a marvelous creation it is. Your skin can serve as a barrier or as an entryway into your body. Your skin is a barrier against penetration and infection. At the same time, your sweat pores and hair follicles serve as pathways for minerals to enter, and there is massive evidence that the body absorbs many minerals through the skin.

Blood is among the most important fluids in the human body. Metals in micro-doses are part of your blood's makeup. Microelements — including these metals — are vital for our well being. The beneficial effect of the "Rolling Bed" begins when the tips of the Rolling Bed's needles are differently charged, producing galvanic current at the contact points on the skin.

In reaction, blood rushes to your skin's surface, repairing and rejuvenating your skin, resolving certain skin problems and stimulating cells with a minuscule current. If these metals are missing from the body, and from the skin cells in particular, they will absorb through the skin.

Trace amounts of copper exist in all body tissues. Copper increases iron assimilation. Iron and copper work together in the formation of hemoglobin and red blood cells. Iron is also vital in keeping blood vessels, skin and connective tissue supple and elastic. Various enzyme reactions also require copper.

Your body needs small amounts of nickel to produce red blood cells. Iron increases your resistance to diseases, firms the skin, fights fatigue, helps in creating new red blood cells, brings oxygen to the tissues, and heals anemia. Copper improves your metabolism. Zinc is vital for new cell growth, strengthening your immune and nervous systems. More than 300 known enzymes need zinc for proper functioning. Copper, iron, and zinc are even present in human milk in the early stages of lactation.

Both copper and silver have been used for centuries for their biocidal properties. Nomads used silver coins to improve the quality of their drinking water. Well water containing copper and silver coins is very bright, owing to the disinfecting influence of these metals. European and Russian villages have been using silver in treating drinking water for generations.

Your skin's condition is a reflection of your internal health. Skin problems such as acne, blemishes, and dryness are signs of an overtaxed system. The "Rolling Bed" device helps your body cure numerous exterior skin problems, summoning your clean fresh blood to the surface.

You can use the "Rolling Bed" not only on your face and scalp, but on any other part of your body. The "Rolling Bed" promotes healing and releases pain. In 1971, *New York Times* columnist James Reston visited China and personally witnessed surgical operations in which acupuncture was the only anesthetic. The "Rolling Bed" works the same way. All you have to do is roll the Bed along an aching area and the pain leaves within minutes.

Use your "Rolling Bed" gently, evenly, smoothly. You'll feel no scratching or gouging — only a warm, tingling sensation. As long as you roll along the surface, the pins touch your skin but never pierce it. Blood comes closer to your skin but never contacts the needles. The "Rolling Bed" is completely noninvasive — there is absolutely no possibility of blood-related infection. Clean in hydrogen peroxide 3% solution.

I carry my "Rolling Bed" with me all the time — at home and on the road. When I have an extra minute, I take it out and use it on my face. Your "Rolling Bed" will give you a young girl's rosy cheeks. I never use blush anymore. I love my "Rolling Bed" so much I refuse to be without it. At home I wear a short apron to carry my essentials — my cell phone, a pen, and a notebook, and lately, my "Rolling Bed of Pins." I use it while I read; when I'm on the phone, when I watch TV. I even use my "Rolling Bed" in the car but *not* while driving.

Those of you who've tried my meridian facial (described in my first book) know the exercise works. The "Rolling Bed" is 100 times more effective. Try the "Rolling Bed" — I know you'll love it!

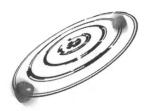

Chapter 39

The Violet Ray

Looking for smooth skin? Voluminous, lustrous hair? Here's a Ray of Hope!

Traveling across the country delivering my message about the virtues of raw food, I stand in front of other people every single day. Before big crowds. And with individuals and small groups. They look. My word, how they look! And what do they see?

At one appearance, I ate a single cookie at the raw food potluck offered by the hosting group. Apparently, whoever made that cookie had failed to use *raw* honey — I developed a blister on my lip. Since becoming 100 percent raw, my body can no longer tolerate processed food. Since I talk about Rawsome Beauty, people are very inquisitive about my looks. Let me tell you, nothing is more uncomfortable than having a blemish on your face when hundreds of people are scrutinizing you.

I was so happy I had my Violet Ray with me. I used a Straight Rod zapping electrode on that unsightly blister several times per day for five minutes and the blemish healed much faster than it would have without the treatment.

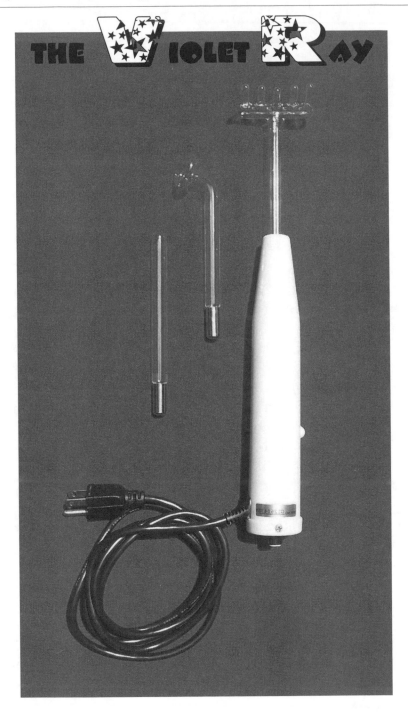

The Violet Ray is great for such emergencies. But it's even better for long-term results. Make it a part of your lifestyle as a means for a beautiful complexion and a full head of hair. I use a Spoon electrode on my face for five minutes after using *Your Right to Be Beautiful™ Facial Cream* generously on my skin. I also use my Violet Ray with a Rake electrode on my scalp for another five minutes every morning.

The Violet Ray is a holistic device that will complement your healthy lifestyle and will provide invaluable assistance in revealing your own *Rawsome Beauty.*

Decades ago, physicians used this device for every imaginable health problem. Today, the FDA approves the Violet Ray's use specifically for various skin and scalp conditions, such as reducing wrinkles, eliminating acne, fighting gray hair, eradicating dandruff, and treating baldness.

The Violet Ray was originally developed by the famous scientist Nikola Tesla. Tesla was successfully experimenting on disease and rejuvenation with ozone in the late 1800s and early 1900s. In the '20s and '30s, oxygen/zone therapy was used in hospitals, sanitariums and clinics. Beginning in the second half of the twentieth century, pharmaceutical companies disparaged all electro-therapies as drug-oriented medicine was taking off. Electro-therapies became unpopular in the United States. Since then, the use of the Violet Ray has declined as a medical tool, just as all non-drug therapies have. It remains FDA-certified for treating signs of aging and skin conditions as well as hair loss. In a time when drug therapies are king and older remedies disparaged, that continuing FDA approval stands as an important recognition of this significant tool's real value.

The Violet Ray uses argon, an inert gas which makes the violet color in the electrode. This hand-held unit comes with three glass electrodes — the Spoon, the Rake, and the Straight

Rod. The Spoon electrode is used anywhere on the skin surface. The Rake is used on the scalp, for hair growth, promoting circulation, and halting hair loss. The Straight Rod electrode is used for zapping acne, warts, moles, and blackheads.

The Violet Ray is a high-voltage, low-current source of high frequency waves in the violet range of the spectrum. Light, heat, and electric energy are produced in each glass vacuum applicator. It generates ozone when an electrode is applied to the skin. It is absolutely safe. In nature, the sun turns oxygen into ozone. In the Violet Ray, this is done though a high-frequency (10,000 Hz), high voltage, *low*-current electrical source. High-voltage is what makes the device work. Low current (low amperage) is what makes it safe. You'll find that the current produces an agreeable tingling on your skin's surface as it increases oxygenation in the form of ozone (O_3) in the blood.

Ozone is so chemically reactive that it constantly wants to become stable oxygen (O_2) by giving up O_1. This reactive form of oxygen is known to chemists as "singlet oxygen." These singlet oxygen molecules are created in a gush of O_1 releases. These O_1 molecules are negatively charged. They are hungry to catch something positively charged. Toxins and pathological bacteria are all positively charged. Because of the active oxygen's negative charge, it combines with all the filth in the body, oxidizing it, so that it may be flushed out in the bloodstream.

All the wastes your body excretes — whether through urination, bowel movements, sweating, spitting, skin particles that sloughed off your body's outer surface — are composed mainly of four basic elements: hydrogen, carbon, nitrogen and sulfur. If combined with oxygen, natural oxidation processes will turn these into H_2O, CO_2, NO_2 and SO_2. These are respectively just the chemical names for water, gaseous carbon dioxide, the toxic gas nitrogen dioxide, and the acidic gas sulphur dioxide. Applying the Violet Ray stimulates this vital "detox" process. When an electrode is applied to aging, diseased, or infected areas, it promotes healing and its sterilizing properties help fight infection.

The fundamental difference between diseased and normal cells is that healthy cells have an army of protective enzymes to protect themselves from oxygen by forming a self-protective antioxidant coating. Strict anaerobes, just like diseased cells, lack these protective enzymes and are killed by oxygen. Anaerobic microorganisms cannot live in the presence of active forms of oxygen. Viruses, fungi, and other human pathogens are drawn out to bind with reactive oxygen. They will be burnt — neutralized by oxygen. Oxygen is your most aggressive free radical scavenger.

Inflamed tissues are swollen. They hold more water, giving the face a puffy look. The ray improves circulation in congested parts, restoring bruised, inflamed, and diseased tissues to normal. Your body will regulate the intensity of the current and when to charge or discharge. Current drops off for healthy tissues because they have a higher resistance than swollen and infected tissues.

You'll find the Violet Ray an excellent tool for diminishing wrinkles, warts, and moles. It also decreases hair loss and promotes new growth. Despite the FDA's refusal to certify the Violet Ray for anything except skin care and hair loss, many people find it beneficial for a wide range of problems. Many users find that the penetrating electrical currents can relieve pain, stimulating cells and organs by enhancing blood flow in the treated area. While electrical currents infuse your body's cells and tissues, they stimulate and strengthen your vital organs, steady your nerves, and help rebuild your sense of vitality and well-being.

Energize your vital organs by moving the electrode along the meridians, producing an effect similar to reflexology. The Violet Ray offers a unique ability to balance *chi* in a manner similar to meditation.

Pain is caused by a build-up of hydrogen in the affected area. Pain is an accumulation of positive ions, which replace the beneficial negative ions. Applying a Violet Ray electrode generates an electro-therapy that oxygenates the effected areas. The high frequency of the Violet Ray's electrical currents transmits active oxygen to the blood, purifying it. This action helps neutralize infected areas containing bacteria, viruses, and fung1 wherever the electrode is used.

The Violet Ray diffuses the healing power of electricity throughout the body — *without pain*. It plugs into an ordinary household electrical outlet. The healing rays are dispersed through glass applicators, called electrodes, in the violet colored stream — hence the name Violet Ray. (Not "ultraviolet" or UV rays, mind you — a different part of the spectrum, outside the visible range.) Violet rays do not produce any significant amount of ultraviolet light and do not cause UV burns.

The substantial voltage is applied to the point of contact without any shock. A pleasant warmth is all you'll feel. Use it in any area where you have discomfort of one sort or another. There is no place on the body that cannot be helped by a suffusion of fresh, oxygenated blood.

You'll find it easy to use your Violet Ray. Used five to ten minutes each time, just twice a day, will give you all the benefit without inconvenience or fuss. Your Violet Ray will require no maintenance. Just remove the electrodes when you've finished your short session, unplug your Violet Ray, and you're done.

Use your Violet Ray sensibly. Used well, used a little each day, it will bring you real benefit. Naturally, however, it's *not* a cure-all. We do not make claims for any cure of injury or disease beyond the specific cosmetic recommendations made here. It's meant for the many cosmetic reasons we've detailed here, and only for those purposes. By no means is this device a substitute for raw food nutrition, exercise, or proper professional health attention.

You can purchase the Violet Ray from
www.beautifulonraw.com

The Violet Ray will be delivered directly from the manufacturer. Your Violet Ray comes with a full one-year warranty, parts and labor included, unless your unit is dropped or abused in any way.

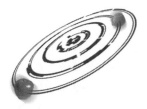

Chapter 40

Conclusion: My Quantum Shield

I sincerely hope that *Quantum Eating* has enriched your reflections about the living foods lifestyle — about sunlight, breathing, sleeping, and thinking. As I wrote, I was aware that every chapter could be a book in itself. I've only scratched the surface.

You have the responsibility to explore. I mention books which can expand your knowledge about the topics that I discuss. The idea of seeing ourselves as quantum beings is itself radically new and has far-reaching significance. What significance this great governing metaphor will have for you individually, *you* must choose. Choose wisely. Beyond knowledge, there is an emotional foundation here. I *live* for every story from my readers telling me how they've been touched by one of my books, speeches, or workshops. My joy comes from making a difference in people's lives through being who I am.

One day I received a most heartening remark from one of the ladies attending my seminar in New York. "You really do have the most beautiful skin I've ever seen. It looks almost transparent," she wrote. Sure, I took it for what it was — another score for the raw food power! But just to be sure that my nose did not rattle the crystals on the chandelier, another email came on the heels of the first:

"I attended your lecture in New York and I bought both of your books. I must admit that I was a little disappointed when I met you. You claim to know how to get rid of bags under one's eyes, when you yourself have bags under your eyes, too. So how do you claim that raw food gets rid of bags under the eyes?" She then continued: "Other than the bags under your eyes, your skin looks amazing!!"

The two exclamation marks are hers, not mine. (Hey, I now have that "poetic license" I couldn't get in Russia — and I'm going to use it).

Have you ever seen a person over forty with bags under their eyes, but "amazing" skin? Look around. I promise you'll have a hard time finding one. These conditions, amazing skin and absence of bags under the eyes, are closely linked to health. And either you'll have them both, or you won't have either. An extended lecture tour in and around New York City is enough to give anyone bags under their eyes. Considering these two reader responses, I'd say one out of two for someone over forty is a good showing under the circumstances — especially from New Yorkers!

I do not have the most beautiful skin and I do have bags under the eyes — or else this is how "no bags under the eyes" looks at fifty. But since reader number two was the only person who's been critical of my appearance among thousands of people I've met in my travels — some of you are kind and haven't written me about my flaws yet! — I'm running a good average. If I get another such response, I'm going to claim it's the lighting. Dear reader, feel free to employ the same excuse.

Still, when I think back to the cruel remark of my old classmate *(I wouldn't want to live)* I feel devastated. And then by turns I'm heartened again. I like to see how much I have changed, how little such negativity effects me now.

This time, reading that email from Ms. Bags-Under-Eyes, I was able to laugh, just as if someone had said I had green hair. Spontaneously, I realized a new and profound self-confidence which adverse criticism does not affect. I took her remark for how it seemed then and seems now: if you're still searching for put-downs to deliver weeks after a lecture, your problems may be bigger than bags under the eyes. In public speaking, ten percent of your audience will like you no matter what you say, no matter how you look. Another ten percent will *dis*like you no matter what. Clearly Ms. Bags wanted it both ways.

After reaching our best health and appearance, what next? For some of us, the mission becomes to promote the raw food lifestyle to everyone. We sometimes have to sacrifice our own health and looks to help you attain yours. For me the crusade sometimes means delivering two presentations a day, driving in congested cities, sitting in gas-fumed traffic for hours. Not getting my food on time, not getting sleep when needed, going through the stress and inconvenience of constant travel.

I wrote a book about beauty. In that very act, I made myself an object of intense scrutiny, even among my own family. The biggest nuisance: During the last ten years that I've been 100 percent raw, my husband has gotten used to my improved looks, my relative lack of aging. During our lecture circuit when I am tired — oh, yes, I do have bad face days! — he worries. He stares fixedly at my face. Unsmiling, he stares. I begin to feel like a bug under a microscope. And then he says it. "Yes," he muses. "A possible wrinkle. One I don't believe was there last time ..."

I haven't actually hit him yet. But I've come awfully close to shrieking "Back off, darling! Have you forgotten: I'm not fifteen anymore, I'm fifty! Adjust your expectations!"

Fortunately, Quantum Eating, along with all the beauty tricks I've shared with you in my books, will bring back my Rawsome beauty in no time.

I wish you the best in finding a good role model in your quest for health. I'm nowhere near perfect, Lord knows. If you are one of the ones inclined to make a laundry list of my flaws, I'll make it easier for you: I'm too short, my face is too round, my gait is not quite even, my legs are scarred from numerous operations, and I have them covered with clothing. I show up in sweat pants at yoga class when other women appear in skimpy outfits. Frankly, I feel like the Swamp Thing on a nudist beach. But I don't care. I am the very best I can be — and I feel beautiful.

Negative comments can't hurt me any more. Even better, everything negative life throws at me I will change to positive. When I was receiving complimentary letters, I might occasionally violate my 2 P.M. curfew during draining weeks of traveling. I kept thinking: *I already eat 100 percent raw. I am already a good girl.* After receiving this negative email, I was able to follow the Quantum Eating regimen to the letter. And now I feel and look better than ever! So go ahead. Bring your magnifying glass next time you see me in person! Keep those negative comments coming!

Dear reader, feel free to adopt the same attitude! To paraphrase: *What does not kill us, makes us beautiful!*

Bibliography

Anderson, Brenda. *Playing the Quantum Field, How Changing Your Choices Can Change Your Life.* New World Library, 2006

Austad, Steven N. *Why We Age: What Science is Discovering about the Body's Journey through Life.* Wiley, 1999

Baker, S.M., M.D. with Baar, K., MPH. *The Circadian Prescription.* G.P. Putnam's Sons Publishers, 2005

Baranov, A., Kidalov, V. *Healing with Cold.* Kemerovo, Russia: Astcl Publishing, 2000, (in Russian)

Batmanghelidj, F., M.D. *You Are Not Sick, You're Thirsty!* New York: Warner Books, 2003

Batmanghelidj, F., M.D. *Your Body's Many Cries For Water.* Global Health Solutions, Inc., 1995

Bernard, Dr. Raymond. *Pythagoras, the Immortal Sage.* Kessinger Publishing Co., 2003.

Bikram, Choudhury. *Bikram Yoga: The Guru Behind Hot Yoga Shows the Way to Radiant Health and Personal Fulfillment.* New York: Collins, 2007

Bragg, Dr. Paul C. and Bragg, Dr. Patricia. *Super Power Breathing for Super Energy, High Health & Longevity.* Bragg Health Sciences, 2006

Brooks, Wiley and Foss, Nancy *Breatharianism: Breathe and Live Forever.* Breatharian International, Inc., 1983

Brothwell, Don and Brothwell, Patricia. *Food in Antiquity, a Survey of the Diet of Early Peoples.* Johns Hopkins University Press, 1998

Callahan, Phillip S., PhD. *Paramagnetism: Rediscovering Nature's Secret Force of Growth.* Acres U.S.A., 1995

Capra, Fritjof. *The Tao of Physics, An Exploration of the Parallels between Modern Physics and Eastern Mysticism.* Shambhala Publications, Inc., 2000

Capra, Fritjof. *The Web of Life, a New Scientific Understanding of Living Systems.* Anchor books, 1996

Collins, Francis S. *The Language of God.* Free Press, a division of Simon & Schuster, Inc., 2006

Daugirdas, John T. *The QUD Diet: Eating Well Every Other Day.* Willowbrook, IL: White Swan Publishing, Ltd., 2006

Davies, Paul and Gribbin, John. *The Matter Myth, Dramatic Discoveries That Challenge Our Understanding of Physical Reality.* Simon & Schuster/Touchstone, 1993

Davies, Paul. *The 5th Miracle, The Search for the Origin and Meaning of Life.* Simon & Schuster Paperbacks, 1999

De Vogel, C. J., PhD. *Pythagoras & Early Pythagoreanism.* Assen: Royal VanGorcum Ltd., 1966

Durant, W. *The Life of Greece.* New York: Simon & Schuster, 1939

Eden, Donna. *Energy Medicine.* Tarcher/Penguin, 1998

Foster, Russel G. and Kreitzman, Leon. *Rhythms of Life: The Biological Clocks that Control the Daily Lives of Every Living Thing.* New Haven and London: Yale University Press, 2004

Gordon, Richard. *Quantum-Touch, The Power to Heal.* North Atlantic Books, 2002

Goswami, Amit, PhD. *The Quantum Doctor, a Physicist's Guide to Health and Healing.* Hampton Roads Publishing Company, Inc., 2004

Groff, James L., Gropper, Sareen S. *Advanced Nutrition and Human Metabolism.* Wadsworth Thomson Learning, 1999

Grout, Pam. *Jumpstart Your Metabolism: How to Lose Weight by Changing the Way You Breathe.* New York: Fireside, a trademark of Simon & Schuster Inc., 1998

Hall, Stephen S. *Merchants of Immortality, Chasing the Dream of Human Life Extension.* Mariner Books/ Houghton Mifflin Company, 2003

Harvey, John R., PhD. *Deep Sleep, Complete Rest for Health, Vitality & Longevity.* M. Evans and Company, Inc., 2001

Hicks, Esther and Jerry. *The Science of Deliberate Creation Journal: the Teachings of Abraham,* "The Amazing Power of Deliberate Intent — Living the Art of Allowing." Hay House, Inc., 2906

Hobday, R. *The Healing Sun, Sunlight and Health in the 21st Century.* Findhorn Press, 1999

Holick, Michael, PhD, M.D., and Jenkins, Mark. *The UV Advantage.* Publishers Group West, 2003

Hotema, Hilton. *Man's Higher Consciousness.* Health Research, 1962

Iyengar, B.K.S. *Light on Life, The Yoga Journey to Wholeness, Inner Peace, and Ultimate Freedom.* Rodale, 1984

Kahn, C. H. *Pythagoras and The Pythagoreans: A Brief History.* Hackett Publishing Company, Inc., 2007

Kervran, C.L. *Biological Transmutations.* Beekman Publishers, Inc., 1999

Koenig-Bricker, Woodeene. *365 Saints, Your Daily Guide to the Wisdom and Wonder of Their Lives.* Harper Collins Publishers, 1995

Lane, Nick. *Oxygen: The Molecule that Made the World.* New York: Oxford University Press Inc., 2002

Le Fanu, James, M.D. *The Rise and Fall of Modern Medicine.* Carroll & Graf Publishers, 2001

Liberman, Jacob, O.D., PhD. *Light: Medicine of the Future: How We Can Use It to Heal Ourselves Now.* Bear & Company, 1947

Lipton, Bryce. *The Biology of Belief: Unleashing the Power of Consciousness, Matter, & Miracles.* Mountain of Love, 2005

Mamonov, Valery, PhD. *Control for Life Extension, a Personalized Holistic Approach.* Long Life Press Co., 2001

McCabe, Ed. *Flood Your Body With Oxygen.* Energy Publications, 2003

McFadden, Johnjoe. *Quantum Evolution: How Physics' Weirdest Theory Explains Life's Biggest Mystery.* W. W. Norton & Company, 2002

McTaggart, Lynne. *The Field, The Quest for The Secret Force of The Universe.* Harper Perennial, 2002

Mednick, C. Sara. *Take a Nap! Change Your Life.* New York: Workman Publishing, 2004

Mindell, Arnold, PhD. *The Quantum Mind and Healing, How to Listen and Respond to Your Body's Symptoms.* Hamilton Roads Publishing Company, Inc., 2006

Moynihan, R., Cassels, A. *Selling Sickness.* First Nation Books, 2005

Nutton, Vivian. *Ancient Medicine.* Routledge, 2004

Olshansky, Jay and Carnes, Bruce A. *The Quest for Immortality,* New York: W. W. Norton & Company, Inc., 2001

Orr, Leonard. *Breaking the Death Habit, the Science of Everlasting Life.* Frog, Ltd., 1998

Pagel, Heinz R. *The Cosmic Code.* Bantam, 1984

Palmer, John D. *The Living Clock: The Orchestrator of Biological Rhythms.* Oxford Press, 2002

Prigogine, Ilya. *Order Out of Chaos, Man's New Dialogue with Nature.* Bantam Books, 2004

Rappoport, L. *How We Eat,* ECW Press, 2003

Reid, Daniel P. *The Tao of Health, Sex, & Longevity, A Modern Practical Guide to The Ancient Way,* Fireside, a trademark of Simon & Schuster Inc., 1989

Riedweg, Christophe. *Pythagoras: His Life, Teaching, and Influence,* translated from German by Steven Rendall and Andreas Schatzmann, Cornell University Press, 2005, (German) Munchen, 2002

Schrodinger, Erwin. *What is Life?: with Mind and Matter and Autobiographical Sketches.* Cambridge University Press, 1992

Seligman, Martin E.P. , PhD. *Authentic Happiness,* Free Press, a division of Simon & Schuster, Inc., 2002

Sell, Christina. *Yoga from Inside Out: Making Peace with Your Body through Yoga.* Prescott, Arizona: Hohm Press, 2003

Smolensky, M., PhD, and Lamberg, L. *The Body Clock Guide to Better Health.* Henry Holt & Co. LLC, 2000

Somers, Suzanne. *The Sexy Years.* Three Rivers Press, 2004

Suzuki, D.T. *Zen Buddhism: Selected Writings Edited by William Barrett.* Three Leaves Press, Doubleday, 1956

Taylor, Thomas. *Iamblichus's Life of Pythagoras.* Rochester, Vermont: Inner Traditions International, Ltd., 1986

Thich Nhat Hanh. *The Miracle of Mindfulness.* Beacon Press, Boston, Massachusetts, 1976

Tompkins, Peter and Bird, Christopher. *The Secret Life of Plants.* Harper Perennial, 1973

Vital, Mony, PhD. *Ageless Living: Freedom from the Culture of Death.* Del Mar, California: Vital Publishing, 2005

Whitehouse, Maureen. *Soul Full Eating: a (Delicious) Path to Higher Consciousness.* Hollywood: Axiom Publishing, 2007

Wiley, T.S. with Formby, B., PhD. *Lights Out.* Pockets Books, 2000

Wilson, Robert Anton. *Quantum Psychology: How Brain Software Programs You & Your World.* New Falcon Publications, 1990

Wolf, Fred Alan. *Taking the Quantum Leap, The New Physics for Nonscientists.* Perennial Library – Harper & Row Publishers, 1989

Zohar, Danah. *Quantum Self: Human Nature and Consciousness Defined by the New Physics,* New York: Quill/William Morrow, 1990

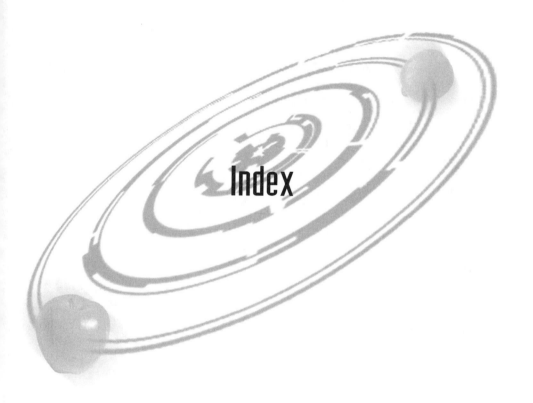

Index

If the order form on the following page has already been used, you may order additional copies of *Your Right to Be Beautiful,* the companion *un*cookbook, *Beautiful On Raw,* and *Quantum Eating,* directly from BR Publishing:

online: *www.BeautifulOnRaw.com*
or
by telephone: *(866) STAY-RAW*

Quick Order Form

Order additional copies of *Your Right to Be Beautiful,* the companion ***un***cookbook, *Beautiful On Raw* and *Quantum Eating* directly from BR Publishing:

online: *www.BeautifulOnRaw.com*

or

by telephone: *(866) STAY-RAW*

Mail Orders *(please photocopy form):*

BR Publishing
P.O. Box 623
Cordova, TN 38088-0623

Please send me _____ copies of *Your Right to Be Beautiful* @ $20.00 each.

Please send me _____ copies of *Beautiful On Raw* @ $20.00 each.

Please send me _____ copies of *Quantum Eating* @ $30.00 each.

Name: _____

Address: _____

City: _____ State: _____ Zip: _____

Please add $5 for 1 to 2 books for shipping.

Payment: Check _____   Money Order _____